$\mathcal{B}_C$

RC 337 .M48 1988

Methods in clinical trials in neurology
: vascular and degenerative brain
disease

METHODS IN CLINICAL TRIALS IN NEUROLOGY

METHODS IN CLINICAL TRIALS IN NEUROLOGY

Vascular and Degenerative Brain Disease

Edited by

R. CAPILDEO

and

J. M. ORGOGOZO

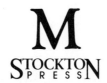

STOCKTON PRESS

First published 1988

Published by
THE MACMILLAN PRESS LTD
Houndmills, Basingstoke, Hampshire RG21 2XS
and London
Companies and representatives
throughout the world

Printed in Great Britain by
Camelot Press Ltd,
Southampton

British Library Cataloguing in Publication Data
Methodology in clinical trials in neurology:
vascular and degenerative brain disease.
1. Neurology   2.   Clinical trials
I.   Capildeo, Rudy   II.   Orgogozo, J. M.
616.8'072   RC346
ISBN 0–333–42305–4

Contents

The Contributors

M. G. Bousser
  Clinique des Maladies du Système
    Nerveux du Pr. Castaigne
  Hôpital de la Saltpêtrière
  47 Bd de l'Hôpital
  Paris 17
  France

R. Capildeo
  Regional Centre for Neurology
  Oldchurch Hospital and Neurosurgery
  Romford
  Essex RM7 0BE
  UK

D. Commenges
  Département d'Informatique
    Medicale
  Université de Bordeaux II
  146 Rue Leo-Saignat
  33076 Bordeaux
  France

J. F. Dartigues
  Département de Neurologie
  Hôpital Pellegrin

  and

  Département d'Informatique
    Medicale
  Université de Bordeaux II
  146 Rue Leo-Saignat
  33076 Bordeaux
  France

L. J. Findley
  Regional Centre for Neurology and
    Neurosurgery
  Oldchurch Hospital
  Romford
  Essex RM7 0BE
  UK

  and

  MRC Neuro-Otology Unit
  National Hospital
  Queen Square
  London
  UK

H. V. Fineberg
  Harvard School of Public Health
  Centre for the Analysis of Health Practice
  Boston
  Mass.
  USA

S. Haberman
  Department of Mathematics
  The City University
  London EC1M 7BB
  UK

M. J. G. Harrison
  Department of Neurology
  Middlesex Hospital
  London W1N 8AA
  UK

R. B. Haynes
  Faculty of Health Sciences
  McMaster University
  Hamilton
  Ontario
  Canada

J. P. Kistler
  Department of Neurology
  Massachusetts General
    Hospital
  Boston
  Mass.
  USA

X. Lataste
  Neurology Department
  Clinical Research
  Sandoz AG
  CH-4002 Basel
  Switzerland

  and

  Bordeaux University
  France

W. Maurer
  Clinical Research
  Sandoz AG
  CH-4002 Basel
  Switzerland

J. Olesen
  Department of Neuromedicine
  Københavns amts Sygehus Gentofte
    and Rigshospitalet
  Copenhagen
  Denmark

J. M. Orgogozo
  Hôpital Pellegrin
  38076 Bordeaux
  France

J. M. S. Pearce
  Department of Neurology
  Hull Royal Infirmary
  Hull HU3 2JZ
  UK

B. S. Schoenberg
  Neuroepidemiology Section
  Office of the Director
  National Institute of Neurological
    and Communicative Disorders and
    Stroke
  Bethesda, Maryland
  USA

  and

  Georgetown University School of
    Medicine
  Washington, DC
  USA

P. Tfelt-Hansen
  Department of Neuromedicine
  Københavns amts Sygehus Gentofte
    and Rigshospitalet
  Copenhagen
  Denmark

M. G. Wallace
  Regional Centre for Neurology
    and Neurosurgery
  Oldchurch Hospital
  Romford
  Essex RM7 0BE
  UK

C. P. Warlow
  Department of Clinical
    Neurosciences
  Northern General Hospital
  Edinburgh EH5 2DQ
  UK

Discussants

A. Alperovich   (Paris)
J. F. Dreyfus   (Paris)
S. Fahn   (New York)
R. Knill-Jones (Glasgow)
J. W. Norris   (Toronto)
R. Salamon   (Bordeaux)

Foreword

The description of the clinical syndromes of disease was the gigantic contribution of physicians in the eighteenth, nineteenth and early twentieth centuries. The scientific basis which lent credibility to descriptive medicine was the correlation between the clinical syndromes and the gross and microscopic tissue changes detected by the anatomists and pathologists of that era. The burgeoning of biochemistry, pharmacology and physiology in the second half of the twentieth century introduced a scientific understanding of disease allowing for early detection and rational treatment. Since then, revolutionary new imaging methods have added immeasurably to our diagnostic precision.

The major benefit for the practice of medicine gained from the application of these scientific disciplines was first observed in dramatic cures which were effected in some acute illnesses. For example, a treatment for a disease such as tuberculous meningitis, known to kill all its victims in less than two months, was very easy to recognise and quickly accorded universal acceptance. A sample-size of two patients was needed to constitute the clinical trial to prove the benefit of streptomycin treatment. The first patient represented the pilot study but the possibility existed that the recovery was due to a diagnostic error or a miracle. A second patient going on to recovery meant that these improbable chances were eliminated, and the therapy had passed the clinical trial stage.

An equally important challenge now is the development of treatment strategies to reduce the impact of chronic illness. Treatment programmes for many of the chronic disorders of the nervous system and those which manifest themselves intermittently have become confused by a variety of putative therapeutic suggestions. The benefit of treatment in chronic illness has been difficult to evaluate and hard answers are dependent on the rigid application of the newest of the advances applied to medicine: the use of methodology and biostatistics.

This monograph focuses on this evolving science, and on the art of its application. It details the early steps which have been taken in coming to grips with the significance of therapeutic advances in several chronic neurological conditions: stroke, threatened stroke and Parkinson's disease, dementia and migraine. Clearly this new science of therapeutic evaluation which combines clinical expertise, epidemiology, methodology and biostatistics is to therapeutics what pathology was to the clarification of disease syndromes.

In the early days of therapeutics, authoritarian medicine allowed for the promulgation of directives, based on the experience, the opinion and the judgement of the gifted teacher. This reverence for tradition and acceptance of authority persists to some extent even today despite the warning from as long ago as the time of Hippocrates that 'experience is misleading'. It is increasingly apparent, however, that patients deserve better from modern scientific medicine.

The next halting step beyond the acceptance of the dicta of the professor was the judgement of therapeutic advance by the comparisons of groups of patients given a new treatment with some historical references to reputedly similar patients who were not given the new treatment. Modern scientific medicine denies the value of this method of 'contrived controls' for a number of reasons, including: the selection process which channels patients into any given treatment milieu; the known or unknown disparity between the treatment and comparative groups in what are now recognised as important risk factors; the changing background of baseline therapy and prognosis; and the process by which decisions to treat or not to treat led to the emergence of the particular and peculiar population which is the subject of the reports. There are many other flaws. Decision making by utilising the observations from historical controls is almost as misleading in modern medical science as is that based on 'clinical judgement'.

The randomised clinical trial emerges as the only way in which convincing answers can be obtained in assaying the value of treatment in chronic disease with few endpoints. It is an expensive process, not only in terms of money, but also in energy and time. The alternative, of remaining equipped with a host of indefinite and vague answers, is infinitely less helpful to our patients.

The editors of this book have been helpful to the international community of clinical neurological researchers by bringing into focus the state of the art of therapeutic evaluation in these selected neurological disorders. The essayists have focused on some of the problems which still exist in this type of disciplined search for clinical answers. The early mistakes should not be used to fuel a flame to destroy these new methods. Rather, the flame should be used to light our way to improvements in these new techniques. In the long run the sharpened tool of clinical evaluation by modern methods will be infinitely superior to previous 'commonsense decisions' and subjective evaluations. To quote from Thomas Huxley: 'The methods of science differ from those of common sense only as far as the guardsman's cut and thrust differ from the manner in which a savage wields a club'.

H. J. M. Barnett, OC, MD
University Hospital
London, Ontario

Preface

At least one aspect of clinical trials is certain. Following publication of the results, there will be criticism. Some authors believe this criticism is proportional to the size of the study. Those clinical trialists who have completed this task will have had many doubts as to whether the whole exercise was worthwhile. The answer to this question must certainly be 'Yes'. Without clinical trials we rely solely on impression, intuition and experience — all variables known to be notoriously inaccurate.

This book is based on a workshop. The members of this workshop were selected because of their special experience in the design and setting up of clinical trials in neurology. Those chapters relating to theoretical aspects are essential prerequisites to the clinical chapters that follow. The principles they employ form the basis of any critique.

Published clinical trials represent the state of the art at that particular point in time. They form the foundations upon which current clinical trials are based. We all think 'we could have done it better'. This desire for excellence forms the basis for those chapters relating to recommendations for future trials. One day, these trials will also be criticised, but with each step our therapeutic knowledge will have increased. This has to be important for the clinician and the people he looks after — the patients.

We wish to thank all the authors and discussants for their contributions to this book. The chapters are based on the presentations and discussions that took place in the workshop. Special thanks are due to Sandoz Switzerland and affiliates in France and the UK for providing the necessary ambience for their workshop, which was held in Aix-en-Provence, France. The Editors wish also to thank two special people whose efforts helped to complete our work — Rita and Ruth.

Finally, any deficiencies in this book are the sole responsibility of the Editors. Even with this proviso we hope that this book will be useful and helpful to all those brave clinicians who embark on clinical trials in neurology.

Romford and Bordeaux, 1987   R. C.
                                                                          J. M. O.

SECTION 1
BACKGROUND TO CLINICAL TRIALS

1
Epidemiological considerations in the design of controlled clinical trials. Part I: Introduction

R. B. HAYNES

DEFINITION OF ANALYTICAL EPIDEMIOLOGY

There is no agreed definition of 'analytical epidemiology' so I will suggest my own *ad hoc* one, borrowing from the traditional definition of epidemiology:

Analytical epidemiology is the study of disease in defined groups of humans, for the purposes of ascertaining the relationships of various characteristics of these groups to the diagnosis, course or prognosis, and causes of their disorders.

For the purpose of discussion, I will arbitrarily exclude studies in which the investigator purposefully intervenes in an attempt to alter the course of a disorder. Thus, clinical trials are specifically excluded from this definition. However, studies of a disorder under usual conditions of treatment or when no experimental protocol is involved (even when a new treatment or diagnostic test is involved) are not excluded.

CASE-CONTROL STUDIES

In these investigations, the investigator tries to gain a greater degree of 'control' on the natural variation that occurs among individuals. First, a group of individuals are selected who have a disease of interest ('cases'). Then, a number of individuals who are free of this disease are 'matched' on as many characteristics as possible with the cases, except for characteristics that the investigator feels may be the cause of the disease or related to this

3

cause (these subjects are then called 'controls'). The investigator then determines whether this putative cause occurs more frequently in the cases. For example, if the cases are stroke victims, the study may attempt to determine whether more cases than controls have hypertension. This sort of study has fewer potential biases than the analytical survey but it is only feasible to control for a small number of characteristics in any one study, whereas there are usually many that one would want to control for.

A variant of the case-control method is often used to define the accuracy of diagnostic tests. In this type of study, the test is performed on individuals who are known, by relatively definitive means such as angiography or biopsy, to have the disease of interest. The results are then compared with the test's results when applied to individuals who are known to be free of the disease. For example, one might compare ultrasound of the carotid with angiography in subjects who have carotid stenosis and compare the results with those in people who are found to be free of carotid disease on angiography.

COHORT ANALYTIC STUDIES

In chapter 2 Drs Schoenberg and Haberman describe this sort of investigation very well: '. . . we begin with a group or cohort exposed to a particular factor(s) thought to be related to disease onset or outcome and a group not exposed to the particular factor(s). The two groups are observed over time and their experience is compared.' They also delineate clearly the limitations of this type of investigation: it is difficult to ensure that the two groups will be comparable to begin with for all the factors that might be important to understanding the results that are observed.

It is worthwhile remarking here on the use of cohort studies to describe new or old treatments. Often the first and last reports in the literature about a treatment appear in the form of 'case series' in which the author reviews his personal experience with the treatment in a series of consecutive cases that have been followed for variable periods of time. The data collected then form a cohort study without a comparison group. To provide a comparison, the author will often cite other reports in the literature ('literature controls') or cases managed previously in a different fashion ('historical controls'). Since the data for such reports have usually been collected in an unstandardised fashion and the controls are selected from different times or places, such studies have all the limitations of formally conducted cohort analytical studies plus many more. An example of how deceiving such reports can be is provided in the history of the gastric freeze for peptic ulcers, in which the initial reports of case series indicated 100% response (Wagensteen *et al.* 1962), whereas a randomised control trial demonstrated that the procedure was completely worthless (Ruffin *et al.*, 1969).

There are a multitude of different study designs employed in analytical epidemiology but these are mainly variations on the themes that I have just described.

ABUSES AND USES OF ANALYTICAL EPIDEMIOLOGY IN THE DESIGN AND EXECUTION OF CLINICAL TRIALS

Because of the limitations of analytical studies alluded to above (and a host of problems that I have not described), these studies are inadequate for the testing of treatments. For example, the numerous analytical investigations showing the relationship between various lipids and cardiovascular disease seem to indicate that lowering low-density lipoproteins in humans would result in large-scale sparing of human lives (Kannel *et al.*, 1979). However, randomised control trials such as the Multiple Risk Factor Intervention Trial (1982) have shown no such benefit, and the large European trial of clofibrate (Committee of Principle Investigators, 1978) indicates that lipid lowering may actually be harmful to life.

Nevertheless, analytical epidemiological investigations do have an indispensable part to play in the design and execution of clinical trials. First, and most important, they generate and partially test hypotheses that then become the basis for the more sophisticated and expensive clinical trials that must take place to confirm or refute these hypotheses. For example, analytical studies of the factors that influence patient compliance with therapeutic regimens led to the formulation of interventions that were subsequently tested in randomised trials (Haynes, 1979a). These trials demonstrated the value of several behaviourally orientated strategies and, equally important, documented the failure of patient instruction to improve long-term compliance (Haynes, 1979b). It would be wasteful and negligent to mount clinical trials to test every idea of therapeutic potential without fairly extensive testing by analytical studies.

Secondly, analytical studies can provide the information that is essential for estimating the number of subjects that will be required to test a treatment properly. All such estimations depend on the accuracy of estimation of rates of event occurrence in the control group, and these estimates are commonly derived from analytical studies.

Thirdly, the measurement properties of various screening and diagnostic tests that are needed in the execution of clinical trials are generally determined in analytical investigations.

Fourthly, the selection of appropriate subjects for clinical trials is aided by analytical studies that have demonstrated subgroups of patients with a given disorder who are at high risk of adverse outcomes. As a rather obvious example, epidemiological investigations have shown that the risk of stroke is proportional to the level of blood-pressure elevation (Kannel *et al.*, 1970).

Thus, early clinical trials of antihypertensive drugs concentrated on subjects with more severely elevated pressures (Veterans Administration Cooperative Study Group, 1967).

Finally, many of the biases that can distort the results of clinical trials can be avoided or at least anticipated if the results of analytical studies are attended to. For example, analytical surveys have demonstrated substantial differences in the health of those who volunteer for clinical trials and those who do not (Cobb *et al.*, 1957).

Of course, the use of the results of analytical studies to design clinical trials is not without pitfalls. In the first place, these studies may be poorly done. Thus, many of the rigorous scientific standards that Drs Schoenberg and Haberman have prescribed for clinical trials must also be applied in analytical studies if their results are to be valid. Furthermore, generalising the results of analytical studies to clinical trial settings can be risky. An important and apocryphal example of this occurred recently in the MRFIT study. The planners of this study utilised data from the Framingham cohort study (Kannel *et al.*, 1979) to estimate the rate of cardiovascular events that would occur in the control group for the trial. However, cardiovascular death rates have dropped dramatically since the 1960s when the Framingham study ended and the event rates for the trial were thus overestimated by 81%, substantially reducing the power of the trial to find a real benefit.

I will end my comments on this cautionary note and with the complementary epithet that analytical studies are often good (but sometimes bad) servants to clinical trialists. No investigator contemplating a clinical trial can afford to ignore analytical epidemiological investigations — but they must be used with due regard for their inherent limitations as well as the rigour with which they have been executed.

REFERENCES

Cobb, S., King, S. and Chen, E. (1957). Differences between respondents and nonrespondents in a morbidity survey involving clinical examination. *J. Chron. Dis.*, **6**, 95.

Committee of Principle Investigators (1978). Co-operative trial in the primary prevention of ischemic heart disease using clofibrate. *Brit. Heart J.*, **40**, 1069.

Haynes, R. B. (1979a). Determinants of compliance. In Haynes, R. B., Taylor, D. W. and Sackett, D. L. (eds), *Compliance in Health Care*. Johns Hopkins University Press, Baltimore, pp. 49–62.

Haynes, R. B. (1979b). Strategies to improve compliance referrals, appointments, and prescribed medical regimens. In Haynes, R. B., Taylor, D. W. and Sackett, D. L. (eds), *Compliance in Health Care*. Johns Hopkins University Press, Baltimore, pp. 121–43.

Kannel, W. B., Wolf, P. A., Verrer, J. and McNamara, P. M. (1970). Epidemiologic assessment of the role of blood pressure in stroke, the Framingham study. *J. Am. Med. Assoc.*, **214**, 301.

Kannel, W. B., Castelli, W. P. J. and Gordon, T. (1979). Cholesterol in the prediction of atherosclerotic disease, new perspectives based on the Framingham study. *Ann. Intern. Med.*, **90**, 85.

Multiple Risk Factor Intervention Trial Research Group (1982). Multiple Risk Factor Intervention Trial, risk factor changes and mortality results. *J. Am. Med. Assoc.*, **248**, 1465.

Ruffin, J. M., Grizzle, J. E. and Hightower, N. C. (1969). A co-operative double-blind evaluation of gastric 'freezing' in the treatment of duodenal ulcer. *New. Engl. J. Med.*, **281**, 16.

Veterans Administration Cooperative Study Group on Antihypertensive Agents. (1967). I. Results in patients with diastolic blood pressures averaging 115 through 129 mmHg. *J. Am. Med. Assoc.*, **202**, 1028.

Wagensteen, O. H., Peter, E. T. and Nicholoff, D. M. (1962). Achieving 'physiological gastrectomy' by gastric freezing: a preliminary report of an experimental and clinical study. *J. Am. Med. Assoc.*, **180**, 439.

2
Epidemiological considerations in the design of controlled clinical trials. Part II: Methodology

BRUCE S. SCHOENBERG AND STEVEN HABERMAN

Unlike the laboratory investigator who is able to manipulate experimental conditions precisely, the clinical epidemiologist studies disease and its treatment or prevention in humans who cannot be subjected to such rigid control available in the basic science laboratory. Special research strategies have therefore been designed to evaluate the efficacy of new treatments for diseases in humans. This report presents a brief review of the available methods, the rationale for their use, and the problems involved in their implementation, with particular reference to neurological diseases.

ANALYTICAL PROSPECTIVE EPIDEMIOLOGY

The study of the outcome of natural experiments is the domain of this branch of epidemiology. During the course of our lives, different individuals are exposed to a variety of factors or conditions, some of which may play an important role (a) in the occurrence of disease, or (b) in the outcome or length of survival in those who have developed disease.

In the prospective approach (figure 2.1), we begin with a group or cohort exposed to a particular factor(s) thought to be related to disease onset or outcome and a group not exposed to the particular factor(s). The two groups are observed over time and their experience is compared. Because such investigations involve the observation of groups or cohorts of individuals exposed or unexposed to specific factors, they are often referred to as cohort studies.

An important consideration in this type of investigation is the comparability between the exposed and unexposed cohorts. As in any good experiment, the epidemiologist attempts to make his or her two groups

9

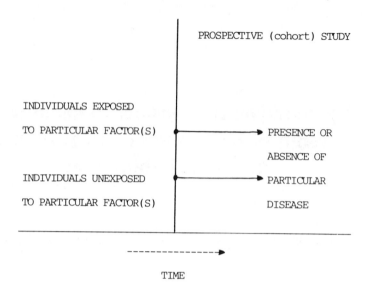

PROSPECTIVE (cohort) STUDY

INDIVIDUALS EXPOSED

TO PARTICULAR FACTOR(S)   PRESENCE OR

                                           ABSENCE OF

INDIVIDUALS UNEXPOSED   PARTICULAR

TO PARTICULAR FACTOR(S)   DISEASE

TIME

Figure 2.1 Format for the design of analytical prospective studies. (Modified and reproduced with permission from Schoenberg, 1978.)

matching in all recognisable aspects which might influence the outcome, except for the variable(s) he or she wishes to measure. If the two cohorts differ in a number of characteristics such as age, race, sex, etc., it may be these very factors (rather than the exposure status) that are responsible for an observed outcome.

For a prospective investigation we begin with a group of individuals exposed to the factor we wish to study (table 2.1). This group is designated as A + B. They are followed over a period of time to determine how many in this cohort will develop disease, represented by A. Thus, we are able to determine the absolute risk of disease in the cohort exposed to the factor. This is calculated as the ratio $A/(A + B)$. One then deals with a comparable cohort unexposed to the factor. This group is labelled C + D. They are also followed over a period of time for the possible development of disease. The group developing disease is designated as C. Just as was done previously, it is possible to calculate an absolute risk of disease in the unexposed group: $C/(C + D)$.

Besides studying the risk of disease in those exposed to a particular factor, one can also utilise the prospective approach to investigate the natural history of disease. By following patients with a specific disease, it is possible to measure the pattern of appearance and/or disappearance of signs or symptoms, disability, survival, etc. Special subgroups of patients can then be compared with regard to outcome. Results of such investigations provide useful information concerning prognosis and the variability in measurements of neurological dysfunction over time in the same patient and among several

Table 2.1 Format for a prospective study (Reproduced with permission from Schoenberg, 1982b.)

Cohort	Develop disease		
	yes	*no*	*total*
With putative aetiological factor	A	B	A + B
Without putative aetiological factor	C	D	C + D

patients with the same disease. These data can be extremely important in designing therapeutic trials of proposed new forms of treatment.

In a prospective study it is possible to measure absolute risk, i.e. the proportion of people exposed or unexposed to a given factor who develop a particular disease. Because exposure status at the very start in such a study is known and a uniform protocol for all people included in the investigation is used, there is little risk of misclassification according to exposure. It is unnecessary to rely on patients' or relatives' memories to gather this information. With such a study it is also possible to obtain data on people who give up the characteristic. For example, if we are interested in smoking as a risk factor for stroke, we can begin with a group of smokers and a group of non-smokers. Smoking status is measured at the beginning of the study, and it can even be quantified. These groups are then followed for changes in their smoking habits as well as for developing stroke. If a smoker stops smoking or otherwise changes his smoking habits, this can be noted and taken into account when calculating absolute risk. It is also possible to measure different diseases related to the characteristic. Once we have a cohort or group of smokers under observation, we can measure their risk of lung cancer or coronary artery disease, in addition to stroke.

Despite these advantages, the prospective study design also presents a number of problems. It is expensive and difficult to keep a large number of individuals under medical surveillance. It is not unusual to lose a substantial proportion of the original cohort. They may move away, lose interest in the study, or simply refuse to provide any required information. Prospective studies are generally unsuitable for investigating uncommon disorders. The study may itself alter people's behaviour. If we are examining the role of elevated blood pressure as a risk factor for subsequent stroke, an increased concern in the study population with regard to hypertension may be created. The concern and desire for medical examination and treatment may markedly change such individuals' blood pressures.

Those who volunteer for a prospective study, and those of the initial volunteers who continue under medical surveillance, may not be representative of all individuals with the characteristic of interest.

Once we have established the study protocol, it is difficult to incorporate new knowledge or new tests later. As an example, suppose we begin a planned 20-year study of certain diets and subsequent dementia. Assume that 15 years later a test is developed to determine blood aluminium levels, and studies indicate that chronic exposure to high aluminium levels is an important factor in subsequent Alzheimer's disease. If we then measure aluminium levels in everyone, these may not reflect levels some 15 years previously. Furthermore, some of the original patients in the study may already have developed Alzheimer's disease or may have died.

With any prospective study we are faced with ethical problems of varying importance. As evidence mounts implicating a particular factor in the aetiology of disease, we are obligated to intervene and, if possible, reduce or eliminate this factor. Finally, with a cohort study, practical considerations dictate that we must concentrate on a limited number of factors possibly related to disease outcome.

Note that the vertical line along the time axis in figure 2.1 is not labelled. Most prospective studies begin in the present and continue into the future. However, under certain circumstances it may be possible to begin the point of observation at some time in the past and look at disease outcome in the present. This is possible if cohorts of exposed and unexposed individuals were examined and questioned in a standardised manner in the past to determine health and exposure status. The two groups must then both be followed in a uniform, standardised manner. Such a study is called a non-concurrent prospective study or a prospective study in retrospect. This approach has the advantage of greatly reducing the time and expense often associated with prospective studies. On the other hand, it is most unusual to find cohorts of individuals who have been examined, questioned and observed in a standardised manner over a number of years. In reality, we must settle for cohorts who are examined and followed in a more or less uniform manner that does not achieve the level of standardisation available with prospective studies beginning in the present and continuing into the future.

EXPERIMENTAL EPIDEMIOLOGY

Experimental epidemiology is similar in approach to prospective analytical epidemiology, except that the investigator controls the assignment of individuals to exposure or non-exposure status with regard to a particular factor or condition. The fact that several neurological disorders are characterised by a pattern of exacerbation and remission introduces complications because it is difficult to evaluate whether an observed response is due to the treatment or to the natural history of the disease or to some combination of the two factors.

Objectives and the selection of subjects

Ethical considerations

Before embarking on an experiment there is a fundamental problem that must be carefully considered and solved. The distinguishing feature of experimental epidemiology is the investigator's control over whether study subjects receive a given form of therapy. The problem concerns whether it is proper to withhold from any patient a treatment that might, perhaps, give him benefit.

In any particular situation, certain general ethical issues must be considered. Some of these issues are given below, together with a brief discussion of each.

(a) Is the proposed treatment safe and therefore unlikely to bring harm to the patient?

The possible dangers of a treatment (and the reversibility of any side-effects) may need to be considered in relation to the dangers of the disease being treated.

(b) In a controlled trial (see below) can a treatment ethically be withheld from any patient in the doctor's care?

If the clinicians have good evidence that one treatment is, on average, superior, then it is problematic whether this treatment can be withheld. However, it is usual that some information is available regarding the conventional treatment but little is known about the new. Thus, it might be that the orthodox treatment is of limited value or is useless.

(c) What patients may be entered into a controlled trial and allocated to different treatments?

It must be ethically possible to give any patient enrolled in the trial either the new therapy or the comparison treatment (active medication or placebo). If the clinician believes that, for the patient's benefit, one particular treatment should be given, then that patient cannot be admitted to the trial. In any event, careful consideration would need to be given to the inclusion of certain categories of patients, e.g. pregnant women, patients with very severe disease, and infants.

(d) It is necessary to obtain the patient's consent to inclusion in a trial.
At least two points should be considered.

   (i) whether the patient will be subjected to discomfort or pain which is not an inevitable outcome of the disease or its orthodox treatment; and

(ii) the state of the clinician's ignorance concerning the relative efficacy of the treatments being tested.

(e) Is it ethical to use a placebo?

There may be no orthodox treatment of known or generally accepted value, so that the use of a placebo is justifiable in attempting to indicate whether the treatment under test is of value.

The aim of the trial

The first practical step in any trial is to decide precisely what it sets out to prove, that is, in statistical terms, to formulate the hypothesis. As a general principle, it is sensible to define precisely the questions to be asked and to limit them to a few.

It will be necessary to define exactly the disease under investigation and in particular its severity, whether incident or prevalent cases are to be entered into the trial, and whether particular subgroups of patients (defined by age, sex or other demographic variables) are to be entered. If prevalent cases are to be studied, it may be necessary to specify the duration of the disease.

Similarly the treatments being compared (including the placebo, if appropriate) require careful definition: the drug, dose, interval of administration, method of administration, period of treatment, etc. It is often the case that, for a new treatment about which little is known, one closely defined regimen is chosen. Sometimes, however, it may be more informative to allow for individual idiosyncrasies during the trial and permit the clinician to vary the dosage to his judgement of the patient's needs.

The number of treatments that a trial can cope with also needs careful consideration. If it is difficult to recruit patients such that the number of individuals within each group is expected to be small relative to the predicted sample size requirements, it is advisable to use only two treatment groups.

The endpoints of a trial should be defined in advance, as should the measurements that are to be made and their timing and frequency. The timing of events should be measured from the initiation of treatment rather than the completion of treatment to avoid bias (for example, affecting the comparison of a short-duration regimen and a long-duration regimen).

Assignment of exposure status

The distinguishing feature of experimental epidemiology is the investigator's control over whether study subjects receive a given form of therapy.

Uncontrolled trials

Following careful testing of potential therapeutic agents in animals to determine efficacy, safety, pharmacology, etc., initial use in humans usually involves an uncontrolled trial with no carefully designed comparison group. Patients with a specific disease are given a new form of therapy in an open trial in order to determine whether the treatment has any potential usefulness. These investigations are also helpful in determining an appropriate dose, in documenting adverse reactions, etc. However, for drugs which do not have a dramatic impact on the course of a disease, a formal comparison group is generally required in the design of studies used to measure therapeutic efficacy. Even for those therapies that radically alter the outcome of a given disease, one is using implied historical controls (i.e. the experience of earlier untreated patients affected by the same disease). Under such circumstances, one must be certain that the natural history of the disease has not been changing over time in untreated patients, and one must ensure comparability between the currently treated patients and those untreated in the past. Since most therapeutic trials deal with drugs that do not produce such remarkably beneficial results, it is becoming increasingly common to employ an experimental design in which the effects of a new drug are compared with some concurrent comparison experience (either placebo or an already accepted therapy).

Selected assignment

In this type of investigation, one or more therapies are compared with the natural history of the disease in untreated patients. The decisions to treat or not, and the specific type of treatment to be employed are usually made by several different physicians in the absence of well defined criteria for assigning the patient to a particular form of therapy. Very often this type of analysis is done in retrospect. For example, the experience of a group of patients with transient ischaemic attacks (TIA) who receive no treatment is compared with the outcome of TIA patients treated with carotid endarterectomy or TIA patients treated with anticoagulants. Although it is theoretically possible to match the groups according to the age, sex and racial distribution of the patients and the length of the observation period, questions of comparability remain. There may be important reasons why a given patient is not treated with anticoagulants or subjected to an endarterectomy (e.g. the patient may have a history of gastrointestinal bleeding or may be a poor candidate for surgery because of the presence of other diseases). It may be these factors which are responsible for an observed outcome rather than the specific form of therapy employed.

Random assignment

As in any experiment, it is important that the study group receiving the treatment and the comparison group not receiving the treatment be as similar as possible. Although it may be theoretically feasible to assure comparability on all factors that are *known* to influence the outcome by matching on these characteristics, there may be other factors whose effect is not recognised or cannot be determined. The random assignment of individuals to the study group and the comparison group is a frequently used strategy for attempting to achieve similarity for both known and unrecognised characteristics affecting outcome.

The use of randomised block designs and other derivatives will be covered in the following chapter. It should be emphasised, however, that randomisation does *not guarantee* comparability: randomisation is a *procedure* not an *outcome*.

Measurement

What to measure

In any therapeutic trial one must first decide what measurement or endpoints will be used to determine whether a specific form of treatment is effective for a particular neurological disease. Should one measure survival, the strength of a certain muscle, the characteristics of the electromyographic examination of a specific muscle, some overall clinical assessment, etc? Whatever one decides to examine, one must be certain that such a measurement is relevant to the clinical course of the disease. For example, let us assume one wishes to study a group of patients with motor neurone disease. The investigator may decide to evaluate the strength of the first dorsal interosseous muscle as one measure of outcome. If the patients under investigation are rapidly declining because of swallowing difficulties, the measurement of muscle strength in the first dorsal interosseous is not very relevant, since it does not adequately reflect the clinical course.

How to measure

In choosing a measurement procedure, one must take into account the accuracy and reproducibility of the method which is selected. The accuracy or validity of a test tells us how well or how closely it measures the 'true' or 'actual' value of what it is intended to measure (Schoenberg, 1982a). One must also consider the reproducibility or precision of the measurement, whether it is carried out repeatedly by the same observer or by multiple observers.

Finally, one must consider the possibility of bias in any measurement procedure or observation. In some situations, such as the self-evaluation of pain or discomfort, the patients themselves must serve as the observers. Patients may subjectively feel better or report improvements if they know they are receiving a new form of therapy. Even the investigator measuring the outcome of a therapeutic trial may be influenced by knowledge of whether or not a given patient is receiving a particular drug. In hopes of finding an effective treatment, the observer-investigator may subconsciously give patients receiving the drug a more optimistic evaluation. Both forms of potential bias can lead to incorrect inferences in an open trial in which individuals are receiving a new drug. To reduce this problem, three procedures for making the required observations have been developed (Lilienfeld and Lilienfeld, 1980).

The first method is termed a single-blind study. With this approach, the patients are not given an indication of whether they are receiving the specific therapy. This is often accomplished by means of a placebo, which for the study subjects must be indistinguishable from the active drug being tested. If two drugs are being compared, the two substances should be indistinguishable to the study subjects. This strategy prevents the patients from introducing bias into the observations. In this situation, however, both those measuring the outcome and those analysing the results are aware of which particular individuals are receiving the new drug.

In the double-blind investigation, neither the study subjects nor those measuring outcome are aware of which individuals are receiving the therapy under consideration. This is the most commonly used approach for current clinical trials. However, with a vast array of statistical tests at their disposal, the data analysts may search and re-examine results until they can demonstrate statistical significance for the new therapy.

To avoid this possibility, some have suggested the triple-blind strategy. With this procedure, the study subjects, the observer, and the data analyst are all unaware of which participants are receiving the drug being evaluated. Critics of clinical trials have facetiously defined triple-blind studies as investigations in which neither the patients nor the observers know who received the new drug and for which no one can figure out the result!

The need for a double-blind trial depends to some extent on the measurement to be taken. When examination of the patients is not necessary to measure the outcome, and an objective test (e.g. an X-ray, an electrocardiogram, a laboratory test) is available, it is a simple matter to assemble records and have them interpreted by someone independent of the trial. When mortality is used as an endpoint, determination of the cause of death may be biased. The same is true of measurement of the degree of disability.

It is fundamental that the same care in measurement and recording should be given to all the participating groups in a double-blind trial. The fact that some are specially treated and some are not is irrelevant. Unless the responses of the groups of patients are noted and recorded equally, any comparisons of them will clearly be of limited value.

Experimental design

Concurrent parallel trials

For controlled clinical trials with a predetermined fixed sample size, one may choose to use a concurrent parallel study design (figure 2.2). In this situation, observations on patients receiving the new therapy are carried out together with observations on patients receiving some other active treatment or placebo. Patients remain in the study group or the comparison group for the duration of the investigation. One way to attempt to achieve comparability is to match on all variables known to affect outcome. Thus, one can obtain pairs of patients of the same age, sex, race, duration and severity of illness, etc., and randomly allocate one to the treated group and one to the comparison group. There may be great difficulties in obtaining patients matched on all of these characteristics, and it may be necessary to wait a considerable period of time before obtaining adequate matched pairs. Another alternative is to assign patients to subcategories (strata) based on their characteristics; patients within each stratum are then randomly allocated to the study group or the comparison group. A third possibility is to assign all the participants in the trial randomly and without prior stratifica-

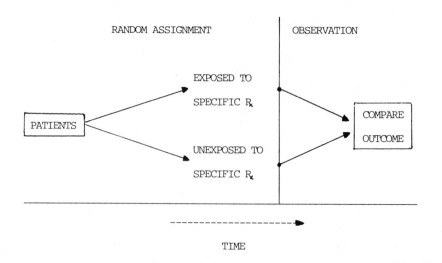

Figure 2.2 Schematic diagram of the design of concurrent parallel controlled therapeutic trials. (Reproduced with permission from Schoenberg, 1982c.)

tion either to the new therapy being studied or to some other form of active treatment or a placebo. In all these situations, it is important that the study group (those receiving the new drug) and the comparison group (those receiving either some other form of active therapy or a placebo) be as comparable as possible.

Cross-over trials

With the cross-over type of study design (figure 2.3) each patient serves as his or her own comparison. As before, patients are randomly assigned to a group receiving the therapy under study or to a group receiving some alternative form of active treatment or a placebo. The two groups are observed over time. Then the patients in each group are taken off their medication or placebo to allow for the elimination of the drug from the body and for the possibility of any 'carry-over' effects. This period is represented in figure 2.3 by the diagonal lines. After this period off medication (the length of this interval is determined by the pharmacological properties of the drug being tested), the two groups are switched. Those who received the treatment under study are changed to the comparison therapy or placebo, and vice versa.

Cross-over studies offer a number of advantages. With such a design, all patients can be assured that some time during the course of the investigation they will receive the new therapy. Such studies generally economise on the total number of patients required at the expense of the time necessary to

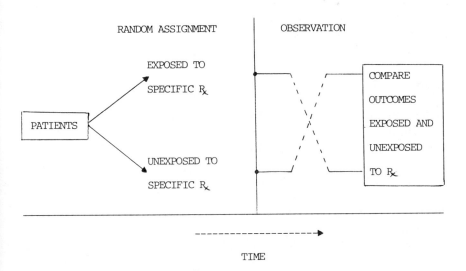

Figure 2.3 Schematic diagram illustrating the format of cross-over controlled therapeutic trials. (Reproduced with permission from Schoenberg, 1982b.)

complete the study (since all study subjects must receive *both* the new therapy and the comparison therapy or placebo). This approach is not suitable if the drug of interest cures the disease, if the drug is effective only during a certain stage of the disease, or if the disease changes radically during the period of time required for the investigation. If patients withdraw from the trial before its completion, they cannot serve as their own controls. These advantages of cross-over trials are at the expense of introducing the variability *within* patients from one time point to another.

Sequential trials

As indicated earlier, ethical considerations usually preclude random alloca-tion in a clinical trial if there is a *strong prior* view that one of the rival treatments is much superior. In the same way it will often be undesirable to continue a trial beyond a point at which one treatment is clearly seen to be better than a comparison treatment. To find when such a situation is reached the investigator must proceed sequentially: the observations will be analysed continuously and the decision to stop the trial will depend on the results obtained to date.

Such sequential designs are possible in clinical trials since patients may be entered into a trial serially, over a period of time, rather than all at the same time.

Other study designs have been advocated for evaluating the usefulness of particular forms of treatment. Some of these methods have special applica-tions, whereas others are controversial. The reader is referred to other reviews for a discussion of these different types of experimental design (Armitage, 1971; Good, 1976).

Sample size determinations

In the planning of controlled clinical trials, one of the most crucial questions concerns the number of patients required to obtain an answer as to whether a particular drug or therapy is effective. Many trials fail to achieve enough patients to provide a reliable treatment comparison.

An an example, consider a trial with two treatments, one new and one standard/placebo. To determine sample size, one must consider the factors outlined in table 2.2. We begin with the null hypothesis, and the statistical tests employed in evaluating the results of the trial provide us with some indication of whether we should accept or reject this hypothesis. There are two types of error we can make in this regard. We may mistakenly decide to reject the null hypothesis even though it is in fact correct. Translated into the results of our therapeutic trial, this decision is equivalent to accepting a new therapy which is of no value (when tested against placebo) or accepting

Table 2.2   Features that determine the estimated minimal sample size required for controlled therapeutic trials. (Reproduced from Schoenberg 1982c with permission.)

Null hypothesis	There is no difference between the effect of a new therapy and either some other form of active therapy or no therapy (placebo)
Type I or α error	Rejecting the null hypothesis when it is indeed correct (i.e. accepting a new therapy which is of no value or accepting that two treatments differ when in fact they do not)
Type II or β error	Accepting the null hypothesis when it is actually incorrect (i.e. rejecting a new therapy which is of value or accepting that two treatments are the same when in fact they are not)
Power	The probability of not making a Type II or β error
Sensitivity of trial	The smallest difference in effect between the new therapy and the comparison 'therapy' (i.e. other form of active treatment or placebo) one wants to detect through the clinical trial
Treatment difference = (in units of standard error*)	$\dfrac{\text{Effect of new therapy} - \text{Effect of comparison 'therapy'}}{\text{Standard error of difference}}$

*Standard error measures the variability of the outcome observation used in the controlled therapeutic trial.

that the new therapy is better than the active comparison treatment when in fact it is not. This is known as a type I or alpha error. On the other hand, we may mistakenly decide to accept the null hypothesis in a situation in which it is indeed incorrect. This is equivalent to rejecting a new therapy which is of value or rejecting a new therapy as not being superior to the active treatment when in fact it is. This is defined as a type II or beta error. This quantity is sometimes expressed in terms of its converse (i.e. the probability of not making a type II error). The converse is referred to as the power of the experiment or trial, and represents the probability of finding a treatment difference if in fact one exists. The remaining variable which we must consider in estimating sample size is the sensitivity of the trial. This is a measure of the smallest drug effect one wants to be able to detect by means of the controlled clinical trial. The smaller the drug effect one is able to detect, the greater the sensitivity of the trial. In general, the sample size is inversely proportional to: (a) the size of the type I error one is willing to tolerate; (b) the size of the type II error one is willing to tolerate; and (c) the

Methods in Clinical Trials in Neurology

size of the drug effect one hopes to detect. With a very large sample, it is possible to detect even relatively trivial treatment effects.

Figure 2.4 illustrates the interaction of these various factors in estimating sample size. The figure assumes that the drug is being tested against a placebo or against a form of treatment that has no effect on the course of the disease. The graphs further assume that we are willing to allow a 5% chance of making a type I or alpha error. The dashed line is for situations in which we are willing to allow a 5% chance of making a type II or beta error. The solid line corresponds to a 20% chance of making a beta error, and the dotted line corresponds to a 50% chance of making a beta error. Let us assume that the smallest drug effect one wishes to be able to detect is a situation in which 30% of the subjects respond. Then if one is willing to allow a beta error of 50% or 0.50, one needs only about 12 patients in the

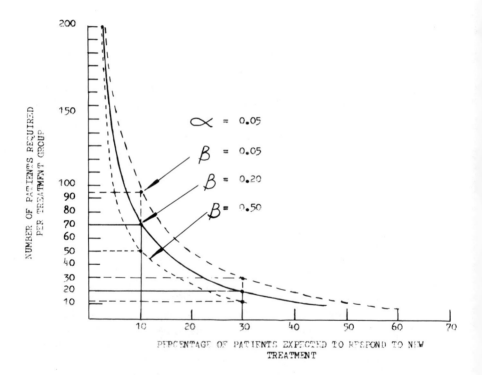

Figure 2.4 Minimal number of patients required in the study group (those receiving the therapy being evaluated) and the comparison group (those receiving some other form of active treatment or placebo) as a function of the size of the beta error one is willing to tolerate and the smallest percentage of patients expected to respond to the new treatment. (Modified and reproduced with permission from Clark and Downie, 1966.)

treated group and 12 patients in the comparison group. If one wants to reduce the beta error to 20%, one requires about 20 patients in each group, and if one wants to lower the allowable beta error to 5%, one needs about 28 patients in each group. If one wishes to design a controlled clinical trial able to detect a smaller drug effect in which 10% of the subjects respond, then the number of patients required increases. In this situation, for a tolerable beta error of 50%, one needs about 50 patients in each group; for a tolerable beta error of 20%, one requires approximately 70 patients in each group; and for a tolerable beta error of 5%, one needs about 93 patients in each group.

The series of graphs in figure 2.4 is applicable for outcome measurements that are all or none. For example, the patient can either be cured or continue to have the disease. For quantitative measurements such as the length of survival, nerve condition velocity, etc., one must also consider the variability of the outcome observation. The standard error provides a measure of this variability. In general, the greater the standard error of the outcome measurement, the larger the sample size required to detect a given treatment difference.

These considerations provide estimates of the theoretical numbers one should have in each group. In reality, however, patients may withdraw from the investigation. Therefore, the sample size projections represent minimal estimates. One must make allowances for withdrawals by beginning with larger groups than those derived from the theoretical figures.

In a practical case, one has to balance the benefits of increased precision (by raising the size of the trial) against the cost of the increased collection, experimentation and analysis.

Problems of implementation

Selection processes and bias

In every controlled clinical trial one is dealing with a sample of all those with the disease in the population. One is further restricted to those volunteering to participate. The selection process may result in a group of study subjects who are not representative of all those with the disease. The results of the investigation are applicable only to those types of patient represented in the study sample. One may purposely decide to restrict the investigation to certain subgroups, such as those with clinical evidence of disease for less than one year. In this instance, if the clinical trial demonstrates the effectiveness of a particular form of therapy, one cannot then assume that the therapy will be effective for all patients. It is essential that investigators state precisely their diagnostic criteria and their rules for the inclusion and exclusion of study subjects (Schoenberg, 1978). This will permit others to replicate the trial or decide whether the results are applicable to their own patients.

Those volunteering for a controlled therapeutic trial are then randomly allocated to a study group and a comparison group. Those assigned to either cohort may later refuse to participate just as the trial is about to begin. Finally, patients may be lost to follow-up or may voluntarily withdraw from the study. The withdrawals may consist of more benign cases but this may be less of a problem with severe neurological illnesses since such patients are highly motivated to participate in a trial of a potentially beneficial therapy. The patients remaining in the study group and comparison group at the end of the trial represent the final result of all of these selection processes, leading to both known and unrecognised sources of bias.

The problem of differences between volunteers and non-volunteers can be dealt with, to some extent, by following the non-volunteers in the same way as the volunteers to determine their outcome. Even if such follow-up is limited to mortality data, the comparisons will provide valuable information on the degree to which the results are generalisable. As with non-volunteers, the problem of withdrawals and refusals to participate can be partially solved by obtaining whatever information is available concerning their characteristics in addition to determining their outcome. It may be possible to follow up intensively a random sample (depending on their size and the difficulty in obtaining information about them). Regarding the losses, attempts should be made to obtain minimal information on this group such as mortality data.

Thus the more we know about how patients in the trial compare with those not included in the investigation, the more information we have concerning these potential biases.

Number of treatments

The number of treatments that any trial can deal with needs careful consideration. In any trial for which patient numbers are liable to be inadequate there should be only two treatment groups. Adequate patient numbers must be available for each group.

If two or more different forms of treatment can be considered in combination as well as separately, then a factorial experimental design may be used (see chapter 3).

If prior information on the standard treatment is substantial, then it may be sensible to reduce the fraction of patients allocated to the comparison group and increase the fraction allocated to the new treatment.

Unexpected outcomes

During the course of the study, patients may experience outcomes which were not anticipated. For example, in a clinical trial for patients with motor neurone disease, the study subjects may develop angina pectoris or die from a myocardial infarction during the course of the investigation. One must decide whether such deaths should be registered as possibly related to the drug or whether such deaths are incidental events unrelated to the therapy. Either choice has important implications for how the results of the investigation are analysed and interpreted.

If a patient develops a serious problem during the course of the trial, it may become necessary to withdraw the individual from the investigation. If such problems continue to occur, the entire study may have to be terminated.

Multicentre trials

Multicentre trials may be needed if the disease under investigation is rare, and the enrolment of several centres would ensure an adequate sample size. Alternatively multicentre trials may be set up to test the reproducibility of the results of a single-centre trial. Unlike infectious diseases, with their well known aetiology and epidemiology, some of the chronic, neurological diseases may be caused by several, different agents (mainly unknown) which may react with therapies synergistically or antagonistically. There is, therefore, a need for study populations chosen from many diverse communities and for collaborative studies between communities with different risks of morbidity.

Stopping rules

In most trials, patient accrual takes time and/or the period of treatment is prolonged so that the data and results build up only gradually. For ethical reasons it is important to undertake interim analyses to see if there are major differences to merit an early termination of the trial.

At the beginning of the investigation one must decide at what point in time the data are to be evaluated. If one looks at the results frequently and applies statistical tests to the data whenever the results appear to be interesting, by chance one may find the treatment effect to be statistically significant (i.e. a false positive conclusion). This is a dangerous approach fraught with error. As described by Macrae (1976): 'The application of significance tests to the data whenever an "interesting" difference is seen is analogous to watching a horse race and stopping it whenever the horse one wishes to win is ahead.'

For interim statistical analyses a stringent significance level, say $p < 0.01$, could be adopted as one's stopping criterion (in fact 10 repeated tests at this level give an overall 5% chance of reaching a false positive conclusion).

One should avoid looking at too many different response variables at each analysis since this will increase the chances of false positive conclusions. There is little advantage in performing several repeat interim analyses. It would be better to ensure a high quality and completeness of interim data before any analysis is carried out and limit the number of interim reports.

Combining of results of several trials

Perhaps the greatest problem plaguing clinical trials reported in the litera-ture is an inadequate sample size. The results look interesting but do not reach statistical significance. As a solution, some have suggested combining the data for all published results with the same drug. Even if one were able to ascertain that the various studies were conducted using the same techniques and the same outcome measurements, integrating the findings of several published studies has a major potential source of bias. The problem arises because therapeutic trials yielding negative results are frequently not published. Studies appearing in the literature tend to be biased in favour of those suggesting a positive value for the drug in question. The selection of such published data would therefore tend to provide an overly optimistic picture. A practical guide to controlled clinical trails for the practising neurologist is provided by Kurtzke (1982).

Organisation of trials

Probably more important than the statistical problems raised so far is the need for a trial to be efficiently organised. The randomisation process must be highly controlled: a simple design should be adopted to ensure that no rules are broken in its implementation. The statistical centre should be active throughout the course of the trial in ensuring the reliable and prompt recording of patient evaluations on well designed forms.

With any clinical trial, particularly those involving multiple centres, one must make special efforts to assure that the measurements are being made according to a standard protocol and recorded properly. If the integrity of the data cannot be maintained, the quality of the entire study will be diminished. One must also devise systems to verify whether patients are actually receiving medication according to the regimen dictated by the protocol. This is a particular problem when the patient or a member of the patient's family is responsible for administration of the drug as scheduled. After checking, the data should be processed with reasonable speed so that comprehensive analyses can be made without undue delay.

Reporting of results

In reporting the results of clinical trials, it is essential to describe the techniques employed, the conditions in which the trial was conducted, and the detailed statistical analysis of the results. Comments should address the various issues discussed in this paper and, in particular, attention should be given to checking the characteristics of the two groups under investigation and to mentioning the statistical power of the trial and the considerations leading to the choice of sample size. Results of a negative nature should be reported alongside positive results: to do otherwise would be to prejudge their significance.

CONCLUSIONS

Many of the difficulties inherent in the design and implementation of controlled therapeutic trials have been briefly reviewed. Future studies must carefully address these issues. Perhaps the most practical advice on how these investigations should be carried out was offered by Cornfield (1959) when he warned: 'Be careful'.

REFERENCES

Armitage, P. (1971). *Statistical Methods in Medical Research*. Blackwell Scientific Publications, Oxford.

Clark, C. J. and Downie, C. C. (1966). A method for the rapid determination of the number of patients to include in a controlled clinical trial. *Lancet*, **ii**, 1357–8.

Cornfield, J. (1959). Principles of research. *Am. J. Ment. Defic.*, **64**, 240–52.

Good, C. S. (1976). *The Principles and Practice of Clinical Trials*. Churchill Livingstone, London.

Kurtzke, J. F. (1982). On the role of clinicians in the use of drug trial data. *Neuroepidemiology*, **1**, 124–36.

Lilienfeld, A. M. and Lilienfeld, D. E. (1980). *Foundations of Epidemiology*. Oxford University Press, New York, pp. 256–74.

Macrae, K. D. (1976). Statistical aspects of trial design. In Good, C. S. (ed.), *The Principles and Practice of Clinical Trials*. Churchill Livingstone, London, pp. 87–92.

Schoenberg, B. S. (1978). Epidemiology of the inherited ataxias. In Kark, P., Rosenberg, R. and Schut, L. (eds), *The Inherited Ataxias: Biochemical, Viral and Pathological Studies*. Raven Press, New York, pp. 15–32.

Schoenberg, B. S. (1979). The epidemiologic approach to Huntington's disease. In Chase, T., Wexler, N. and Barbeau, A. (eds), *Huntington's Disease*. Raven Press, New York, pp. 1–11.

Schoenberg, B. S. (1982a). The scope of neuroepidemiology: from stone age to Stockholm. *Neuroepidemiology*, **1**, 1–16.

Schoenberg, B. S. (1982b). Hypothesis testing in neuroepidemiology: experiments of nature and experiments of man. *Neuroepidemiology*, **1**, 85–101.

Schoenberg, B. S. (1982c). Neuroepidemiologic definitions of disease: critiquing criteria. *Neuroepidemiology*, **1**, 197–200.

3
Choice and analysis of judgement criteria

W. MAURER and D. COMMENGES

INTRODUCTION

In neurology the assessment and comparison of efficacy of different treatment strategies is based largely upon subjective observations by investigators, hospital staff (nurses or psychologists), staff of rehabilitation centres (physiotherapists), staff of homes for the elderly, relatives of the patients and — especially in the field of migraine — also by assessment of the degree of pertinent symptoms by the patients themselves (Capildeo and Clifford-Rose, 1978).

Direct 'objective' measurements of physiological dimensions in neurology, for example the size of an ischaemic lesion by CT scan in stroke patients or the pattern of cerebral blood flow or EEG in demented patients, are often complex and seem to have a restricted association with the clinical symptomatology of the patients. Besides, such measurements, although useful in confirming a diagnosis, are not necessarily good indicators of 'clinical change', be it drug induced or representing the natural course of the disease. In addition the symptomatology is most often multidimensional, a fact any assessment of improvement of the state of the patient must take into account.

The choice (or construction) of judgement criteria or rating scales to be used in a clinical trial should be guided by properties of measurements often mentioned (but less often defined in a rigorous way), namely *validity, reliability, sensitivity* and *practicability* (or economy). The first two of these concepts for describing the general properties of scales and tests have been developed mainly by psychologists for the measurement of mental abilities, and a vast literature exists on them. (We will refer to the more recent one in the next section, where different well-known concepts of them are presented.)

Not nearly as much has been written about sensitivity, a property that is of great importance when the measurement is not used primarily as a diagnostic tool but as a means to assess changes (preferably improvements) caused by treatment strategies. We will propose an operational definition of sensitivity, discuss some well-known relations between validity and reliability, and present some (probably) new relations between these properties on the one hand and sensitivity on the other. They will help the reader to understand the means by which the sensitivity of a scale can be increased.

Practicability needs few comments: it is self-evident that assessment of judgement criteria should be as simple to perform as possible and that the raters (especially hospital staff or the patients themselves) must clearly understand what is asked of them. Practicability is closely related to validity and reliability: a scale consisting of too many items will result in a decrease of attention paid to the items towards the end of the scale (and, hence, will decrease reliability); a test battery that is too long may measure the perseverance of a patient rather than what is really intended to be measured (and, hence, will decrease its validity). In the third section of this chapter we will give a short account of how to estimate different types of validity and reliability, together with examples of possibilities for determining the construct and concurrent validity of a psychogeriatric scale by means of factor and cluster analysis.

In the final section we will discuss ways of estimating changes induced in judgement criteria by treatments and statistical tests, comparing these changes between treatment groups. Since judgement criteria and total scores from rating scales are in most cases 'only' ordinal-scaled variables (and not interval-scaled measurements, e.g. weight, blood flow, pulse), estimates and test must necessarily be invariant under monotone transformations of the scale. Rank-based tests and measures have this property. Among them special attention will be paid to possibilities of performing 'non-parametric analyses of convariance', that is, adjusting for factors (e.g. the pretreatment values) that cannot be balanced out completely between groups in a randomised trial. A new test of this type will be proposed that is closely related to an estimate for the conditional probability that a patient in the active treatment group improves more than one in the control group given that they have the same 'baseline conditions'.

Some consideration will also be given to the problem of performing multiple tests on various judgement criteria, and finally the problem of how to take into account the dynamical dimension of the process by means of life-table methods will be discussed.

PROPERTIES OF JUDGEMENT CRITERIA

The purpose of clinical ratings and the scope of this treatise

The purpose of measurements or observations on a patient may be either to diagnose his disease (to classify the patient nosologically) or to search for discriminating properties between different classes of patient (whether this be, for example, with respect to sex, age or various habits). Another aim may be to measure changes induced by natural causes such as age, or by artificial ones such as various treatment strategies. Although many considerations with respect to the appropriateness of the tests, judgement criteria or rating scales (i.e. collections of judgement criteria) are independent of their purpose, some are not. We want to discuss only the last mentioned case: the choice of criteria that provide a picture as clear cut as possible of the efficacy of a new treatment strategy in comparison with a standard one or a placebo.

Each discipline within neurology has developed its own instruments for the assessment of efficacy. In some of them, for example geriatrics, there already exists a certain choice of method — especially psychogeriatric scales — with well-known properties that are compiled and described in handbooks such as the ECDEU *Assessment Manual for Psychopharmacology* (1976), or its German equivalent the CIPS manual *Internationale Skalen für Psychiatrie* (1981); a review of such scales is given by Kochansky (1979). Nevertheless the development of new rating scales in this area is still in progress whereas in other areas of neurology, for example stroke, the first large steps have just been made (see, for example Orgogozo *et al*. 1983). The main goal of a rating scale is the assessment of the course of the *primary* symptoms of a disease under different treatments and of *secondary* symptoms that are possibly induced indirectly (e.g. depression caused by the loss of former abilities). However, criteria related to the long-term effects of treatments, e.g. the length of life of the patient and its quality before and after release from hospital (dependence on help by relatives, professional life) and criteria of socio-economic importance such as the number of days spent in hospital are also taken into consideration with increasing frequency. Although the criteria of the latter type are not free from problems (they may be culture dependent or heavily influenced by 'hospital policy'), they are relatively straightforward; 'number of days absent from work', for example, has face validity and can be observed exactly, i.e. it has high reliability.

In order to narrow the scope of this paper we shall now concentrate on questions related to the choice and analysis of criteria that must be rated on a subjective basis and hence cannot be measured on an interval-based scale, for instance the flicker-fusion frequency or the dominant frequency in a patient's EEG. In addition we shall try to expose problems and to describe ways of attacking them common to all disciplines of neurology from a *biometrical point of view*.

The neurological dimensions and their measurement

Most often in neurology the possible primary causes of a disease (be it a stroke, a progressive loss of neurones, vasoconstriction or a dopamine deficit) lead to losses of former abilities such as motor, verbal and cognitive skills or to affective disturbances. This may happen directly or it may be induced indirectly or connected with symptoms distressing for the patient such as headache and tremor. The prime goal of any therapy must be at least to alleviate or possibly suppress these symptoms, to stop further deterioration and possibly to restore former abilities. This may be achieved partly by symptomatic treatment (analgesics in migraine), by the removal of primary causes or by improvement of the functioning of intact or only little impaired parts of the brain to compensate for other irreversible damage.

If an underlying dimension affected is defined narrowly enough (e.g. the walking ability of a patient), it may be observed directly and in this case the criterion or test is said to possess *face validity*. Whenever possible, criteria with this property should be chosen. For more fundamental and complex dimensions (for example cognitive function) it is, however, rarely possible to measure them directly. Only certain of their aspects are observable. It is an important task of a clinical investigator to define a collection of such aspects (criteria) that are in close connection with the dimension of interest, i.e. that have a high *validity* with respect to the unobservable construct (dimension). A suitable mathematical function (mostly linear combinations are used) may then possess a higher validity than each single item (see p. 34). The question of how to define validity operationally and how to estimate it from empirical data has been dealt with in the literature on psychological measurement, especially in the context of determining mental abilities (see, for example, Lord and Novick, 1968; Lienert, 1969; Bock and Wood, 1971; Levy, 1973).

Validation of a scale is actually a circular and practically unending process. The initially only vaguely defined dimension of interest will also become less fuzzy than it was initially by the empirical evidence gained from validation experiments with a potential scale consisting of a large number of tentative items — especially with respect to its connection to other dimensions (think of the possible interactions between motor and mental skills or between affect and soma). We will give a practical example later.

The reliability of measurements

Even an essentially valid criterion is of little use if it is unreliable, i.e. blurred by a large and random error of measurement. There are many sources of such errors.

First, the dimension to be measured may vary over time in a patient. An interview or a test performed at a clinical visit then represents a random 'picture' cut out from a temporally continuous flow of fluctuating states (this is especially true in diseases with interchanging remissions and relapses or with relatively short episodes of symptoms). In this case a 'smoothed' assessment of a longer period of observation or the count and description of the episodes respectively by persons who attend the patient may provide a more reliable account of the actual state than a 'flashlight' picture — even if the rater's recollection introduces a new source of error. In most cases the rater himself represents the largest source of error when he tries to 'map' the patient's state — as he perceives it — on to an ordinal scale.

To estimate the size of this error empirically is not as straightforward as the estimation of a physical instrument's error of measurement. In the latter case, measurements performed under the same experimental conditions need just be repeated several times. The empirical variance or standard deviation of the observed values then represents a consistent estimate of the 'true' variance or SD of the instrument. This is possible, since each measurement can be considered as being statistically independent of the others. If the 'instrument of measurement' is a person, this is not true anymore. One cannot ask a rater to assess the same patient twice (or more) within a short time on the same scale, because he will remember the rating he gave earlier and simply repeat it. If each measurement is repeated only when the preceding ones have been forgotten, the patient (i.e. the measurement condition) may have changed considerably in the meantime.

In special cases (e.g. in geriatrics) where the rating is based on an interview exclusively, the use of videotaped interviews may be an answer (see, for example, Andreasen *et al.* 1982). In clinical trials the ratings are sometimes done by several investigators (not only in multicentre trials). This, of course, introduces new sources of error. With respect to a clinical trial, validity and reliability are of importance only in so far as they affect the sensitivity of a scale. Sensitivity could be measured, e.g. by the probability with which a true difference of treatment effects in a certain dimension can be detected by an appropriate statistical test with a fixed number of patients, or equivalently by the number of patients that are needed to detect such a difference with a fixed predetermined probability (power). Before we discuss this question in more detail, another will be addressed.

How many score values should a judgement criterion have?

There are two extremes for the number of possible scores, namely 2 at the one end (for a dichotomous item with codes, e.g. 0 for no or absent and 1 for yes or present) and a continuous scale at the other end. In between, usually three to ten different score steps (points) are chosen for ordinal criteria. Clearly there is no general answer to the question of what choice is best.

For the self-rating of mood, pain or more generally symptoms whose intensity cannot be described unequivocally, preference might be given to a 'visual-analogue' scale or 'thermometer' scale. Here the patient marks graphically the degree of the symptom on a 10 cm scale between two extreme states as 'alert' and 'drowsy', for example (Bond and Lader, 1974).

For ratings done by a second person it seems advisable to choose only as many scores as can be described unequivocally in words. It may be true that the sensitivity of a scale increases when the number of possible scores is increased, for example from three to five steps. But this is hardly the case if the error of observation is already of the same size as the step width. The effect may even be reversed if the choice of possible scores is too large because of the 'trend to the middle', the tendency to avoid extreme judgements. An alternative to a judgement criterion with many score values is the construction of several dichotomous items that have different 'difficulty' with respect to the underlying dimension. The sum of such items will then have a sensitivity comparable to that of an item with many score steps.

It is not necessary that all items of a scale have the same number of points. But if the items are to be summed up to a total score, due consideration should be given to the question of weighing. McKenna *et al.* (1981) present an example of how to use Thurstone's method of paired comparisons of items in order to achieve an objective weighing scheme.

A mathematical model and its implications

Some remarks and a warning

In this section we will attempt to derive some well-known and some possibly new relations between coefficients for validity, reliability and sensitivity. The less mathematically orientated reader might prefer to read just the italicised definitions.

We shall follow by and large the lines of Lord and Novick (1968) for the 'classical model' and for the definitions. However, we will enlarge the model on the one hand so that it suits the more general framework we are dealing with, but simplify on the other hand the derivations of the formulae by assuming (without loss of generality) that all observed scale or item values are standardised to unit variance. The same assumption will be made for all random variables that may contribute to an observation. The definitions given should also help the reader to understand better the concepts of inter- and intrarater reliability.

Coefficients of validity and reliability

Let S be a random variable defined over a population of patients and representing the *score* of a scale or of a single judgement criterion. A realisation of S, i.e. an actual observation on a certain patient, will, as in all other cases, be denoted by the respective lower case letter (in our case s).

Let X be the *unobservable neurological dimension* of interest, Y be a *combination of other dimensions* that may contaminate the observation of X (e.g. mood may contaminate an observation of mental alertness) and E the random error of the observation performed by a specific rater R.

The score S of a randomly chosen patient rated by R may then be written as:

$$S = \sigma_x X + \sigma_y Y + \sigma_e E \tag{3.1}$$

where σ_x, σ_y and σ_e are real numbers such that:

$$\sigma_x^2 + \sigma_y^2 + \sigma_e^2 = 1 \tag{3.2}$$

Usually the following assumptions (criticised by Bock and Wood (1971) as being somewhat platonic) are made

$$E(E) = 0$$
$$\text{Cov}(X,Y) = \text{Cov}(X,E) = \text{Cov}(Y,E) = 0 \tag{3.3}$$

where $E(\cdot)$ denotes the expectation, Cov the covariance and Var the variance. In addition we assume

$$\text{Var}(X)\,\text{Var}(Y) = \text{Var}(E) = 1 \tag{3.4}$$

By (3.2) and (3.4) we also have $\text{Var}(S) = 1$.
The validity of S with respect to the unknown dimension X is then defined as the correlation r_{tc} *between S and X.*

As an immediate consequence we have

$$r_{tc} = \sigma_x \tag{3.5}$$

Proof (given as an exception)

$$r_{tc} = \text{Corr}(S,X) = \text{Cov}(S,X)/\sqrt{\text{Var}(S) \cdot \text{Var}(X)} = \text{Cov}(S,X);$$
$$\text{Cov}(S,X) = \sigma_x\text{Cov}(X,X) + \sigma_y\text{Cov}(Y,X) + \sigma_e\text{Cov}(E,X) = \sigma_x \qquad \text{Q.E.D.}$$

Let S_1 be a rating independent of the first one on the same patient by rater R (e.g. by the videotape approach) then

$$S_1 = \sigma_x X + \sigma_y Y + \sigma_e E_1, \text{ where } \text{Cov}(E,E_1) = 0$$

The (intrarater) reliability of S is defined as the correlation r_{tt} *between S and* S_1. (One can show that this definition is equivalent to the one proposed by Lord and Novick, namely r_{tt} being the squared correlation between S and the 'true score' $(\sigma_x X + \sigma_y Y)$.)

It implies

$$r_{tt} = \sigma_x^2 + \sigma_y^2 = 1 - \sigma_e^2 \qquad (3.6)$$

and

$$|r_{tc}| = \sqrt{r_{tt} - \sigma_y^2} \qquad (3.6')$$

From (3.6') follows immediately the well-known formula

$$\boxed{|r_{tc}| \leqslant \sqrt{r_{tt}}} \qquad (3.7)$$

which says essentially that a criterion with a low reliability necessarily also possesses a low validity.

Consider now a second rater R' assessing the same criterion as R on the same patient as R. His score then is:

$$S' = \sigma_x' X + \sigma_y' Y' + \sigma_e' E'$$

that is, his perception of the true dimension X is contaminated by a factor Y' that may be the same as Y or different from it. Rater R's intrarater reliability $r_{t't'}$ then is $\sigma_x'^2 + \sigma_y'^2$. We can now *define the interrater reliability as the correlation $r_{tt'}$ between S and S'.* This implies

$$r_{tt'} = \sigma_x \sigma_x' + \sigma_y \sigma_y' \, \mathrm{Cov}(Y, Y') \qquad (3.8)$$

An inequality similar to (3.7) can now be derived from (3.6) and (3.8):

$$\boxed{r_{tt'} \leqslant \sqrt{r_{tt} \cdot r_{t't'}}} \qquad (3.9)$$

This formula tells us that if the interrater reliability is high (and of about equal size) the intrarater reliabilities must be at least of about the same size.

On sums of scores

Let us assume now that a dimension X (e.g. cognitive dysfunction) is assessed by two different criteria S and S^* (for example 'confusion' and 'reduced mental alertness'). Each measures partly X but is contaminated by different other factors Y and Y^* and affected by different errors:
$$S^* = \sigma_x^* X + \sigma_y^* Y^* + \sigma_e^* E^*, \, r_{tc}^* = \sigma_x^*.$$

If we sum S and S^* (as is often done in scales) then $\Sigma = S + S^*$ has the validity

$$r_{tc}(S + S^*) = \text{Cov}(X, S + S^*)/\sqrt{\text{Var}(S + S^*)}.$$

Since the numerator is $(\sigma_x + \sigma_x^*)$ and the denominator cannot be larger than $\sqrt{4}$, on using (3.5) we obtain

$$r_{tc}(S + S^*) \geq (r_{tc} + r_{tc}^*)/2 \qquad (3.10)$$

Especially if the reliability of each of the two criteria is low (i.e. σ_e and σ_e^* are large) and if the two contaminating factors Y and Y^* are either only or even slightly negatively correlated, the validity coefficient of the sum of the two criteria can be considerably higher than the mean of the validity coefficients of each single criterion (this can be seen easily if one derives the exact expression for $\text{Var}(S + S^*)$).

An immediate and important consequence of inequality (3.10) is that for a complex dimension many criteria should be selected which measure different aspects of it and which all have about the same validity. The sum of these criteria will then have higher validity than each single item. Since — as we will show — validity is influencing directly the sensitivity, the latter can be considerably increased by using weighted sums of the scores of items that are well correlated with the underlying dimension of interest.

For a scale that covers different dimensions, a factor analysis on the pretreatment scores, or on a different sample, gives a guide as to which items should be summed up to 'factors'.

This, of course, only proves a fact that has been recognised already experimentally for a long time.

Sensitivity

As already mentioned, sensitivity is closely related to the detection of a difference σ between treatment time effects on the dimension X of interest. We propose the following model:

That in a controlled clinical trial, the actively treated group is compared with a placebo group of the same sample size. The 'latent trait' X is assessed by a scale with score S. The treatment effects δ_1 and δ_2 in the two groups are fixed with difference $\delta = \delta_1 - \delta_2$ (a more realistic model would assume these effects to be random).

By S_1 and S_2 we now denote the random post-treatment scores in the two groups, respectively, i.e.

$$S_1 = \sigma_x(X + \delta_1) + \sigma_y Y + \sigma_e E$$

and

$$S_2 = \sigma_x(X' + \delta_2) + \sigma_y Y' + \sigma_e E' \tag{3.11}$$

$((X,Y,E)$ has the same distribution as (X',Y',E').)

Let u_p denote the p-quartile of the standard normal distribution, μ_1 and μ_2 the expected scores after active and placebo treatment respectively, and σ_1 and σ_2 the variance of the scores S_1 and S_2 in both groups. Then the sample size n necessary to detect a (small) difference $(\mu_1 - \mu_2)$ of the expected values by means of a two-sample t-test on the post-treatment values (we assume asymptotic normality of the means for large samples) can be computed by

$$n = (u_{1 - \frac{\alpha}{2}} + u_{1 - \beta})^2 \cdot (\sigma_1^2 + \sigma_2^2)/(\mu_1 - \mu_2)^2 \tag{3.12}$$

where α is the level of significance and $1-\beta$ the power of the test.

For model (3.11) we have $\sigma_1^2 = \sigma_2^2 = 1$ and $\mu_1 - \mu_2 = \sigma_x \delta = r_{tc}\delta$; hence

$$n = c/r_{tc}^2 \tag{3.13}$$

where $c = 2(u_{1 - \frac{\alpha}{2}} + u_{1 - \beta})^2/\delta^2$. The *coefficient c is independent of the scale's properties*, except that δ is measured in SD of X. We *define the sensitivity*, sens(S), *of a scale S* (in relation to a test on the post-treatment scores) *by*

$$\boxed{\text{sens}(S): = c/n \text{ (or equivalently)} \ n = c/\text{sens}(S)} \qquad = \tag{3.14}$$

To our knowledge, up to now no explicit coefficient of sensitivity has been proposed in the literature. The one defined by (3.14) has the property that it is low when the sample size needed to detect δ is large, and vice versa. For our model we get, from (3.13) and (3.14)

$$\boxed{\text{sens}(S) = r_{tc}^2} \tag{3.15}$$

If we define similarly the sensitivity sens* *(S) with respect to a two-sample test on the change from baseline* within each patient, we get

$$\text{sens}^*(S) = r_{\text{tc}}^2/2(1-r_{\text{tt}}) \qquad\qquad (3.16)$$

At least within this model, sensitivity is a simple function of validity and reliability.

Let us assume that we assess the dimension X = 'walking ability' by the dichotomous criterion S with the two scores $S = 0$, if the patient cannot walk 50 m without help, and $S = 1$ if the patient can walk without help. Then the reliability of S may be quite high but the validity is low when X is essentially a continuous variable. The reason is that the correlation between a continuous and dichotomous variable cannot be large (≤ 0.8, if X is normal). By formulae (3.15) and (3.16), sensitivity then must be low as well. Admittedly, under these assumptions the error term is negatively correlated with X and the formulae are not exact anymore, but still describe the trend. A much more valid and hence more sensitive criterion S for X would be, for example, the 11-point scale proposed by Hazama *et al.* (1976).

Comparing (3.14) and (3.15) shows that

$$\text{sens}^*(S)/\text{sens}(S) = 1/2(1-r_{\text{tt}}) \qquad\qquad (3.17)$$

This confirms the old wisdom that testing for treatment effects between groups by means of changes from baseline (instead of only post-treatment values) may result in a considerable gain of sensitivity which is equivalent to a reduction of sample size needed to detect a true effect. This gain, however, can be realised only if the ratio in (3.17) is larger than 1 or equivalently if the reliability coefficient is larger than $\frac{1}{2}$.

ESTIMATING VALIDITY AND RELIABILITY

Validity

It is obvious that the theoretical coefficient of validity as defined on p. 34 in most instances cannot be estimated directly, since only certain aspects of the underlying dimension X may be observable.

Concurrent validity

There are, however, cases where there exists for X a generally accepted measure, as for example the total score of the Hamilton Depression Scale for the dimension 'depression', or the Wechsler Adult Intelligence Scale (WAIS). The use of a scale designed for diagnostic purposes in psychiatry or of a relatively time-consuming psychometric test that in addition cannot be repeated at relatively short intervals of time may be impractical within the scope of a clinical trial in neurology.

Subsets of such a scale, of a psychometric test or of entirely new scales designed specifically to cover the needs in a special population (for example a depression scale for geriatric purposes) *can* then *be validated with respect to the already established scales* by assessing the new scale and the reference scale simultaneously on a sample population.

The empirical correlation coefficient between them is a measure of the *concurrent validity* of the new scale (Oswald, 1979). We shall not deal here with the problem of what correlation coefficient is appropriate; in general a non-parametric version such as Spearman's ρ or Kendall's τ is a good choice (see, for example, Kruskal, 1958). Correlating 'old' with 'new' scales is not without pitfalls since an established scale in general is not error-free and hence is not 100% valid or is designed for a completely different population.

Criterion-related validity

Criterion-related or predictive validity is the circumscription for a validation procedure in which the scores of the new scales are compared between extreme groups of a population that can be clearly distinguished clinically. This of course can only give an answer to the question 'does the scale have any validity at all', and does not really measure the degree of validity.

Construct validity

An internal method of validation for a multidimensional scale is subsumed under the term 'construct validity'. It tries to answer the question of how many and what dimensions (constructs) account for the variability of the scale's items. Construct validity is studied ordinarily by examining the empirical correlations among the items comprising the scale.

If the data reveal correlations among the items not in accord with the *a priori* conceptualisations (or constructs), or if relationships between the items do not provide any inferential evidence for revision of the *a priori* conceptualisation, the scale is declared to lack construct validity (Hamot, 1974). Factor analysis of the items comprising the scale is the usual method for establishing construct validity. An alternative method where no implicit or explicit assumption on the relationships between the underlying factors as in factor analysis is necessary in a cluster analysis on the items with absolute correlation as a measure of similarity between items.

A concurrent visualisation of the results of both methods is often helpful. An example is given in figure 3.1. It depicts the results of a factor analysis (varimax rotation of the first five principal components) and of the average linkage cluster algorithm (Hartigan, 1975) on the absolute correlations between the 18 items (seven-point scaled) of the SCAG (Sandoz Clinical

Factor
loadings   Dendrogram

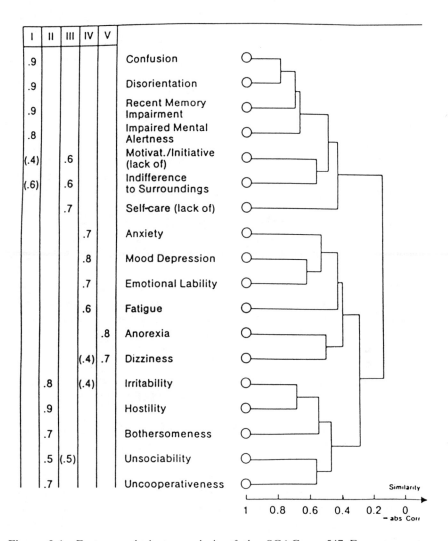

Figure 3.1 Factor- and cluster-analysis of the SCAG on 547 European cases. Loadings (on the left) in brackets indicate that item loads are still higher on another scale; loadings less than 0.4 are suppressed. (In the American sample 'fatigue' belongs to factor V and 'unsociability' to factor III.) Comparing the 'clusters' of items with high loadings on one factor with those visualised in the dendrogram on the right (computed with the average linkage algorithm, BMDP 1981, program P1M) reveals a high coincidence. This is always the case if the factors are immanently orthogonal, i.e. uncorrelated.

Assessment Scale: Geriatric). The sample on which the correlations are based is a pooling of the pretreatment scores of 547 geriatric patients from different European countries. Since, along with the English original of the scale, German and French translations were used, before the pooling separate factor analyses were performed on the respective subsamples and compared with the results of a similar analysis of 1165 cases from 21 American trials. Essentially, in all but one sample, a structure with five factors emerged (Maurer *et al.*, 1982; Hamot *et al.*, 1983), namely I = cognitive dysfunction, II = interpersonal relationships, III = apathy, IV = affect, and V = somatic functioning.

Reliability

The estimation of reliability is much less controversial than that of validity. An example of the set-up of a trial designed to estimate the interrater reliabilities of a new neurological scale is described by Orgogozo *et al.* (1983).

Often the interrater reliability is estimated by taking into account the ratings of more than two raters and using measures of concordance or various coefficients of intraclass correlation. The latter rely on estimates of mean sum of squares from two-way ANOVAs with investigators and patients as blocks. Here also differences between mean scores of the investigators can be taken into account if this seems necessary (in an ordinary correlation coefficient they are of no importance). For details see Shrout and Fleiss (1979) and Cho (1981).

STATISTICAL ANALYSIS OF JUDGEMENT CRITERIA AND RATING SCALES IN CLINICAL TRIALS

In the sequel we shall discuss a few points that are of importance with respect to a confirmatory and explanatory analysis of a rating scale and the items of which it consists.

If possible the properties of the main scale used to assess efficacy should be known already before a trial, especially with respect to its dimensionability. If the scale is unidimensional, the total sum score is the most sensitive measure for efficacy. In this case a non-parametric test between groups on the post- minus pretreatment total score or on the ratios between post- and pretreatment total score is a sensible way of testing the null hypothesis of no treatment effect. Non-parametric analogues of analysis of covariance with the pretreatment values as covariate (or other prognostic factors) as described by Koch *et al.* (1982) should also be considered. If the scale is multidimensional (e.g. the SCAG with five factors), it is preferable to test simultaneously the score sums of items belonging to the same factor (confirmatory for those factors where a treatment effect is to be expected and wanted, and exploratory by just giving *p*-values or confidence intervals for treatment differences for those factors where no treatment effect is expected or wanted). Clearly, if more than one factor is tested, due consideration is to be given to the problem of multiple testing. If the factors are essentially orthogonal (i.e. uncorrelated), the sequentially rejecting procedure proposed by Holm (1979), a generalisation of the well-known Bonferroni procedure, is to be recommended. Otherwise again a multivariate test on the factors might be considered.

Especially when the control group is treated with a standard drug, it may be of greater importance to compare between groups the course of disease during the trial period than to compare the patients' state at the end of the trial (for example to answer the question as to whether the beneficial effect occurs earlier in the active treatment group than in the control group). Here a multivariate test between groups on the measurements at different visits or their change from baseline might give a global answer to the question of the existence of a main effect and time–treatment 'interaction'. If the total scores are approximately normally distributed at the visits, a Hotelling's T^2 test in the two-sample case or a more general MANOVA in the *k*-sample case can be used. In general, however, a non-parametric multivariate analogue of the Kruskal-Wallis test as proposed by Puri and Sen and described in detail by Koch (1969) is a more robust alternative to a parametric test.

In the next section we describe in detail a non-parametric procedure that can be used if the treatment effect on a single (ordinal) judgement criterion (e.g. an overall assessment of the patient's status) is to be estimated and tested for difference between two groups.

A Measure and a Test for Difference of Change in a Judgement Criterion

The problem

Assume that a judgement criterion is observed before (pre) and after (post) treatment in two treatment groups (numbered 1 and 2) in a randomised trial with *N* patients resulting in *m* and *n* patients in the two groups respectively ($m + n = N$). Campbell (1978) has reviewed several possibilities for testing the treatment difference if the scores are essentially normally distributed. Among them are *t*-tests (or more general one-way ANOVA for more than two treatments) on the pre–post differences, blocked ANOVA on blocks of subjects with similar initial scores, and analysis of covariance. All these methods have the disadvantage that they are not invariant under monotone transformations of the measurement scale. Hence, they may be applied properly only to interval-scaled variables.

If tests are based on the ranked observations after treatment, however, as, for example, in a Mann-Whitney U-test (or equivalently the Wilcoxon two-sample rank test), they do have this property, but in most instances much power is wasted by not taking into account the values before treatment. It is well known from parametric statistics that pre–post differences may have a drastically lower variability than the post- (or pre-) treatment values within groups since, in the former, between-patient variation is eliminated and only the measurement error and within-patient variation account for the observed variability. The same is true for analysis of covariance (ANACOVA), which in addition (compared with tests on differences) adjusts for possible imbalance of the pretreatment values by assuming a linear relationship between the expected pre- and post-treatment values (or equivalently between expected pretreatment values and the pre–post difference). This assumption of linearity is unrealistic or even nonsensical for a discrete single judgement criterion with relatively few possible score (say up to seven) values. Let $(X_{b,i}, X_{a,i})$ denote a pair of scores before and after treatment of patient i in group 1 (e.g. new active drug) and $Y_{b,j}, Y_{a,j}$ the respective pair of (random) scores for a patient j of group 2 (placebo or standard treatment). Then the model underlying ANACOVA is:

$$X_{a,i} = \alpha + \gamma \cdot X_{b,i} + \epsilon$$

$$Y_{a,j} = \alpha + \beta + \gamma \cdot Y_{b,j} + \epsilon$$

with ϵ being the random error of measurement with expectation 0 (normally distributed), α the overall effect of the standard, and β the additional effect of active treatment.

Clearly for extreme pretreatment scores (be it minimum or maximum), the model may ask the expected post-treatment scores to be even larger or smaller, which is impossible. In addition, the discreteness of the scale implies the same for the error of measurement – violating the assumption of normality. Finally and most importantly, as already mentioned, the model is not invariant under monotone transformations. An alternative that has all the advantages and none of the disadvantages of 'classical' analysis of covariance will be explained with the help of an example.

Example

The data stem from a double-blind clinical trial lasting 8 weeks comparing a new chemical entity with placebo in 2×25 geriatric patients suffering from senile mental deterioration. Among other measures of efficacy (as psychometric tests before and after treatment), the patients had to be rated by the investigator before, during and at the end of the trial on a psychogeriatric scale (the SCAG, see earlier). Just for the purpose of illustration of the method we will pick out one of the items of the factor 'cognitive dysfunction', namely 'impairment of mental alertness', which had to be rated on a 7-point scale ranging from 1='absent' to 7='severe' (as for the other items). In table 3.1 the respective ratings before and after treatment for all 50 patients are presented.

Obviously the mean score difference between groups after treatment (0.2 points) is very small, and a one-sided Mann-Whitney U-test (with correction for ties) yields a p-value of $p = 0.27$, i.e. no statistically significant difference.

Table 3.1 Impairment of mental alertness.

	Active drug (group 1)				Placebo (group 2)		
Patient no.	*Before* X_b	*After* X_a	Δx $X_a - X_b$	*Patient no.*	*Before* Y_b	*After* Y_a	Δy $Y_a - Y_b$
1	3	2	−1	2	3	3	0
3	2	2	0	6	5	4	−1
4	5	4	−1	8	4	3	−1
5	5	5	0	9	3	3	0
7	6	2	−4	10	4	4	0
11	3	3	0	13	4	3	−1
12	3	3	0	14	5	4	−1
17	7	6	−1	15	2	2	0
19	5	3	−2	16	3	3	0
20	6	5	−1	18	6	5	−1
23	3	2	−1	21	5	4	−1
26	3	2	−1	22	2	2	0
28	5	4	−1	24	3	3	0
29	4	3	−1	25	2	2	0
32	4	3	−1	31	4	3	−1
33	5	4	−1	35	2	2	0
34	5	4	−1	38	6	5	−1
36	3	3	0	39	5	5	0
37	6	4	−2	40	6	6	0
41	6	5	−1	43	4	4	0
42	6	4	−2	45	4	3	−1
44	4	4	0	47	5	5	0
46	4	3	−1	50	5	5	0
49	4	4	0	54	6	5	−1
51	4	4	0	55	5	5	0
Mean	4.44	3.52	−0.92		4.12	3.72	−0.4
Median	4.0	4.0	−1.0		4.0	4.0	0.0
Minimum	2	2	−4		2	2	−1
Maximum	7	6	0		6	6	0

The picture changes if we look at formal score changes Δ (post- minus pre-) and compare them between groups; here the mean difference is 0.52 since the baseline values in the active treatment group are 4.44 and 4.12 in the placebo group. A formal U-test on Δ between groups yields (one sided) $p = 0.01$, i.e. the decrease in the first group is statistically significantly larger than in the second. Nevertheless this result is questionable since in its calculation it is implicitly assumed that a decrease, say from 3 to 2, is the same as a decrease from 6 to 5, and furthermore that the difference in baseline values is of no importance. As we shall see in the sequel, it seems to be easier to improve from a bad initial state (say 6) than from a good one (say 2), and hence a group with worse average starting values than the other one will have some advantage. This is an observation that can be made quite often but in some cases it may also be reversed (e.g. for irreversible damage). What actually can be compared with respect to the degree of improvement are only the post-treatment scores of those patients with the same baseline values. They can be easily summarised as in table 3.2. In this table we have as the first column the pretreatment scores k ranging from 2 to 7. They define the strata (or blocks) within which we can compare the post-treatment scores between the two treatments. (It is quite obvious that these strata could also be based on other concomitant variables such as sex, age groups, or groups with different severities of the disease.)

Table 3.2 shows that the main reason why the distribution of post-treatment scores is not very much different between groups (see sum*) is that, in particular, patients with little impairment (score 2) who do not improve further (down to 1) in either group are more prevalent in the placebo group. Good improvements in the active treatment group can be seen, especially in patients with pre-scores 5 and 6, whereas in the placebo group there is either no or only little improvement by one point.

Combining data from several blocks

A Mann-Whitney test statistic U_k may be computed within each of the strata defined by a pretreatment score k where both subsample sizes n_k and m_k are different from 0. (U_k is as usually defined as the number of post-treatment scores in group 1 larger than scores in group 2 plus half the number of pairs of scores from both groups with equal values. The number of comparisons to be made is that of all $m_k \cdot n_k$ possible pairs of scores between both groups. U_k therefore always takes a value between 0 and $m_k \cdot n_k$. Under the null hypothesis of no treatment effect, H_0, the expected value of U_k, $E(U_k)$, is $n_k \cdot m_k / 2$.)

An observed value of U_k smaller than $m_k \cdot n_k / 2$ therefore shows that within stratum k the post-treatment scores in group 1 are 'in the average' smaller (i.e. in our example 'better') than those in group 2.

Table 3.2 Number of patients with a given combination of pre- and post-treatment scores per treatment group and summary statistics.

Group	Pretreatment k	Post-treatment scores						m_k / n_k	N_k	U_k	Uw_k	Vw_k
		2	3	4	5	6	7					
Active Placebo	2	1 4						1 4	5	2	0	0
Active Placebo	3	3 4	3					6 4	10	6	−2.5	2.43
Active Placebo	4		3 4	3 2				6 6	12	21	1.0	3.18
Active Placebo	5		1	4 3	1 4			6 7	13	11	−3.095	3.71
Active Placebo	6	1		2	2 3	1		5 4	9	3	−3.15	2.78
Active Placebo	7				(1)			(1) 0	(1)	—	—	—
Sum* Active Placebo		5 4	7 8	9 5	3 7	(1) 1		24 25	49		−7.745	12.11

Note: To improve readability of the contingency table, 0s have been removed. The right part of the table contains m_k and n_k (the sizes of subsamples with pretreatment score k), $N_k = m_k + n_k$, the ordinary Mann-Whitney test statistic U_k, the weighted statistic Uw_k, and its estimated variance Vw_k.
*The sum goes only over those subsamples with m_k and n_k both different from 0.

It is not a new idea to obtain a 'global' statistic for comparison of the 'overall' improvement between the two groups in the framework of blocked randomised designs — k denoting then the block number — by combining the centred statistics

$$U'_k = U_k - m_k \cdot n_k/2 \qquad \text{(with } E(U'_k) = 0)$$

in a weighted sum

$$U^* = \sum_{k=1}^{K} c_k \, U'_k/\sigma$$

where the c_k are deliberate weights and σ is the variance of the numerator under H_0.

Various choices (sometimes implicitly) for c_k have been proposed, the first one with $c_k = 1, k = 1, \ldots, K$ (probably) by Benard and Van Elteren (1953), then Van Elteren (1960) with $c_k = 1/(N_k + 1)$, and Mantel (1963) with $c_k = 1/N_k$ (see also Noether, 1963). Van Elteren's proposal is optimum with respect to power of the resulting test, if the same treatment effect is to be expected in all strata, an assumption that, as we have shown, is hardly realistic for our case where the strata are defined by the (random) pretreatment scores.

A conditional measure of superiority

A measure of *superiority* of the active treatment over placebo *within stratum* k (defined by the pretreatment scores X_b and Y_b being k) is

$$\pi_k = P(X_a > Y_a \mid X_b = Y_b = k) + \tfrac{1}{2} P(X_a = Y_a \mid X_b = Y_b = k)$$

essentially the probability that after treatment a randomly selected patient with pretreatment score k has higher score after active treatment than after placebo (Lehmann, 1975). π_k is $1/2$ under H_0, larger than $1/2$ if high scores indicate a better state and smaller if low scores do so (as in our example) under the alternative hypothesis H_1 of a beneficial effect of the active treatment.

$$\pi = P(X_a > Y_a \mid X_b = Y_b) + 1/2\, P(X_a = Y_a \mid X_b = Y_b)$$
$$= \sum_{k=1}^{K} \pi_k \cdot P(X_b = k \text{ or } Y_b = k)$$

then is a *realistic measure for the overall superiority*, a measure that in addition is invariant under monotone transformation of the scale and hence ideal for ordinal scores. $(1 - \pi)$ is essentially the *probability that an actively treated patient is better off than another one with the same baseline value but treated with placebo*.

A new conditional rank test

It can be shown that a test unbiased to alternatives of the type $H_1 : \pi < 1/2$ (small scores are 'good' scores) vs. $H_0 : \pi_k = 1/2, k = 1, \ldots, K$, can be gained by choosing $c_k = N_k/(m_k \cdot n_k)$. For this choice of c_k, U_k is denoted by Uw_k and U^* by Uw. If σ_k^2 denotes the usual variance corrected for ties of the Mann-Whitney statistic U_k (or U'_k), then $Vw_k = (\sigma_k N_k/(m_k \cdot n_k))^2$ is the variance of Uw_k. U_k, Uw_k and Vw_k are given for our example in table 3.2.

We therefore propose

$$Uw = \frac{\sum_k^* (U_k - m_k \cdot n_k/2) \cdot N_k/(m_k \cdot n_k)}{\sqrt{\sum_k^* (\sigma_k \cdot N_k/(m_k \cdot n_k))^2}}$$

as a new test statistic (which can be shown to be asymptotically standard normal under H_0). $\sum_k^*$ goes over those strata with m_k and n_k *both* different from 0.

In our example we compute for Uw the value

$$Uw = \sum_k^* Uw_k / \sqrt{\sum_k^* Vw_k} = -7.745/\sqrt{12.11} = 2.23$$

yielding (from the standard normal table) $p = 0.013$.

Estimation of the conditional measure of superiority

An important advantage of the test proposed is that it is closely linked to the measure of superiority π. π can be estimated unbiasedly by

$$\hat{\pi} = \sum_k^* Uw_k / \sum_k^* N_{k.} + {}^1/_2$$

with $\sum_k^*$ again denoting the sum over those strata with m_k and n_k both different from 0.

For our example we find $\pi = -7.745/49 + 0.5 = 0.34$ or $1 - \hat{\pi} = 0.66$. This means (roughly) that the probability for a patient to be better off with respect to impairment of mental alertness after active treatment than after placebo is about 0.66, and this estimate is statistically significantly different from $^1/_2$ at the 5% significance level. This statement remains true even if we had chosen to test the two-sided alternative H_1': $\pi \neq {}^1/_2$ vs H_0: $\pi \neq {}^1/_2$, since in that case we have just to double the 'one-sided' p-value: $p' = 0.026$.

Taking into account the dynamic dimension of the process

In the method described in the preceding section we have considered only the observations performed at baseline and at the end of the study. Most often, as already noted in the introduction, observations and measurements are performed repeatedly during the trial. One way to use this information has already been mentioned. Another way of taking advantage of it is to compute the time from beginning of treatment until the point in time when a certain grade of rehabilitation is reached. Especially in the field of stroke the regaining of abilities such as consciousness, walking or more generally the reaching of say 60 points on the Barthel scale can be considered essentially irreversible. The time to this event or to 'loss of follow-up' (mostly the end of the study or death unrelated to treatment) can then be evaluated statistically according to the well-known 'life-table' methods for censored data.

Besides the possibility of depicting graphically the difference between treatment strategies by drawing the 'survival' or rather 'regain of ability' curves, differences between them can be tested by an appropriate method, e.g. the log-rank test. It has the additional advantage that the test statistic can be adjusted relatively easily for discrete prognostic variates in a similar way as has been done in the test proposed on p.49. This technique is very well described in non-technical terms by Peto *et al.* (1977).

For continuous or discrete covariates the use of Cox's model (Cox, 1972; Kalbfleisch and Prentice, 1980) may be indicated if the assumptions on which the model is based can be verified. This model is specified by the form of hazard function $\lambda(t)$ which is the 'probability density' for an individual of 'dying' at time t knowing that he is still alive just before t. The model assumes that $\lambda(t)$ can be written as follows.

$$\lambda(t) = \lambda_0(t) \exp (a_1x_1 + a_2x_2 + \ldots + a_px_p)$$

where $x_1, \ldots, x_p$ are the variates and covariates, and $a_1, \ldots, a_p$ are the regression coefficients. This model is called the proportional hazards model because the functions $\lambda_1(t)$ and $\lambda_2(t)$ corresponding to different values of the variables are proportional.

The hypotheses $a_i = 0; i = 1, \ldots, p$ can be tested, although only asymptotic results exist, i.e. the tests are reliable only for a 'sufficiently large' sample size. The model can be used in therapeutic trials in the following manner. Suppose that there are two treatments. The variable x_1, for example, is chosen as the label of the treatment groups: $x_1 = 0$ if the patient has treatment 1, $x_1 = $ if the patient has treatment 2. The hypothesis $a_1 = 0$ is then equivalent to the hypothesis of no difference between the two treatments. If there are no covariates, the test based on Cox's model is equivalent to the log-rank test.

Introducing covariates enables one to adjust for factors which are a cause of heterogeneity of the sample. It is as if the sample were homogeneous with respect to the introduced covariates, and this leads to a much more powerful procedure.

We illustrate this method with a simulation of a therapeutical trial and an example with real data. Using computer programs that allow us to generate pseudorandom numbers from various distributions we simulated

(a) a random allocation to two treatment groups, $x_1 = 0$ for treatment 1, $x_1 = 1$ for treatment 2; each patient was allocated to one or the other treatment with probability $^1/_2$

(b) three covariates x_2, x_3, x_4 having standard normal distributions

(c) an exponentially distributed survival time with constant hazard function:

$$\lambda(t) = \exp\,(0.7x_1 + 0.1x_2 + 0.2x_3 + 0.9x_4)$$

(d) a random censoring time independent of the survival time with hazard function:

$$\lambda(t) = \exp\,(-0.7 - 0.1 - 0.2 - 0.9)$$

Among the 100 observations generated this way, 57 'patients' were allocated to treatment 1, 43 to treatment 2 and 10 were censored.

The hypothesis of equivalence of the two treatments was tested first by means of the log-rank test. This yielded $p = 0.11$. We then used Cox's model introducing the three covariates and tested the hypothesis $a_1 = 0$, and found $p = 0.007$.

This example demonstrates that the power of a test procedure can be increased dramatically whenever good prognostic factors are known and used in the statistical analysis.

We illustrate the idea of using life-table methods in the field of stroke by means of an example taken from a study more thoroughly described in Dartigues *et al.* (1985). It stems, however, not from a clinical trial but from a retrospective study which aims at detecting prognostic factors. Hence, the aim was not to detect a possible treatment effect but to give an answer to the following question: 'Is age a prognostic factor influencing the outcome of a stroke?'. We studied a population of 111 stroke patients who were admitted to the Département de Neurologie at Pellegrin Hospital (Bordeaux). Afterwards they were admitted to the rehabilitation centre, Les Grands Chênes. The functional level of these patients was regularly assessed and the Barthel Index (BI) calculated at days 15, 30, 60, 90, 180 and 360. The mean follow-up time was 6.7 months. For each patient the BI was always increasing and the regain of walking was irreversible. There were 26 censored observations for the BI and 36 for the walk. We compared two groups: namely 70 'old' (more than 65 years old) and 41 'young' (less than 65 years old) patients. The survival curves were drawn (figures 3.2 and 3.3) for the two criteria walk and BI > 60. The log-rank test yielded for the criterion 'walk' $\chi^2 = 6.4$ $(p = 0.012)$ and for 'BI > 60' $\chi^2 = 7.93$ $(p = 0.005)$.

An analysis using Cox's model was undertaken in order to determine whether age is still a prognostic factor when other factors are taken into account. The factors considered were: nature of the stroke, affected cerebral hemisphere, volume, sensory deficit, level of consciousness and speech deficit. The coefficient of the age factor was found to be significantly different from zero for both criteria ($p = 0.004$ for walk and $p = 0.002$ for

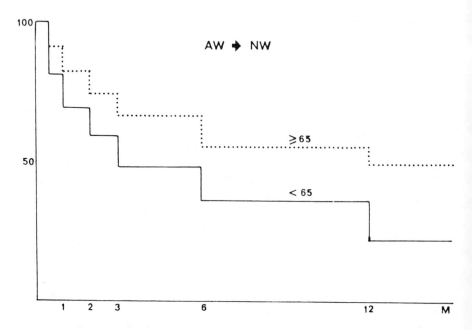

Figure 3.2 Survival curves of the 'young' and 'old' groups for the criterion 'regain of normal walk' (NW).

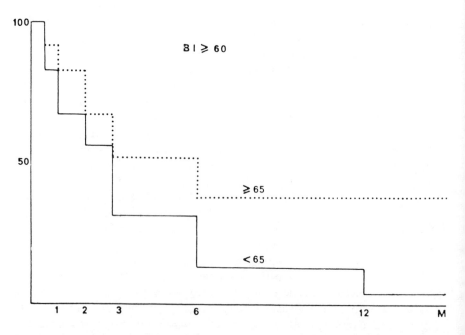

Figure 3.3 Survival curves of the 'young' and 'old' groups for the criterion 'BI > 60'.

BI). These values are better than those found with the log-rank test. The reason is that the variables introduced are almost independent of age, i.e. we have a situation similar to that of the clinical trial. This is not always necessarily so, and the effect of adjusting for concomitant variables in general is in clinical trials not the same as in retrospective studies. Whereas in the latter type of studies it may easily happen that a factor appears to have a significant effect when tested alone and no significant effect after adjustment, in clinical trials, on the contrary, the p-value tends to decrease after adjustment for prognostic factors that are balanced with respect to the treatment groups.

In conclusion the major advantages of the method proposed in this section are the use of the information carried by the dynamic dimension of the data and in censored observations. Similarly, as in more conventional methods, we have the possibility of adjusting for concomitant factors either non-parametrically as explained in Peto *et al.* (1977) or parametrically by the use of Cox's model which may be more powerful in the case of continuous covariates.

One drawback of using Cox's method is that the assumptions on which the model is based should be verified. Although some procedures to this effect have been proposed, it is difficult to have complete confidence in the validity of the model because there are several possibilities of departure from it. Moreover the tests are based on asymptotic results and thus are valid only for large samples.

Finally we must notice that taking the dynamic dimension into account means sacrificing the semi-quantitative character of the scale. Optimal methods should consider both the dynamic and the semi-quantitative characters of the data. Although some ideas may be borrowed from growth-curve theory, such methods have still to be developed.

ACKNOWLEDGEMENT

We would like to thank Dr A. Yotis and Dr J. M. Moeglen for their helpful comments.

REFERENCES

Andreasen, N. C., McDonald-Scott, P., Grove, W. M., Keller, M. B., Shapiro, R. W. and Hirschfeld, R. M. A. (1982). Assessment of reliability in multi-center collaborative research with videotape approach. *Am. J. Psychiat.* **139**, 876–82.

Benard, A. and Van Elteren, P. (1953). A generalization of the method of *m* rankings. *Indagationes Mathematicae*, **15**, 358–69.

Bock, D. R. and Wood, R. (1971). Test theory. *Ann. Rev. Psychol.* **22**, 193–224.

Bond, A. and Lader, M. (1974). The use of analogue scales in rating subjective feelings. *Brit. J. Med. Psychol.*, **47**, 211–18.

Campbell, M. E. (1978). Estimation of treatment effect and measurement of change. *Perceptual and Motor Skills*, **46**, 387 92.

Capildeo, R. and Clifford-Rose, F. (1978). The design of an acute stroke trial. In Jukes, A. M. (ed.), *Baclofen: Spasticity and Cerebral Pathology*. Cambridge Medical Publications, Northampton, 85–94.

Cho, D. W. (1981). Inter-rater reliability: intraclass correlation coefficients. *Educ. Psychol. Meas.*, **41**, 223–6.

Collegium Internationale Psychiatrae Scalarum (CIPS) (1981). *Internationale Skalen für Psychiatrie*. Beltz Test GmbH, Weinheim.

Cox, D. R. (1972). Regression models and life tables (with discussion). *J. Roy. Stat. Soc. B*, **34**, 187–220.

Dartigues, J. F., Krassinine, G., Commenges, D., Orgogozo, J. M., Salamon, R. and Mazaux, J. M. (1985). Analyse longitudinale de la récuperation de la marche après une hemiplegie par accident vasculaire cerebral. *Ann. Réadapt. Med. Phys.*, **27**, 207–14.

Guy, W. (Ed.) (1976). *ECDEU Assessment Manual for Psychopharmacology*, Revised Edn. Department of Health, Education and Welfare, Rockville, Maryland.

Hamot, H. B. (1974). Estimating the reliability and validity of rating scales. Unpublished manuscript. Sandoz Inc., East Hanover, NJ.

Hamot, H. B., Patin, J. R. and Singer, J. M. (1983). Factor structure of the SANDOZ Clinical Assessment Geriatric (SCAG) scale. *Psychopharmacol. Bull.*

Hartigan, J. A. (1975). *Clustering Algorithms*. Wiley, New York.

Hazama, T. *et al.* (1976). *Japan. J. Clin. Exp. Med.*, **53** (12), 3781.

Holm, S. (1979). A simple sequentially rejective multiple test procedure. *Scand. J. Statist.*, **6**, 65–70.

Kalbfleisch, J. D. and Prentice, R. L. (1980). *The Statistical Analysis of Failure Time Data*. Wiley, New York.

Koch, G. G. (1969). Some aspects of the statistical analysis of 'split-plot' experiments in completely randomized layouts. *J. Am. Stat. Assoc.*, **64**, 485–505.

Koch, G. G., Amara, I. A., Davis, G. W. and Gillings, D. B. (1982). A review of some statistical methods for covariance analysis of categorical data. *Biometrics*, **38**, 563–95.

Kochansky, G. E. (1979). Psychiatric rating scales for assessing psychopathology in the elderly: a critical review. In Raskin, A. (ed.), *Psychiatric Symptoms and Cognitive Loss in the Elderly*. Hemisphere, New York, pp. 125–56

Kruskal, J. B. (1958). Ordinal measures of association. *J. Am. Stat. Assoc.*, **53**, 814–61.

Lehmann, E. L. (1975). *Nonparametrics, Statistical Methods Based on Ranks*. Holden-Day, San Francisco.

Levy, P. (1973). On the Relation between Test Theory and Psychology. In Kline, P. (ed.), *New Approaches in Psychological Measurement*. Wiley, New York, pp. 1–42.

Lienert, G. A. (1969). *Testaufbau und Testanalyse*. Verlag Julius Beltz, Berlin.

Lienert, G. A. (1982). *Verteilungsfreie Methoden in der Biostatistik. Band II. 2. Auflage*. Verlag Anton Hain, Meisenheim am Glahn.

Lord, F. M. and Novick, M. R. (1968). *Statistical Theories of Mental Test Scores*. Educational Testing Service/Addison-Wesley, New York.

McKenna, S. P., Hunt, S. M. and McEwen, J. (1981). Weighting the seriousness of perceived health problems using Thurstone's method of paired comparisons. *Int. J. Epidemiol.* **10**, 93–7.

Mantel, N. (1963). Chi-square tests with one degree of freedom. Extensions of the Mantel–Haenzel procedure. *J. Am. Stat. Assoc.*, **58**, 690–700.

Maurer, W., Ferner, U., Patin, J. and Hamot, H. B. (1982). Sandoz Clinical Assessment Geriatric Scale (SCAG): eine .transkulturelle faktorenanalystische Studie. *Z. Gerontologie*, **15**, 26–30.

Noether, G. E. (1963). Efficiency of the Wilcoxon two-sample statistic for random-ized blocks. *J. Am. Stat. Assoc.*, **58**, 894–8.

Orgogozo, J. M., Capildeo, R., Anagnostou, C. N., Juge, O., Péré, J. J., Darti-gues, J. F., Steiner, T. J., Yotis, A. and Clifford-Rose, F. (1983). Mise au point d'un score neurologique pour l'évaluation clinique des infarctus sylviens. *Presse Med.*, **12**, 3039–44.

Oswald, W. D. (1979). Psychometrics as a method of testing drugs. *Sandorama*, **IV**, 26–31.

Peto, R., Pike, M. C., Armitage, P., Breslow, N. E., Cox, D. R., Howard, S. V., Mantel, N., McPherson, K., Peto, J. and Smith, P. G. (1977). Design and ana-lysis of randomized clinical trials requiring prolonged observation of each patient. II Analysis and examples. *Brit. J. Cancer*, **35**, 1–39.

Shrout, P. E., and Fleiss, J. L. (1979). Intraclass correlations: uses in assessing reliability. *Psychol. Bull.*, **86**, 420–8.

Van Elteren, P. (1960). On the combination of independent two-sample tests of Wilcoxon. *Bull. Inst. Int. Stat.*, **37**, 351–61.

4
Evaluation of diagnostic tests and the role of diagnosis in therapeutic trials

HARVEY V. FINEBERG

INTRODUCTION

The proper evaluation of new and existing diagnostic tests is a continuing challenge for medical researchers. The practice of neurology has been and will continue to be influenced by the advent of new imaging techniques, such as computed tomography, positron emission tomography, and nuclear magnetic resonance. As new tests become more sophisticated, often more expensive, and on occasion more risky, a careful assessment of the impact of different tests is needed for rational decision making about the care of patients and for sensible allocation of health resources. Diagnostic tests are thus important subjects for evaluation. Proper diagnosis also lays the foundation for studies to compare different therapies.

This chapter has two objectives. The first is to review key considerations in the design of studies to evaluate diagnostic tests. These considerations include specifying the test or test system being analysed, defining the purposes of evaluation, selecting appropriate objectives and measures of test performance, and proper collection, analysis and interpretation of evaluative data. The second purpose of the chapter is to provide a quantitative estimate of the benefits of more accurate classification of patients in studies intended to compare alternative therapies. Understanding diagnostic performance and the consequences of incorrect classification of patients can aid in the design and analysis of studies to compare the effectiveness of different treatments.

DEFINITION OF A TEST

For the purposes of our discussion, we can define a test as any source of information about the presence, nature and extent of disease in a patient. This broad definition applies to any kind of information gathered from the patient (such as history and physical examination) as well as to all types of imaging, and laboratory and physiological-function tests. This definition also cuts across a number of clinical purposes, including the diagnosis of disease in patients suspected of having disease, screening for disease among the population believed to be healthy, and monitoring the course of illness and recovery during treatment. A test provides information that enables clinicians to revise their understanding of the likelihood of disease. A precise quantitative expression called Bayes' formula relates the probability of disease prior to a test, the performance of the test, and the revised probability of disease after the test.

DESIGN OF STUDIES TO EVALUATE DIAGNOSTIC TESTS

Three important questions in planning a study to evaluate diagnostic tests are:

(1) What is the test system, and what are its key components?
(2) What, exactly, are the purposes of the evaluation?
(3) What are the objectives of the test (or test system) that will serve as the basis for judging its performance?

The test system

The context of performing a diagnostic test constitutes a system that typically includes patients, physicians, technicians, diagnostic equipment, a clinical environment, and a larger social milieu (Fineberg and Sherman, 1981). All of these together determine the net clinical performance of a diagnostic procedure, and changing any of them may alter the apparent performance of the test. For example, physicians with different levels of experience may achieve quite different accuracy in diagnosis with the same test and same pool of patients (Fineberg, 1979). Advances in the technology of equipment, like increased experience on the part of clinicians, also tend to improve test performance (Fineberg *et al.*, 1986).

For a study to be valid, the patients to be included in the evaluation should be representative of the clinical population in whom the test will be employed in practice. Numerous sources of bias threaten the validity of a test evaluation (Ransohoff and Feinstein, 1976). Changes in the population being tested, due either to shifts over time in the frequency or severity of disease or to differential forces of selection, can have profound effects on apparent test performance. In part these effects are matters of natural evolution, in part they are matters of selection bias, and in part they are due to the mathematical properties of probabilities. Though these properties are thoroughly described in the literature, many physicians do not adequately appreciate, for example, how a change in the prior probability of disease in a group of patients can sharply alter the predictive value of a test (Berwick *et al.*, 1981). I shall examine how this works quantitatively in the section on measures of diagnostic performance.

A subtle source of bias in patient selection arises when tests are compared only among patients for whom there is definitive proof of diagnosis. Indeed, many measures of test performance require independent proof of the presence or absence of disease, as might be obtained, for example, from surgery or from post-mortem examination. If the relative accuracy of the tests being compared is different among patients who do not die or undergo surgery, the apparent performance in the study population will not be matched in clinical practice. In general, whenever the spectrum of patients in a study is narrower, wider, or in any systematic way different from the clinical population, the applicability of study results to practice is weakened.

Another subtle source of selection bias arises from differences in the ability of tests to produce interpretable results. (A variation of the same problem is that tests may also differ in the likelihood of an interpretable result in different groups of patients.) If a comparison of two tests is limited to patients in whom both tests produce an interpretable result, this will wrongly enhance the expected clinical performance of the test that is less often interpretable. Patient selection biases, if unappreciated, can thus lead to erroneous estimates of the clinical performance of a test.

Purpose of evaluation

Assessments of a single test or comparisons of two or more tests are frequent goals in a diagnostic evaluation. Other possible purposes include comparing diagnostic performance of different physicians, evaluating a combination of tests, and assessing different sequences of tests. For example, one recent study attempted to determine what, if any, would be the best sequence of non-invasive tests before proceeding to angiography in patients with suspected extracranial cerebrovascular disease (Sumner *et al.*, 1982). A different study may be aimed at evaluating diagnostic performance of equipment that is capable of providing tests in patients with a variety of clinical conditions. For example, some studies of cranial computed tomography have attempted to measure the overall impact of the device on clinical decision making (Fineberg *et al.*, 1977). Yet other studies may examine the optimal timing of tests in relation to the stage of disease. Each of these different purposes affects the design of an evaluation study.

Performance objectives

Regardless of whether one is evaluating a single test, a combination of tests, or a piece of diagnostic equipment, one must decide on the performance objectives of the test system. In other words, if you ask, 'How good is the test?', you should be prepared to define 'Good at doing what?' For the purposes of setting performance objectives for diagnostic tests and test systems, I find it convenient to think in terms of three clusters of objectives: clinical, economic and scientific. Though these do not exhaust all legitimate objectives for medical care evaluation, they are sufficiently inclusive to cover most types of studies of diagnostic tests.

Clinical objectives

The clinical objectives of diagnostic tests can be visualised along a hierarchy of clinical efficacy (Sumner *et al.*, 1982). At the most basic level are technical performance features of the test. For example, in evaluating a computed tomography scanner: how reliable is the device in day-to-day operation? What are the smallest two-point discrimination and least detectable difference in tissue density? What is the amount of radiation? And so forth. At the second level of efficacy is the production of diagnostic and prognostic information. This information may affect the use of other tests. Prognostic information can be of direct psychological and material benefit to the patient even if no action can alter the course of disease (Fineberg *et al.*, 1977). For the most part, however, diagnostic information exerts its effect by influencing decisions about treatment. Therapeutic decisions thus influenced constitute the third level of efficacy. Different therapy can potentially alter the clinical outcome, and a change in health outcome is the fourth and final level of this efficacy hierarchy. Tests may be evaluated in terms of their performance at any one or more of these four levels of clinical efficacy, depending on the aims of assessment.

As we proceed down the efficacy hierarchy, we may expect that the impact of a test will tend to dissipate because each subsequent level introduces factors that are extraneous to the test and that tend to degrade its value. For example, a test may be technically perfect yet produce little increment in diagnostic information because the correct diagnosis was already highly suspected clinically. Or a test may provide a considerable amount of new information that produces no changes in treatment because the proper therapy had already been instigated. In our study of computed cranial tomography at the Massachusetts General Hospital, for example, we found that approximately half of all CT scans produced a substantial amount of new diagnostic information, yet a consequent change in therapy occurred in only about 15% of cases (Fineberg *et al.*, 1977). Even the best new therapy may not improve clinical outcome, and this contingency further dissipates the clinical impact of a test at efficacy level IV. If we require a new test to improve clinical outcome, we are setting a very demanding standard. Yet, that standard is the common denominator for evaluating all of medical care.

The level of efficacy by which to evaluate a test depends on the investigator's preferences and on the purpose of the evaluation (Sox *et al.*, 1981). Most clinical evaluations of diagnostic tests concentrate on their ability to diagnose disease, level II in the efficacy hierarchy. When I discuss quantitative measures of test performance later in this paper, I will likewise focus on measures of diagnostic information.

Economic objectives

Evaluating the net economic consequences of a diagnostic system involves measuring the economic requirements of the test system itself, tracking induced effects in other parts of the medical care system, and assessing any economic impact on society at large.

The resources consumed by a test system include the direct components of labour, equipment and supplies, plus overhead or indirect costs for resources such as space, light, heat and maintenance. Computation of even these straightforward resource costs may not be so simple. In particular, for a variety of accounting and policy reasons, the price charged for a test may not reflect the resources actually consumed in producing the test (Fineberg, 1983). This is especially true of hospital-based diagnostic equipment.

The induced effects of a test in terms of reductions or additions in other tests or consequent changes in treatment also have economic consequences. It has been argued, for example, that investment in CT scanners has been partly or wholly offset by savings in the use of other tests such as radionuclide scans and pneumoencephalography. While reductions in other tests are well documented, the accounting of economic effects is tricky. Investment in new diagnostic equipment entails both fixed and variable costs, whereas reducing the use of existing test equipment yields near-term savings only in variable costs (Fineberg, 1983). Thus it is quite difficult for new diagnostic equipment to effect net savings from reduced reliance on existing tests.

If a diagnostic system produces changes in health status, its economic effects extend beyond the health-care system to society at large. Healthier people can return to work and be economically productive. On the other hand, social security payments and services such as special education for the handicapped, although obviously necessary and desirable, represent an expenditure of society's resources that should properly be counted as economic costs.

Scientific objectives

New diagnostic procedures may serve at least two types of scientific objective apart from improved detection and characterisation of disease in the tested population. First, improved diagnosis may contribute to advances in basic medical science about the aetiology and pathophysiology of disease. Secondly, improved diagnosis can facilitate evaluation of new treatments. In serving the ends of basic medical or therapeutic research, a diagnostic test is aimed at helping future patients rather than the current population being tested. In a later section of this paper, I will discuss the effects of improved diagnosis on the performance of clinical trials to test new therapies.

Special features of studies to evaluate diagnostic tests

A number of special features apply to evaluations of diagnostic tests that do not necessarily pertain to evaluations of therapy. First, in so far as a test induces changes in the use of other tests and treatments, these induced effects need to be traced if the full impact of the initial test is to be measured. Secondly, because a test is typically more remote than treatment from health outcome, measures of test performance in terms of outcome may be difficult to obtain. Even if they are concerned about health outcome, investigators may be forced to rely on the more accessible measures of diagnostic information and effects on choice of therapy. Thirdly, a test system may have multiple uses in a variety of patients. Consider, for example, diagnostic equipment such as a CT scanner. If the objective is to evaluate the diagnostic ability of the device, then a number of parallel studies covering uses in different groups of patients would need to be undertaken and their results synthesised.

Any evaluation of a test or of a treatment occurs at a particular point in time. If technology is rapidly evolving, as is much diagnostic technology, then studies may soon be outdated, perhaps even at the time they appear in print. The clinical contribution of a test is relative to the clinical perform-ance of alternative tests and also depends on the state of therapeutic technology. Evolution in the primary test or gains in experience and insight in use of the test would naturally affect its net clinical value. Similarly, advances in competitive diagnostic technologies and in therapy can affect the clinical perfotmance even of a stable diagnostic technology. Further-more, shifts over time in the patterns of disease among the population being tested and evolution in basic scientific knowledge can also impinge on the value of a diagnostic test.

An important consideration in planning a clinical trial to evaluate a diagnostic test is the opportunity to employ a randomised design. In such a design, patients would be randomly assigned either to receive or not to receive the test. Randomisation has the advantage of controlling both for known and for unsuspected sources of bias, and a few randomised trials of diagnostic tests have been conducted.

A randomised trial comparing a new test with an older test may be difficult to rationalise because in clinical practice different tests are typically not mutually exclusive. If we are comparing alternative treatments in a randomised trial, part of the rationale is that we can use only one treatment in each future patient. We would like to be able to ascertain the better treatment to benefit all future patients. With diagnostic tests, in general, we can if we like perform all available tests in each patient, so it is difficult on clinical grounds to justify withholding a test from a patient who might benefit from it.

On occasion, a new test constitutes a scarce resource for some period of time after its introduction. A current example may be nuclear magnetic resonance. A scarce resource cannot be made available to everyone who might need it, and this means that some patients will gain access to the test whereas others, of necessity, will not. The only issue is the mechanism by which eligible patients will be selected for examination. In such circumstances, random allocation would be both desirable from a scientific standpoint and ethically justifiable. A reasonable evaluation cannot begin until there is a degree of medical consensus about the methods for using and interpreting a new diagnostic technology. Some new diagnostic technologies will achieve a degree of consensus about the method of use while remaining scarce relative to the potential number of eligible patients. Diagnostic technologies that satisfy these conditions present an ideal opportunity to undertake a randomised clinical trial.

Measures of test information

Assessment of the clinical and economic impact of tests can be approached through the techniques of clinical decision analysis and cost-effectiveness analysis (Weinstein and Fineberg, 1980). A general discussion of these important techniques is beyond the scope of this chapter. In this section, I will introduce selected principles and methods for measuring the diagnostic information of tests. Diagnostic information is the measure of primary concern in most test evaluations. This discussion will also serve as a prelude to assessing the impact of diagnostic imprecision on studies to compare different therapeutic regimens.

Tests as separators

In order to visualise how a test produces diagnostic information, it may be helpful to think of a test simply as a separator: a test produces diagnostic information in so far as it helps to separate the population with disease from the population without disease. Figure 4.1 depicts schematically two population distributions (with the area under each curve normalised to 1.0)

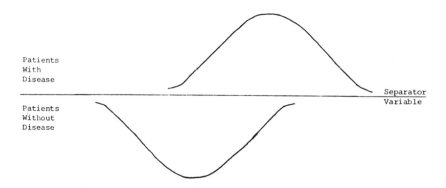

Figure 4.1 Patients with disease/without disease. Population frequency along separator variable.

arrayed along a separator. The separator represents possible results of a test, and the scale of the separator might be any ordinal or interval scale, such as CNS pressure, white blood cell count, serum glucose concentration, degree of positivity on a CT scan, and so forth. One of the two populations has the disease of interest (this population is located above the separator) and the other population (located below the separator) does not have the disease.

The placement of each patient in such an array implies knowledge of the correct diagnosis and knowledge of the test result. Knowledge of the correct diagnosis enables us to place a patient above the horizontal line (if the patient truly has disease) or below the horizontal line (if the patient truly does not have disease). The test result tells us the point along the horizontal axis to which a patient belongs. Nature (i.e. the presence or absence of disease) separates the populations above and below the horizontal axis. The diagnostic test separates the populations by pulling one to the left and the other to the right along the axis of test results.

Typically, the populations with and without disease will be arrayed along the separator with some overlap. In other words, some patients with the disease and some patients without the disease will have the same test results. The best test is one that produces the least overlap in the two populations. Although the degree of separation depends on the quality of the test, the actual sizes of the populations with and without disease depend on the epidemiology of the disease, not on the test.

Cutoff levels

Any test result has associated with it a likelihood that patients have the disease and a likelihood that patients do not have the disease. It is possible, then, to assess the diagnostic information from each particular test result. In everyday clinical use of tests, it is more customary to establish a cutoff level that separates a range of test results considered positive for disease from a range considered negative for disease. Figure 4.2 shows such a cutoff level, with higher results (further to the right) considered positive for disease and lower results (further to the left) considered negative for disease.

Selection of a cutoff level defines four classifications of test results:

True positives (TP): patients with disease and with a positive test
False positives (FP): patients without disease and with a positive test
True negatives (TN): patients without disease and with a negative test
False negatives (FN): patients with disease and with a negative test

Sliding the cutoff to a more stringent level (to the right) reduces true positives and false positives, and increases true negatives and false negatives. Sliding the cutoff to a less stringent level has the opposite effects. The relative rates of increase or decrease in each classified group of patients depend on the shapes and degree of overlap in the distributions of the populations with and without disease. The optimal placement of a cutoff level depends upon the prior probability of disease in the tested population, the performance of the test as a separator, and the consequences of correct versus incorrect classification (Weinstein and Feinberg, 1980, pp. 121–6).

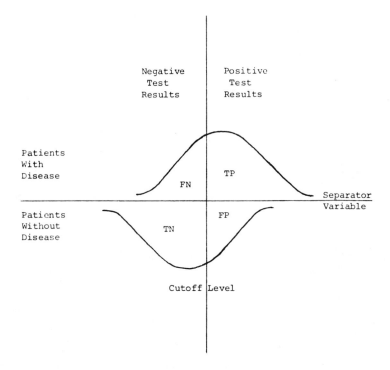

Figure 4.2 Patients with disease/without disease for negative and positive test results. Population frequency along separator variable.

Two-by-two tables: sensitivity, specificity and predictive values

A two-by-two table is a convenient way to represent performance of a diagnostic test using a specified positivity criterion (figure 4.3). Numerous ways have been devised to describe the diagnostic information produced by a test, but four basic measures evident from the two-by-two table are particularly noteworthy: sensitivity, specificity, predictive value positive, and predictive value negative (figure 4.4).

> *Sensitivity* (SE) is the frequency of positive test results among those with disease: TP/(TP + FN)
> *Specificity* (SP) is the frequency of negative test results in those without disease: TN/(TN + FP)
> *Predictive value positive* (PVP) is the frequency of disease among those with positive test results: TP/(TP+FP)
> *Predictive value negative* (PVN) is the frequency of non-disease among those with negative test results: TN/(TN+FN)

In principle, the measures of test sensitivity and specificity are independent of the prior probability or prevalence (PR) of disease. This key feature makes sensitivity and specificity attractive experimental measures of test performance.

A clinician caring for patients is usually most directly interested in predictive values: if a patient has a particular test result, what is the likelihood of disease? The predictive values depend on prevalence of disease

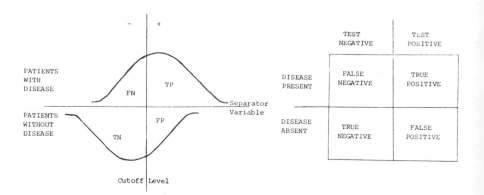

Figure 4.3   Two ways to represent test results.

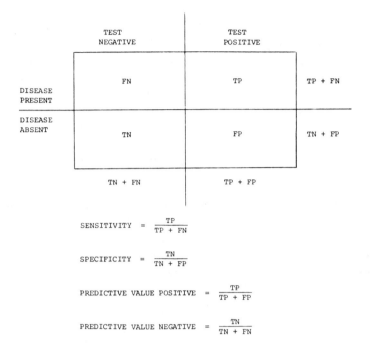

	TEST NEGATIVE	TEST POSITIVE	
DISEASE PRESENT	FN	TP	TP + FN
DISEASE ABSENT	TN	FP	TN + FP
	TN + FN	TP + FP	

$$\text{SENSITIVITY} = \frac{TP}{TP + FN}$$

$$\text{SPECIFICITY} = \frac{TN}{TN + FP}$$

$$\text{PREDICTIVE VALUE POSITIVE} = \frac{TP}{TP + FP}$$

$$\text{PREDICTIVE VALUE NEGATIVE} = \frac{TN}{TN + FN}$$

Figure 4.4 Test performance: 2 × 2 table.

in the target population as well as on the sensitivity and specificity of the test. According to Bayes' formula:

$$PVP = (SE \times PR)/[SE \times PR + (1 - SP) \times (1 - PR)]$$

and

$$PVN = [SP \times (1 - PR)]/[SP \times (1 - PR) + (1 - SE) \times PR]$$

It may be surprising how great the variation in predictive value will be with changes in the prevalence of disease (Vecchio, 1966). For example, suppose you want to evaluate a new biochemical test for multiple sclerosis. You test 100 patients with known multiple sclerosis and 100 patients with a variety of other neurological diseases, and you find the test has a sensitivity of 0.95 and a specificity of 0.95. Since half the patients in your study population have multiple sclerosis, the apparent predictive value positive for the test is, from Bayes' formula:

PVP = (0.95 × 0.5)/(0.95 × 0.5 + 0.05 × 0.5) = 0.95

This seems like a very good test indeed. Yet what would happen if general internists applied the same test to their patients with neurological symptoms vaguely suggestive of multiple sclerosis, in whom only 1% actually have the disease? In this setting, the predictive value would decline drastically:

PVP = (0.95 × 0.01)/(0.95 × 0.01 + 0.05 × 0.99) = 0.16

A positive test now leaves a patient with less than one chance in six of having multiple sclerosis. The clinician and patient might both benefit from learning that the chance of multiple sclerosis now appears to be 16 times greater than previously, though still with odds of five to one against the disease. Such a test, if properly interpreted, could be useful as a screening procedure. The risk is that the 95% positive predictive value found in the initial study will be unthinkingly adopted by practitioners. Researchers should be cognisant of the effects of changes in the prior probability of disease in reporting the results of test evaluations, and clinicians should be similarly aware when seeking to apply tests to their clinical practices.

Likelihood ratios

Another useful measure of the ability of a test to predict disease is the likelihood ratio (LR). The likelihood ratio is the probability of observing a particular test result or range of results (T^*) in the population with disease (D) divided by the probability of observing the same result (T^*) in the population without disease (D). Symbolically,

LR = $p[T^*|D]/P[T^*|\bar{D}]$

The likelihood ratio is a convenient summary of the relation between the odds favouring disease after a test result is known and the odds favouring disease before the test result is known:

LR = Post-test odds/pre-test odds

Sometimes the likelihood ratio is defined to reflect the performance of all positive test results, essentially comparing the area under the curve for the population with disease with that for the population without disease located to the right of the cutoff level. At other times, the likelihood ratio is used to indicate the performance of a particular test result, essentially comparing the height of the curve for the population with disease with the height of the curve for the population without disease at the particular test result in question.

Receiver operating characteristic (ROC) curves

The measures of sensitivity and specificity require selection of a particular cutoff level. If the cutoff selected for one test is better than that for another, the results of a comparative evaluation could be misleading. A different measure of test information, called the receiver operating characteristic (ROC) curve, displays the performance of a test over the range of all possible cutoff levels (figure 4.5).

The ROC curve plots, for each possible cutoff level, the sensitivity or true positive rate [TP/(TP + FN)] on the vertical axis versus (1 − specificity) or the false positive rate [FP/(TN + FP)] on the horizontal axis. As the cutoff level slides from more to less stringent, this defines an ROC curve that arcs from lower left to upper right (figure 4.5).

In general, tests that are better separators will have ROC curves that arc higher and more to the left (figure 4.6). The area under an ROC curve indicates the overall discriminating ability of a test. This area can vary from 1.0 for a perfectly discriminating test to 0.5 for a test that is utterly undiscriminating.

Sumner *et al.* (1982) used ROC curves to examine the accuracy of non-invasive tests in identifying patients with extracranial cerebrovascular disease. Their standard of truth was X-ray arteriography, and among the tests they assessed was ultrasonic arteriography. The ultrasonic imaging was increasingly accurate (i.e. it had an ROC curve that was higher and more to the left) in detecting patients with progressively greater degrees of stenosis demonstrated on X-ray arteriograms. The ROC curves provide a vivid and quantifiable summary of test performance.

ROC analysis was introduced by psychologists who were devising ways to evaluate radar technicians during the Second World War. The idea was to see how well the technicians could discern enemy planes from flying geese.

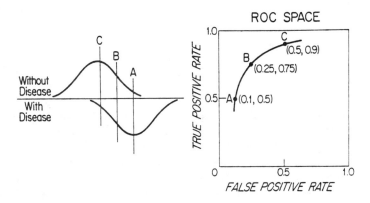

Figure 4.5 Receiver operating characteristic curves (see text).

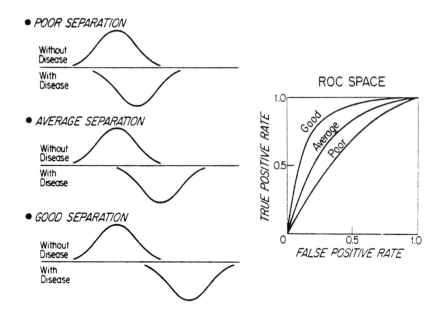

Figure 4.6   Receiver operating characteristic curves (see text).

ROC assessments have become popular means of evaluating imaging tests in medicine, and they are in principle applicable to any diagnostic test. ROC curves are particularly suited to comparing the performance of different diagnostic tests. Both parametric and non-parametric techniques are available to analyse whether differences in ROC performance are statistically significant (Hanley and McNeil, 1982; Swets and Pickett, 1982).

Requirements for different measures

All the measures of test information discussed above (sensitivity, specificity, predictive values, likelihood ratios and ROC curves) require proof of the correct diagnosis independent of any of the tests being evaluated. ROC curves (and likelihood ratios defined for particular test results) do not require specification of a cutoff level, whereas the other measures do. The predictive values are dependent on the prior probability or prevalence of disease, whereas the other measures are not. These features and requirements of the various measures are summarised in table 4.1.

Table 4.1   Requirements for selected measures of test performance.

	Require independent proof of diagnosis	*Require selection of cutoff point*	*Dependent on prevalence*
Sensitivity Specificity	Yes	Yes	No

Predictive value
  positive
Predictive value
  negative
	Yes	Yes	Yes

Likelihood ratio ROC curve	Yes	No	No

Measures for multiple tests

Efforts to evaluate multiple diagnostic tests introduce additional methodological possibilities. For example, some investigators have employed various forms of discriminant analysis to assess the predictive value of multiple tests (Ryback *et al.*, 1982). Other studies have successfully used a technique called recursive partitioning to assign patients to correct diagnostic categories (Goldman *et al.*, 1982). If the degree of statistical dependence among tests is known, or if they are assumed to be independent, Bayes' formula or a two-by-two table can be used to calculate the revised probability of disease from multiple tests (Diamond and Forrester, 1979). In examining repeat tests, the pattern of results, apart from their absolute levels, may have diagnostic value. The diagnostic information from test patterns depends on differences in test–retest correlation between the populations with and without disease (Polister, 1982).

Summary

A number of considerations that bear on the design and conduct of studies to evaluate diagnostic tests have been discussed. Most of the discussion has focused on measuring the diagnostic information produced by tests. An investigator should think carefully about and describe the components of the test system under study and the specific purpose of evaluation. An investigator should be aware of the place of diagnostic information in the efficacy hierarchy, and recognise that the apparent value of tests under experimental conditions may not be matched in the clinic where additional information may be available about patients and where on-line performance may deviate from that observed in the experimental setting. The processes of evolution in technology and disease make it more difficult to achieve pertinent and accurate results.

A good study of diagnostic test information typically demonstrates the following features:

(1) an appropriate spectrum of patients and disease, matching the expected clinical population;
(2) avoidance of selection bias in the patients studied;
(3) delineation of the baseline state of knowledge about the diagnosis at the time of performing and interpreting the test;
(4) proof of correct diagnosis independent of any test being investigated;
(5) use of comparably advanced technologies in comparisons of two or more tests;
(6) assessment of each test in a comparison study independent of knowledge of other test results;
(7) selection of suitable measures of information, with each measure clearly defined;
(8) appreciation of the effects of changes in prevalence and shifts in the selected positivity criteria;
(9) acknowledgement and quantification of the variability in measured parameters; and
(10) discussion of the relation between study findings and expected clinical performance in various settings.

EFFECTS ON THERAPEUTIC TRIALS OF IMPERFECT CLASSIFICATION OF PATIENTS

Analytical questions

Classification of patients into incorrect categories adversely affects the ability of a therapeutic trial to detect differences between treatments. When patients are improperly classified with respect to disease, the treatment group in a study contains some patients who do not have disease along with patients who do have disease. This heterogeneity dilutes the apparent strength of any actual therapeutic effect. The main purpose of this section is to estimate the impact of incorrect disease classification on the observed results and on statistical conclusions of clinical trials intended to compare two treatments. Put positively, the purpose is to suggest the extent to which improved diagnosis of disease can enhance the performance of therapeutic trials.

Diagnosis of the presence and extent of disease enters at two stages of a therapeutic trial. The first is in establishing the population eligible for admission to the trial, a necessary component of any clinical trial. The second is in the determination of a study's outcome. The aims of treatment may include eliminating or containing pathological evidence of disease and improving the physical, cognitive, emotional and social function of patients. At the stage of measuring outcome in a study, more precise diagnosis can produce a more exact measure of the effectiveness of treatment to eradicate, reverse, retard or halt the disease process.

Diagnostic heterogeneity is one of several sources of variability in therapeutic trials. Others include variation in adherence to experimental protocols, in physician acuity or skill, in patient behaviour, in the pharmacodynamics of therapeutic agents, and in the response of disease to treatment. The reasons for focusing specifically on the contribution of diagnostic error are twofold. First, diagnostic imprecision is a source of variability that is potentially reducible by advances in diagnostic technology. For example, nuclear magnetic resonance will conceivably provide more precise diagnoses for some neurological conditions than are possible today using computed tomography and other available modalities (Doyle *et al.*, 1981). Secondly, the degree of diagnostic homogeneity sought in a particular study is, to some degree, under the control of the investigator. Other sources of variability tend to be less susceptible to modification.

The class of therapeutic trials considered here are those intended to compare the success rates (S) of two treatments (A and B) in a population with disease (P_D). In general, an effective experimental treatment will most likely be shown to be effective if the study population is restricted to the spectrum of disease for which the treatment is most efficacious. The analysis compares this ideal situation with that when an imperfect diagnostic system identifies a test-positive population (P_d) that is eligible for the trial. This test system is characterised by a sensitivity and specificity that are each less than 1.0. Hence the study population defined by the imperfect test system (P_d) is more heterogeneous than the population with the disease (P_D).

The major analytical questions to be considered are the following:

(1) In a study to compare the effectiveness of two treatments A and B, how will the expected success of each treatment using the currently available tests to identify eligible patients compare with what would be expected to be observed if available diagnostic tests were perfect?
(2) How will the expected, observed difference between the two treatments compare with the difference that would be expected if the diagnostic classification were perfect?
(3) How does the likelihood of obtaining statistically significant results compare with what would be expected if the available tests were perfect?
(4) How does the needed number of subjects compare with the number that would be needed if the diagnostic tests were perfect?

(5) Are there circumstances in which an investigator might rationally refrain from seeking technically attainable diagnostic precision in a study population?

Scenario

I will discuss the first four questions mainly in the context of a hypothetical study scenario. In a clinic population referred to you because of symptoms suggestive of disease (D) you know from long-term follow-up of previous patients that one-third will in fact have the disease. The disease is serious, and if untreated it invariably leads to death. Patients falsely suspected of disease will recover uneventfully. At the present time, your available diagnostic procedures are good, though imperfect, for the early diagnosis of disease. The sensitivity (SE) of the available test system is 0.8 and the specificity (SP) is 0.9.

Your current baseline treatment, B, has a success rate among patients with disease of 60% survival ($_BS_D = 0.60$). A new, more risky treatment, A, has an anticipated success among patients with disease of 80% ($_AS_D = 0.80$). However, the new treatment also has a 10% risk of death among patients without disease ($_AS_D = 0.90$).

In the coming year you expect to see 180 patients referred for the possibility of this disease. Among the subgroup who test positive for disease (P_d) you are contemplating a randomised clinical trial comparing treatments A and B. You would like to enter appropriately identified patients into the trial over the next two years, though the entry phase could extend over a longer period if necessary.

Potential value of a therapeutic trial

Before beginning to answer the specific questions raised earlier, we might want to verify that such a clinical trial could be worth while: if we did find that the new treatment, A, performed as expected, would we be better off using it? Relying on the available test to classify patients over the next year, we would expect to find a distribution like that shown in the following two-by-two table:

	Disease present	Disease absent	
	D	$\bar{D}$	
Test positive, d	48	12	60
Test negative, $\bar{d}$	12	108	120
	60	120	180

Of the 180 patients expected to come to your clinic, one-third, or 60 patients on average, will actually have disease. The 80% sensitivity of the current test yields 48 patients with a positive test among the 60 with disease. The 90% specificity yields 108 patients with a negative test out of 120 without disease. At the present time, a clinician would be well advised to use the available treatment (B) on all 180 patients regardless of whether or not they test positive. Among those testing negative $(P_{\bar{d}})$ the expected survival using treatment B is $12 \times 0.6 \times 108 = 115.2$ lives; no treatment of group P_d yields $0 + 108 = 108$ lives saved. If the new treatment (A) is as successful as hoped, then treatment A and treatment B would each yield 156 survivors if they were each applied to all 180 patients:

Survivors with B $= 60 \times 0.6 + 120 = 156$
Survivors with A $= 60 \times 0.8 + 0.9 \times 120 = 156$

Even better, however, would be applying the new treatment A to those patients who test positive (P_d) and using treatment B on those who test negative $(P_{\bar{d}})$, as this would lead to more than 164 expected survivors $(48 \times 0.8 + 12 \times 0.9 + 12 \times 0.6 + 108 \times 1.0 = 164.4)$. Thus, an experiment to demonstrate the benefits of treatment A does offer the potential of additional lives saved in the future, and a trial comparing treatments A and B among those who test positive for disease (P_d) appears warranted.

Questions 1 and 2: Expected survival

If it were possible to identify correctly all 60 patients with disease (D), the difference (Δ) in expected survival for treatment A and treatment B would be:

$$\Delta = {_A}S_D - {_B}S_D = 0.8 - 0.6 = 0.2$$

The expected survival under each treatment for patients who test positive (P_d) depends on the fraction of such patients who actually have disease.

From the two-by-two table, we can see that the PVP for the current test system is 48/60 = 0.8. The expected survival among test-positive patients using treatment A is: $_AS_d = \text{PVP} \times {_AS_D} + (1 - \text{PVP}) \times {_AS_{\bar{D}}} = 0.8 \times 0.8 + 0.2 \times 0.9 = 0.82$. Similarly, the expected survival among test-positive patients of treatment B is: $_BS_d = \text{PVP} \times {_BS_D} + (1 - \text{PVP}) \times {_BS_{\bar{D}}} = 0.8 \times 0.6 + 0.2 \times 1 = 0.68$. The difference ($\delta$) in survival for the two treatments now is:

$$\delta = {_AS_d} - {_BS_d} = 0.82 - 0.68 = 0.14$$

This difference (δ) is less than the difference (Δ) that would have been expected if the classification of disease had been perfect. In general, this result ($\Delta > \delta$) will be found with any imperfect classification system so long as the two treatments have larger differential effects among patients with disease than among patients without disease.

Question 3: Likelihood of obtaining statistically significant results

To calculate the likelihood of obtaining statistically significant results in our clinical trial, we proceed in three steps:

(1) we specify a significance level (alpha error) that we seek to achieve;
(2) we estimate the magnitude of the difference in treatment effects that would be required to achieve the specified level of significance; and
(3) we calculate the probability of observing the required difference in the study.

The calculations are based on formulae for standard statistics (z) in comparing two proportions from independent samples (Mosteller *et al.*, 1970; Colton, 1974). The calculations assume that the experimental and control groups each contain 60 patients. If we began instead by testing the 180 clinic patients expected annually, then randomly assigning those who test positive to the experimental or control groups, the likelihood of obtaining statistically significant results would be smaller than calculated here because of additional variability in the number who would be eligible for the trial.

In our study, the proportions of interest are the rates of survival from treatment A and from treatment B. We calculate first the likelihood of a statistically significant result for the study population identified by our imperfect diagnostic system. Then we make a similar computation for circumstances in which the disease classification of patients would be flawless.

In all cases, we choose a significance level (alpha error) of 0.05. This means that we will reject the null hypothesis of 'no difference between treatments A and B' if the likelihood of obtaining the observed result under the null hypothesis is less than 5%.

In response to question 1, we saw that $_AS_d$ is 0.82 and $_BS_d$ is 0.68. The average expected survival (S_d) is $(0.82+0.68)/2 = 0.75$. At a 5% alpha error level, $z_\alpha = 1.96$. The difference in survival (S'_r) required to be observed to achieve statistical significance is then:

$$S'_r = z_\alpha \times [S_d \times (1 - S_d) \times (1/n + 1/n]^{1/2}$$
$$= 1.96 \times [0.75 \times 0.25 \times (1/60 + 1/60)]^{1/2}$$
$$\simeq 0.155$$

The probability of observing a difference as great as or greater than required is the area under the normal curve outside of the standard deviate (z_β) given by the equation:

$$z_\beta = (S'_r - \delta)/[_AS_d \times (1 - _AS_d)/n + _BS_d \times (1 - _BS_d)/n]^{1/2}$$
$$= (0.155 - 0.14)/[0.82 \times 0.18/60 + 0.68 \times 0.32/60]^{1/2}$$
$$\simeq 0.19$$

This area is approximately 0.425; thus, the likelihood of observing a statistically significant result in the study is approximately 43%. Put another way, the study has less than one chance in two of yielding a statistically significant conclusion.

If the classification of disease were perfect, the average expected survival (S_D) would be $(0.8 + 0.6)/2 = 0.7$. The difference in survival (S'_R) required to achieve statistical significance at the 5% level is given by the equation:

$$S'_R = z_\alpha \times [S_D \times (1 - S_D) \times (1/n + 1/n)]^{1/2}$$
$$= 1.96 \times [0.7 \times 0.3 \times (1/60 + 1/60)]^{1/2}$$
$$\simeq 0.164$$

The probability of observing a difference as great as or greater than required is the area under the normal curve outside the standard deviate (z_β):

$$z_\beta = (S'_R - \Delta)/[_AS_D \times (1 - _AS_D)/n + _BS_D \times (1 - _BS_D)/n]^{1/2}$$
$$= (0.164 - 0.2) / [0.8 \times 0.2/60 + 0.6 \times 0.4/60]^{1/2}$$
$$\simeq -0.44$$

This yields an area of approximately 0.67, the likelihood of observing a statistically significant result when all patients in the study truly have disease. A perfect test system would thus convert the likelihood of a statistically significant result from less than one chance in two to about two chances in three.

Question 4: Required size of a study

The required number of subjects in a study depends upon four parameters:

(1) the desired level of statistical significance;
(2) the desired likelihood of detecting a difference if one is present;
(3) the level of difference in treatments the investigator seeks to be able to detect; and
(4) the expected performance of the baseline treatment.

Let us maintain a criterion of 5% for statistical significance. This sets $z_\alpha = 1.96$. If treatment A is as much as 20% better than treatment B in patients with disease, let us suppose we would like to be 90% certain that we will conclude that A is better than B (i.e. that we will reject the null hypothesis of no difference). This sets $z_\beta = -1.28$. We also assume the expected performances of treatments A and B are as given in the scenario and in the response to question 1.

The required number of subjects for the study based on our imperfect diagnostic system (n_δ) is:

$$n_\delta = (\{z_\alpha \times [2 \times {}_BS_d \times (1 - {}_BS_d)]^{1/2} - z_\beta[{}_AS_d \times (1 - {}_AS_d) + {}_BS_d(1 - {}_BS_d)]^{1/2}\}/\delta)^2$$
$$= (\{1.96 \times [2 \times 0.68 \times 0.32]^{1/2} - (-1.28) \times [0.82 \times 0.18 + 0.68 \times 0.32]^{1/2}\}/0.14)^2$$
$$\simeq 218$$

The required number of subjects for the study if our classification of patients were perfect (n_Δ) would be:

$$n_\Delta = (\{Z_\alpha \times [2 \times {}_BS_D \times (1 - {}_BS_D)]^{1/2} - z_\beta[{}_AS_D \times (1 - {}_AS_D) + {}_BS_D(1 - {}_BS_D)]^{1/2}\}/\Delta)^2$$
$$= (\{1.96 \times [2 \times 0.6 \times 0.4]^{1/2} - (-1.28) \times [0.8 \times 0.2 + 0.6 \times 0.4]^{1/2}\}/0.2)^2$$
$$\simeq 118$$

Thus, imprecise diagnostic classification imposes a need for nearly 85% more patients to achieve similar expectations for statistically significant conclusions about differences in the two treatments.

In making these calculations we have not considered the number of clinic patients who would need to be screened in order to obtain the required number for the study. Because the presence of disease is in itself probable (prevalence of one in three in our example), even with a perfect diagnostic system we would need to screen more than 180 clinic patients to be reasonably sure of finding 60 with disease. For example, if the probability of disease is one in three and we want to be 80% certain of finding at least 60 patients with disease, we would need to examine 197 patients.

Question 5: Purposeful imprecision in diagnosis

On occasion, seeking the most accurate, technically attainable diagnosis may not be the best strategy in defining a study population. In some clinical evaluations, for example, an investigator may wish to study patients who represent the range of disease typically encountered by the practitioner who may use the new treatment. This may require a spectrum that is broader than the most narrowly definable disease group. Apart from concerns about matching a study population to the anticipated clinical population, an investigator may intentionally stop short of technically attainable precision in diagnosis because additional diagnostic manoeuvres are impracticable in the study setting, too expensive, too risky, or too aversive to the patient.

As discussed earlier, a study population that includes some erroneously diagnosed patients will weaken a clinical trial's ability to demonstrate the effectiveness of treatment. As we have also seen, the handicap of diagnostic heterogeneity can be offset by expanding the size of the study population, and in particular circumstances an investigator can weigh the costs and risks of more precise diagnosis against the feasibility, costs and added duration of a larger trial.

For example, migraine is one of the clinical problems discussed in this book. This problem may illustrate a situation where less than maximal diagnostic accuracy could be preferred in a clinical trial. Drs Olesen, Larsen and colleagues have found characteristic changes in cerebral blood flow at the time of an attack among patients with symptoms of classic migraine (Olesen *et al.*, 1981a, b). In their studies to date, they have not found similar changes in any patients who have common migraine, i.e. who lack the characteristic visual prodrome of classic migraine. Their clinical impression is that the presence of a classical visual prodrome is virtually pathognomonic for classic migraine as defined by cerebral blood flow changes (personal communication).

Suppose we would like to evaluate a hypothetical new drug for classic migraine that we believe would be effective in halting 90% of attacks. We would like to compare the new drug with current treatment (or placebo) which we can assume would be effective in 70% of attacks. We also assume that either the new drug or the current drug would be effective in 70% of cases of common migraine.

According to our earlier discussion, we expect to be able to carry out a clinical trial with fewer patients if we restrict the study population to those with characteristic cerebral blood flow changes, since this would represent the most homogeneous study population. However, the diagnostic procedure requires injection into the carotid artery, and hence entails some risk. In addition, the test procedure typically induces an attack of migraine, an unpleasant experience for the patient. Therefore, we would like to consider foregoing the cerebral blood flow studies and carrying out the clinical trial among all patients with characteristic symptomatology. The choice is between a smaller, possibly less expensive and more feasible clinical trial versus a larger study that spares all patients some discomfort and risk.

In describing the setting for the proposed study, we can assume that a careful clinical history will produce a diagnosis of classic migraine with a sensitivity of 0.96 and a specificity of 0.98. We also expect that 20% of a typical clinical population with migraine will have classic migraine, and that 80% will have common migraine.

Using these assumptions and the methods developed earlier in this chapter, we can calculate the required sample sizes if all patients with characteristic symptoms are eligible for study, and compare that with the (smaller) required sample size if the study is restricted to patients with diagnostic cerebral blood flow changes. If we wish to be 90% certain of concluding that the new treatment is better when it is in fact as superior as supposed, and select a 0.05 level of statistical significance, the required sample size is approximately 18% larger in a trial using patients with characteristic symptoms compared with a trial restricted to patients who have diagnostic blood flow changes. Because a slightly higher proportion of patients will have characteristic symptoms than will have diagnostic changes in cerebral blood flow, a study using all patients with characteristic symptoms would require only 14% more time to obtain the needed number of subjects. The investigator can judge whether the burden of this added duration outweighs the risk and cost of cerebral blood flow studies in all patients.

SUMMARY

Some effects of imprecise disease classification on therapeutic trials are as follows:

(1) The apparent efficacy of treatment will be altered in a way that depends on the predictive value of the available diagnostic system, the probability of successful treatment of patients with disease, and the probability of successful treatment of patients without disease who are erroneously believed to have disease.
(2) In general, the apparent difference between two treatments will be diminished by inaccurate disease classification. Conversely, a more accurate diagnostic system will increase the apparent difference between treatments.

(3) Statistically significant differences will be less likely to be detected when disease classification is inaccurate. Conversely, more accurate diagnosis will enhance the probability of rejecting the null hypothesis when differences in treatment are actually present.

(4) The required number of subjects in a study will be increased when disease classification is inaccurate. Conversely, a better diagnostic system will reduce the required number of subjects.

In some situations, an investigator may have a choice about the degree of diagnostic precision to seek in a study population. Traditional advice, usually sound, is to seek, as far as possible, definitive proof of disease as is attainable in the study population. The advantages of more accurate diagnosis may be offset by risks or costs incurred in the process of diagnosing a more homogeneous study population. The desirability of seeking a more accurately diagnosed study group depends on the predictive value (i.e. on the prior probability, sensitivity, and specificity) of current classification systems, on the expected effects of each treatment in patients with and without the target disease, on the feasibility, cost and risk of more accurate diagnosis, and on the feasibility and the cost to current and future patients of expanding the study size and duration. Quantitative estimates of the likelihood of obtaining a statistically significant result and of the required size of study groups, as described in this chapter can help an investigator weigh these considerations in the design of a controlled clinical trial to compare different treatments.

REFERENCES

Berwick, D. B., Fineberg, H. V. and Weinstein, M. C. (1981). When doctors meet numbers. *Am. J. Med.*, **71**, 991–8.

Colton, T. (1974). *Statistics in Medicine*. Little, Brown & Co., Boston, pp. 163–9.

Diamond, G. A. and Forrester, J. S. (1979). Analysis of probability as an aid in the clinical diagnosis of coronary artery disease. *New Engl. J. Med.*, **300**, 1350–8.

Doyle, F. H., Pennock, J. M., Orr, J. S., Steiner, R. S., Young, I. R., Burl, M., Clow, H., Gilderdale, D. J., Bailes, D. R. and Walters, P. E. (1981). Imaging of the brain by nuclear magnetic resonance. *Lancet*, **2**, 53–7.

Fineberg, H. V. (1979). Assessing the diagnostic contribution of imaging tests: computed tomography and ultrasound of the pancreas. In Alperovitch, A., DeDombal, F. T. and Gremy, F. (eds), *Evaluation of Efficacy of Medical Action*, North-Holland, Amsterdam, pp. 149–64.

Fineberg, H. V. (1983). Impact of technological investment on the cost of the health care system. *J. Neuroradiol.*, **10**, 199–204.

Fineberg, H. V. and Sherman, H. (1981). Tutorial on the health and social value of computerized medical imaging. *IEEE Transactions on Biomedical Engineering, B.M.E.*, **28**, 50–6.

Fineberg, H. V., Bauman, R. and Sosman, M. (1977). Computerized cranial tomography: effect on diagnostic and therapeutic plans. *J. Am. Med. Assoc.*, **238**, 224–7.

Fineberg, H. V., Wittenberg, J. and Ferrucci, J. T. Jr (1986). The clinical value of body computed tomography over time and technologic change. *Am. J. Roentgenol.*, in press.

Goldman, L., Weinberg, M., Weisberg, M., Olshew, R., Cook, E. F., Sargent, R. K., Lamas, R. G., Dennis, C., Wilson, C., Deckelbaum, L., Fineberg, H. and Stiratelli, R. (1982). A computer-derived protocol to aid in the diagnosis of emergency room patients with acute chest pain. *New Engl. J. Med.*, **307**, 588–96.

Hanley, J. A. and McNeil, B. J. (1982). The meaning and use of the area under a receiver operating characteristic (ROC) curve. *Radiology*, **143**, 29–36.

Mosteller, F., Rourke, R. E. K. and Thomas, G. B. Jr (1970). *Probability with Statistical Applications* (2nd edn). Addison-Wesley, Reading, Mass.

Olesen, J., Larsen, B. and Lauritzen, M. (1981a). Focal hyperemia followed by spreading oligemia and impaired activation of rCBF in classic migraine. *Ann. Neurol.*, **9**, 344–52.

Olesen, J., Tfelt-Hansen, P., Henriksen, L. and Larsen, B. (1981b). The common migraine attack may not be initiated by cerebral ischemia. *Lancet*, **2**, 438–40.

Polister, P. (1982). Reliability, decision rules, and the value of repeated tests. *Med. Decision Making*, **2**, 47–69.

Ransohoff, D. F. and Feinstein, A. R. (1976). Problems of spectrum and bias in evaluating the efficacy of diagnostic tests. *New Engl. J. Med.*, **299**, 1259–63.

Ryback, R. S., Eckardt, M. J., Rawlings, R. R. and Rosenthal, L. S. (1982). Quadratic discriminant analysis as an aid to interpretive reporting of clinical laboratory tests. *J. Am. Med. Assoc.*, **248**, 2342–5.

Sox, H. C., Margulies, I. and Sox, C. H. (1981). Psychologically mediated effects of diagnostic tests. *Ann. Intern. Med.*, **95**, 680–5.

Sumner, D. S., Russell, J. B. and Miles, R. D. (1982). Are non invasive tests sufficiently accurate to identify patients in need of carotid angiography? *Surgery*, **91**, 700–6.

Swets, J. A. and Pickett, R. M. (1982). *Evaluation of Diagnostic Systems: Methods from Signal Detection Theory*. Academic Press, New York, pp. 208–32.

Vecchio, T. J. (1966). Predictive value of a single diagnostic test in unselected populations. *New Engl. J. Med.*, **274**, 1171–3.

Weinstein, M. C. and Fineberg, H. V. (1980). *Clinical Decision Analysis*. W. B. Saunders, Philadelphia.

SECTION 2
CLINICAL TRIALS — PAST AND FUTURE

5

Methodology of clinical trials in migraine

JES OLESEN and PEER TFELT-HANSEN

INTRODUCTION

Migraine is a condition characterised by recurrent attacks lasting from a few hours to a few days. If attacks are comparatively rare, patients are advised to take symptomatic medication such as ergotamine, aspirin and antinauseants at each attack. If patients suffer two or more severe attacks a month, prophylactic therapy may be indicated.

Clinical trials in migraine are hampered by many problems which will be described in this chapter. Unfortunately the need for methodological studies has not manifested itself strongly in previous publication activity. A few older methodological studies must be regarded as obsolete. From the last ten years there is a valuable review (Hübbe, 1975) and occasionally drug studies have included methodological comments. We have used one of our previous prophylactic trials as a basis for an extensive methodological discussion. In other papers we have dealt less extensively with the methodology of how to treat the individual migraine attack. In the present chapter past experience is combined with an analysis of previous drug trials.

ANALYSIS OF PROPHYLACTIC DRUG TRIALS IN MIGRAINE

The number of such trials is so large that it precludes a detailed analysis of every trial. We have therefore decided to evaluate only papers published in the two specialised headache journals: *Headache* from 1977 onwards, and *Cephalalgia* from its start in 1981. We finally include our own most recent study (Tfelt-Hansen and Olesen, 1984) because of its methodological aspects (tables 5.1–4).

ANALYSIS OF DRUG TRIALS DEALING WITH TREATMENT OF THE ACUTE ATTACK

In recent years relatively few such studies have been published. We have therefore included all trials from the past 10 years (tables 5.5–7).

DISCUSSION: PROPHYLACTIC STUDIES

Clinical selection criteria (table 5.1)

Most studies deal with both common and classic migraine. Previously these disorders have been regarded as two variants of the same condition, but increasing evidence from studies of regional cerebral blood flow (Olesen, 1981a, b) indicates that the two disorders are pathophysiologically different. Are results from clinical trials without distinction between the two forms of migraine therefore relevant to classic migraine, common migraine or both? Future trials should study either common or classic migraine according to a generally accepted definition.

An *Ad Hoc* Committee on Classification of Headache of the US National Institute of Health and a committee under the World Federation of Neurology (1970) have produced essentially identical definitions. The NIH definition is as follows.

> Vascular headaches of the migraine type: recurrent attacks of headache, widely varied in intensity, frequency, and duration. The attacks are commonly unilateral in onset; are usually associated with anorexia and, sometimes, with nausea and vomiting; in some are preceded by, or associated with, conspicuous sensory motor and mood disturbances; and are often familial. Evidence supports the view that cranial arterial distension and dilatation are importantly implicated in the painful phase but cause no permanent changes in the involved vessel. Listed below are particular varieties of headaches, each sharing some, but not necessarily all, of the above-mentioned features.

It is obviously impossible to know how such a definition has been interpreted by the individual investigator. Only two of the studies in the table have commented on the problem (Olesen *et al.*, 1981c; Tfelt-Hansen *et al.*, 1984). In seven studies no definition was used. We have previously given a more operational definition of common migraine as recurring idiopathic attacks of headache associated with nausea and one or more of the following characteristics: unilateral pain location, pulsating pain quality, phonophobia or photophobia. This definition may be improved as follows by adding duration of attacks as a typical feature. Common migraine can then be defined as: *recurring idiopathic attacks of headache lasting 3 hours to 3 days and associated with nausea and one or more of the following characteristics: unilateral pain location, pulsating pain quality, phonophobia or photophobia.*

Operationally we suggest the following definition of classic migraine: *recurring idiopathic attacks of gradually developed reversible focal neurological symptoms followed or accompanied by headache.*

The NIH *Ad Hoc* Committee (1962) has defined a subgroup of migraine patients with *combination headache*. This syndrome is particularly ill-defined. It includes patients with a combination of migraine attacks and muscle contraction type headache. We have previously demonstrated that most patients with frequent common migraine attacks virtually always have significant amounts of interval headache, and that increased frequency of migraine attacks correlates with increased frequency of interval headaches (Olesen *et al.*, 1981c). More research is needed to evaluate whether interval headaches and migraine attacks share the same pathophysiology and response to drugs. Until then we advocate that the term 'combination headache' should not be used, but rather symptoms should be grouped as common migraine or muscle contraction headache with a description of the less prominent other headache component. It is apparent from table 5.1 that several previous studies have used no definition of migraine at all, and that our proposal of using an operational definition has not yet gained support by others. Finally, even if most previous studies have described the proportion of classic migraine to common migraine, they virtually all include both types in the final analysis of results.

With or without a proper definition of migraine, all studies should describe the important clinical characteristics of patients entering the trial in quantitative terms to enable comparison with other material. This has unfortunately been done in only a few previous studies.

Patients should have at least two severe attacks a month for prophylactic medication to be indicated, and two attacks a month should therefore be the lower limit for inclusion in a trial. Patients with very frequent attacks have large amounts of interval headache, often misuse drugs, are often treatment resistant and often comply unsatisfactorily. They should probably be excluded, and we have used an upper limit of six attacks a month. Other studies have either had no upper limit or have not described such a limit. To enter a trial, patients should have had migraine for at least one year to assure a relatively stable condition.

A more important but also more difficult problem is interval headaches. If an upper limit of migraine frequency is used, most patients with very frequent interval headaches are automatically excluded. In addition we have excluded patients with daily but not weekly interval headache.

Age limits have been a selection criterion in only a minority of studies, but most studies have given the age range of patients included. In order not to

Table 5.1　Patient selection criteria and clinical characteristics.

	Reference*						
	a	b	c	d	e	f	g
Definition { NIH or WHO / other non-operational / other operational							
No. classic/common			+				+
Migraine attacks (mean/month)		24/26				4/20	10/40
Limits for inclusion		3.94					
Mean duration of migraine disorder (years)	≥2	≥1	≥4			2–10	≥2
Limits for inclusion			15.75				
Interval headaches (mean/month)							
Limits for inclusion							
Age limits (years)			16–64			23–56	19–58
Sex ratio (M/F)		14/36		30/25	70/5	5/19	10/40
Basis population defined: 0 = not defined; 1 = demography selected; 2 = general practice; 3 = specialist practice; 4 = migraine clinic; 5 = hospital	0	0	0	0	0	0	5
Psychiatric illness exclusion +/–							
Narcotic use exclusion +/–							
Ergotamine abuse exclusion +/–							
Previous participation in prophylactic trials exclusion +/–							

*Key to references: a, Herrmann et al., 1977; b, Kallanranta et al., 1977; c, Lawrence et al., 1977; d, Steig, 1977; e, Sulman et al., 1977; f, Anthony et al., 1979; g, Kangasneimi, 1979; h, Mørland et al., 1979; i, Stensrud and Sjaastad, 1979; j, Stensrud and Sjaastad, 1980; k, Lindegaard et al., 1980; l, Louis, 1981; m, Olesen et al., 1981c; n, Capildeo and Rose, 1982; o, Gelmers, 1983; p, Tfelt-Hansen et al., 1984.

Table 5.1 (*continued*)

	Reference[*]								
	h	i	j	k	l	m	n	o	p
Definition { NIH or WHO		+	+	+		+	+	+	+
other non-operational	+								
other operational						+		+	+
No. classic/common			6/29	6/22	18/40	0/33	8/9	12/48	0/96
Migraine attacks (mean/month)				6	1	3.2	10		5.7
Limits for inclusion		≥3	≥3	≥3	≥1	≥2 / ≤8		≥2	≥2 / ≤6
Mean duration of migraine disorder (years)				16.5			10	10	21
Limits for inclusion					≥3	≥2			
Interval headaches (mean/month)						9,5			
Limits for inclusion						<15			<15
Age limits (years)	20–50	20–60	25–60	16–30		21–70	18–60		18–65
Sex ratio (M/F)	2/21	11/27	11/24	9/19	29/29	9/21	1/16	19/31	25/71
Basis population defined: 0 = not defined; 1 = demography selected; 2 = general practice; 3 = specialist practice; 4 = migraine clinic; 5 = hospital	0	0	0	5	2	5	5	0	5
Psychiatric illness exclusion +/–	+								
Narcotic use exclusion +/–								+	+
Ergotamine abuse exclusion +/–						+			+
Previous participation in prophylactic trials exclusion +/–									

Key to references: a, Herrmann *et al.*, 1977; *b*, Kallanranta *et al.*, 1977; *c*, Lawrence *et al.*, 1977; *d*, Steig, 1977; *e*, Sulman *et al.*, 1977; *f*, Anthony *et al.*, 1979; *g*, Kangasneimi, 1979; *h*, Mørland *et al.*, 1979; *i*, Stensrud and Sjaastad, 1979; *j*, Stensrud and Sjaastad, 1980; *k*, Lindegaard *et al.*, 1980; *l*, Louis, 1981; *m*, Olesen *et al.*, 1981c; *n*, Capildeo and Rose, 1982; *o*, Gelmers, 1983; *p*, Tfelt-Hansen *et al.*, 1984.

exclude too many patients we have found wide age limits necessary and we have also decided to study both sexes even if migraine is much more frequent in women and often relates to the menstrual cycle.

It is advisable to describe the recruitment procedure and in particular to state whether patients are recruited from the population at large, general practice, specialist practice, migraine clinic or hospital, but this has only been done in less than half of previous trials.

It is customary to exclude patients with severe heart, liver or renal disease or other severe somatic diseases. Many have excluded females on contraceptive medication, but since most migraine patients are females in the fertile age this would exclude far too many patients. In a previous trial we have excluded females on contraceptive medication. During the trial three undesired pregnancies occurred with resulting drop-out. Contraceptive medication should not be an exclusion criterion, but it must be kept constant because of the well-known hormonal effects on migraine.

In a few previous trials, symptomatic treatment of the individual attacks has been regulated, but we have found this too difficult and believe that the symptomatic medication should simply be recorded and used as an effect parameter.

Patients with severe psychiatric illness and constant psychotropic medication should be excluded, because they comply poorly and because a change of psychotropic medication may influence the migraine condition. The use of narcotic drugs for migraine makes it difficult to treat the condition prophylactically and in later trials we have elected not to include such patients unless they could discontinue narcotics. The same is true of patients with ergotamine abuse.

There is a tendency for patients to come back to a clinic or a specialist if they have had no benefit from previous treatment. Thus most centres have a hard core of patients who have gone through most existing therapies without success. Such patients are ill-suited for drug trials. The same goes for patients who previously participated in several other trials. They are also likely to get to know 'the game', with a higher risk of their breaking the code, and they are likely to be treatment resistant. We suggest that patients should at the most participate in two prophylactic drug trials, preferably with drugs of different class, and it should be stated how many previous prophylactic drugs they have tried. None of the previous trials including our own has commented satisfactorily about these problems.

Trial design (table 5.2)

All trials evaluated were double blind. The high placebo effect and subjective nature of migraine invalidates open trials and even single-blind trials. The triple-blind design, i.e. with individual doses according to plasma level, is a very complicated design which has been used in epilepsy. The implementation of it in migraine research must await evidence of a close correlation between plasma levels and clinical effect.

Four studies utilised group comparison, whereas the other studies used a cross-over design. In two studies a triple cross-over was used comparing a new drug with an established drug and with placebo. This latter design is optimal but requires a long trial period. The advantage of the group comparison method is that the trial period becomes shorter, blindness can more easily be preserved and the problem of carry-over effect is avoided. On the other hand we have calculated that the cross-over design is much more powerful than the group comparison method, the latter requiring up to 28 times as many patients to obtain the same power. In the cross-over design the effect of treatment in one period must not affect the results in the other period. Since drug effects are often slow in onset and wane gradually, a drug-free period must be interposed between the two trial periods (the so-called 'wash-out' period). The length of this period must exceed not only the time taken to eliminate the drug but also the time to eliminate the effect of the drug, which is often unknown. We have suggested one month. Only two other studies have used such a long wash-out period, and in a triple cross-over study we had to accept two weeks in order not to extend the study too much. Some studies have used no wash-out period or one week, which must be regarded as clearly insufficient. Before the trial, a drug-free pretreatment period should be included, and we have used four weeks. This period serves to objectivise the baseline migraine characteristics, thus enabling a calculation of the placebo effect, to reinforce the protocol and to exclude patients who do not comply. Only four other studies have reported a drug-free pretreatment period, but we consider it indispensable. The duration of treatment periods should be quite long since it is important for the power of the trial and because very short-lasting effects are not practically important in therapy. A recent study (Capildeo and Rose, 1982) has shown that placebo effect and real drug effect could only be separated after the first month of treatment and that the difference increased further from the second to the third month. On the other hand, too long treatment periods increase the risk of drop-outs and the amount of labour required to do the trial. Six of the previous trials had treatment periods of six weeks or less, which must be considered insufficient, and one study did not report the length of treatment periods.

The severity of the migraine condition decreases with time in most published materials, even on placebo therapy. As a minimum the same number of patients must therefore start with placebo and active drug, but preferably there should be a balance within small numbers, e.g. six patients, because patient selection may vary with time. For triple cross-over the 'Latin square method' should be used.

Drug compliance has only been evaluated in one previous study. The most generally accepted method is counting residual tablets before the next bottle of tablets is delivered.

Table 5.2 Trial design

	Reference*							
	a	b	c	d	e	f	g	h
Cross-over design (+/−) triple cross-over (*)	−	+	−	+	+	+	+	+
Duration of treatment periods (weeks)	12	4	12	2		4	14	9
Duration of wash-out (weeks)		1		0		0	4	2
Drug-free pretreatment period (weeks)				0		0	4-14	0
Entry balance: 0 = none or not stated; 1 = equal number started on placebo and active; 2 = balance within small number	1	1	0	0	0	0	0	0
Drug compliance evaluation: 0 = none; 1 = asking; 2 = counting residual tablets; 3 = plasma drug levels	0	0	0	0	0	0	0	0
Patient information described								
Number of centres	21	1	3				1	
Number of investigators								
Change of investigators								
Drug identity: 0 = not stated; 1 = stated; 2 = tested		1	1			1	1	0
Placebo included		+	+	+	+	+	−	+
Number of patients included	253	50	36	76	75	24	50	24
Number of patients completed	125		28	55		19	34	14

Key to references: as table 5.1.

Table 5.2 *(continued)*

	Reference*							
	i	j	k	l	m	n	o	p
Cross-over design (+/−) triple cross-over (*)	+	*	+	−	+	+	−	*
Duration of treatment periods (weeks)	4	6	6	12	14	9	13	12
Duration of wash-out (weeks)	4	1	1		4	0		2
Drug-free pretreatment period (weeks)	4		8		4	0	2	4
Entry balance: 0 = none or not stated; 1 = equal number started on placebo and active; 2 = balance within small number	0	0	0			0	1	2
Drug compliance evaluation: 0 = none; 1 = asking; 2 = counting residual tablets; 3 = plasma drug levels	0	0	0	0	2	0	0	0
Patient information described					+			+
Number of centres					1	1	1	4
Number of investigators					1			4
Change of investigators					−			−
Drug identity: 0 = not stated; 1 = stated; 2 = tested	0	1	0	0	1	1	1	1
Placebo included	+	+	+	+	+	−	+	+
Number of patients included	38	35	28	58	33	17	96	96
Number of patients completed	34	29	28	58	30	17	83	83

Key to references: as table 5.1.

It is important to know whether patient information was described and what it contained. This was done in only two of the previous studies.

It is known from many multicentre studies that an important source of variability is within centres, and similarly if there is a large number of investigators and if there is a change of investigator, i.e. the same doctor should follow his patients through the whole trial.

Drug identity is required for double blindness, but is often not described. The preparations should be tested by a small panel of investigators to assure that they are really identical, or as a minimum a specific statement should be made about the identity of the preparations with regard to size, colour, smell and taste.

If a new drug is compared with an established drug without the inclusion of placebo, no significant difference may simply mean that the patient material has been very resistant to therapy, e.g. old hard-core cases. Thus, a drug should either be compared directly with placebo or with placebo as well as with an established drug.

We have found it very difficult to state the number of patients assessed because they are usually recruited from several different sources. Only two previous papers have stated the number assessed. The number included as well as the number completed should be given, and this was so for all trials except two.

If two active drugs are to be compared, it is important that equipotent doses are used. Since information about dose–effect relations in migraine is lacking, doses are often determined on the basis of other effects (e.g. for beta-blockers the pulse-slowing effect). In fact this appeared to be relevant in our recent study of beta-blockers since equipotent doses of propranolol and timolol as determined from their pulse-slowing effect gave an equivalent result on the migraine parameters and an equal proportion of side-effects (Tfelt-Hansen *et al.*, 1984).

Important factors in the evaluation of results (table 5.3)

A headache diary should be used to objectivise the patient's observations. As will be apparent from the rest of this discussion, the headache diary should probably be modified again, with inclusion of the patient's global evaluation of each attack. All data should be quantifiable. Frequency of migraine attacks has been used as an effect parameter by all previous papers except three. It appears to be a good and simple parameter but unfortunately its use entails many problems. Some studies have used all headaches as migraine attacks, i.e. they also include interval headaches. Other studies have asked the patients to record only what they considered migraine attacks. In one study (Herrmann *et al.*, 1977) doctors decided how many attacks the patients had had on the basis of the headache diary! Should continuous migraine interrupted by sleep be recorded as one or two attacks?

Another problem is temporary relief caused by symptomatic treatment. We suggest counting each day with migraine as one attack.

Interval headaches should ideally be separated from migraine attacks. This is extremely difficult since headache, nausea and other accompanying symptoms may vary somewhat independently from episode to episode. We have arbitrarily analysed patients with mild pain or with medium pain without nausea as interval headache in one trial (Olesen *et al.*, 1981c) and in a subsequent trial we have analysed attacks without nausea compared with attacks with nausea. However, any subdivision has to be arbitrary.

The duration of attacks has been used as an effect parameter in about half of the previous publications reviewed. In our latest study (Tfelt-Hansen *et al.*, 1984) this parameter showed a large variability, probably because it is difficult for patients to state exactly when an attack starts and ends, particularly if it ends with sleep.

The severity of attacks is usually scored from 0 to 3, and has been used as an independent effect parameter in six out of 16 papers. It is important that this grading is clearly defined. The most widely used grading is the following: '0' means no pain, '1' means a mild pain, which may be bothering but does not eliminate working capacity, '2' is a headache of medium severity, which makes it impossible to work, and '3' is a very severe headache, which causes the patient to go to bed. However, this grading not only scores pain but rather reflects a global evaluation of the attack. A visual analogue scale might be used for a more specific evaluation of pain intensity.

Traditionally frequency, duration and severity have been combined in a so-called headache index. This has been calculated in different ways: number of days with headache times severity, frequency of attacks times severity, and frequency times duration times severity. The latter would seem to reflect suffering best, but in our two studies it varied more than the others. To multiply such factors, they have to be independent, which is clearly not the case with duration and severity, whereas severity and frequency are more independent. This finding also favours the omission of duration in calculating the headache index.

Effective prophylactic treatment should result in a lower consumption of symptomatic medication. Since it has been impossible to standardise the symptomatic treatment, it becomes somewhat difficult to obtain a comparable estimate of patients' drug consumption. Usually weak analgesics are sold in equipotent tablets so that the same number of tablets may be used, but ergotamine preparations are of an entirely different group as are the narcotic analgesics. We have tried to split medication into these three groups but found that under such circumstances each parameter becomes very variable and not useful. If consumption of symptomatic drugs is to be used, one must use some sort of equation to equalise different medications and obtain a single digital estimate.

Patients' preference can obviously only be used in cross-over trials, and here the risk of impairment of blindness is very large if patients are informed

Table 5.3 Endpoints and other important factors in the evaluation of results.

	Reference*							
	a	b	c	d	e	f	g	h
Frequency of attacks	+	+	+		+	+	+	+
Duration of attacks	+	+					+	
Severity of attacks	+							
Headache index (frequency × severity)			+			+		+
Headache index (frequency × duration × severity)			+	+				
Drug consumption								+
Patients' preference		+					+	
Patients' global evaluation							+	
50% reduction as responders	+					+	+	
Separate evaluation of interval headache +/–							+	
Systematic prospective recording of side-effects +/–	+	+				+	+	+

Key to references: as table 5.1.

Table 5.3 (continued)

	Reference*							
	i	j	k	l	m	n	o	p
Frequency of attacks	+	+	+	+	+			+
Duration of attacks			+		+			+
Severity of attacks	+				+			+
Headache index (frequency × severity)	+	+	+		+	+		+
Headache index (frequency × duration × severity)					+		+	+
Drug consumption					+			+
Patients' preference			+					
Patients' global evaluation				+				
50% reduction as responders							+	+
Separate evaluation of interval headache +/−					+			+
Systematic prospective recording of side-effects +/−			+		+		+	+

*Key to references: as table 5.1.

about details of the protocol. Patients should know that they will obtain different drugs in different periods including placebo, but they should not know how many periods there are and how they change. This precludes the use of patients' preference.

The number of patients with 50% reduction of various headache parameters has been used in five of the studies. Generally, this is not a good parameter for the measurement of effect, but it may be used to identify subgroups of responders.

Systematic prospective recording of side-effects has been done in more than half of the reviewed studies and is of course absolutely necessary.

Statistics (table 5.4)

This is in general a very neglected field in migraine research. Thus six out of 16 studies did not even mention which statistical test they used and in one study there were no statistical calculations at all. Only three of the studies had in advance determined the level of significance, and only two of the studies had in advance determined which test variables to use.

We and others have demonstrated that migraine frequency and derived headache indices decrease with time (Olesen *et al.*, 1981c), and have thus identified a so-called time effect independent of treatment. Migraine is a fluctuating condition with bad periods and good periods. If recruitment of patients requires a fairly severe migraine, patients are likely to be selected during one of their worst periods and will therefore improve spontaneously. Another explanation is of course the medical attention given during a trial and the placebo effect. Despite the good reasons for its existence, a time effect has not always been observed. It is, however, necessary in each trial to analyse for a separate time effect, and, if it is there, then to separate it from the drug effects. We have described how this can be done (Olesen *et al.*, 1981c). If the time effect is not separated from the drug effect, statistical testing will become too weak. Obviously the separation can only be done in cross-over trials. Often two presumably active drugs have been compared without any significant difference. Subsequently migraine parameters during treatment have been compared with pre-study values and it has been concluded that both drugs were effective. This is obviously invalid because of the time effect. To demonstrate that a new drug is as effective as an established drug, triple cross-over with placebo and a demonstration of sufficient power is necessary.

Confidence limits and power were only calculated in two of the previous reports (Olesen *et al.*, 1981c; Tfelt-Hansen *et al.*, 1984). The importance of these parameters is most obvious in trials where no significant difference between a test drug and placebo or between a test drug and an established drug has been demonstrated. What could the reason be for such a lack of significance? Unfortunately most authors have concluded that no significant difference means no real difference. In a small and poorly conducted trial the chance of finding a statistical significance is very small even if the test drug is vastly superior to placebo. Thus a clinical trial can be an accurate or an inaccurate tool depending on the patient selection criteria, number of patients included, length of trial periods, number of drugs, etc. Therefore the burning issue in cases of no significant difference is: how good was the study? This is reflected by the confidence limits which are wide if the study is poor. The calculation of power is an expression of the same phenomenon. The power to detect a 25% difference between test drug and placebo means: what are the chances of identifying such a difference? Conventionally a power of 0.80 is considered satisfactory (Cohen, 1977). We have previously calculated that sufficient power to detect a 25% difference was obtained in a one-centre, one-investigator study with 30 patients in a cross-over design utilising test periods of three months each provided the time effect was separated from the drug effect (Olesen *et al.*, 1981c). In a later multicentre trial (Tfelt-Hansen *et al.*, 1984) power was less satisfactory. We have also demonstrated that many more patients — probably at least ten times as many — are necessary in a group comparison trial to obtain the same power. Power can probably be improved in group comparison trials by stratification, but this has not been done. With these figures at hand we can conclude that the majority of previous trials have had insufficient power. How can we then explain how 11 out of 16 studies showed a significant difference? It is likely that large numbers of trials are conducted and a lot with negative results are published. This has been called 'publication significance'. We suggest that some kind of international body, probably under the World Health Organization, should register all drug trials that remain unpublished.

Since we have demonstrated that large patient materials and long-lasting trials are necessary for sufficient power, it becomes more and more pertinent to identify the best possible effect parameters. Previously we have asked: which parameters best reflect the condition of the patients? One might justifiably ask: which parameters are most likely to discriminate between an active drug and placebo? Such information can quite easily be obtained by power calculations on the different test parameters. We have done that in two trials, but results were not consistent and more work is required along these lines.

Handling of drop-outs is important, especially in group comparison trials where drop-outs can quite easily make a study worthless. The basic principle here must be that intention to treat makes it necessary to include patients in calculations. Thus drop-outs should somehow be included, but this is by no means easy and sometimes impossible. As a minimum, a thorough description of reasons for drop-out and their statistical handling should be given. This was only found in two of the previous reports.

Table 5.4 Statistics.

| | \multicolumn{9}{c}{Reference*} | | | | | | | | |
	a	b	c	d	e	f	g	h	i
Name of test				Covariance				Wilcoxon	t-test
Drug/time effect separation									
Level of significance predetermined									
Test variables predetermined									
Confidence limits									
Power									
Handling of drop-outs: 1 = excluded; 2 = excluded if unrelated to trial; 3 = regarded as failures; 4 = assigned a relative value; 5 = not stated	5	5	5	5	5	5	5	5	5
Conclusion of study: 1 = active better than placebo; 2 = active equal to or worse than placebo; 3 = active equal to active; 4 = active better than active; 5 = no conclusion	3	1	1	1	1	2	3	1	5

*Key to references: as table 5.1

Table 5.4 *(continued)*

	Reference*						
Name of test	j	k	l	m	n	o	p
	Wilcoxon, t-test	Wilcoxon, t-test	Mann-Whitney	Analysis of variance		Analysis of variance	Analysis of variance
Drug/time effect separation				+			
Level of significance predetermined		0.05		+			0.05
Test variables predetermined		+					+
Confidence limits				+			+
Power				+			+
Handling of drop-outs: 1 = excluded; 2 = excluded if unrelated to trial; 3 = regarded as failures; 4 = assigned a relative value; 5 = not stated	5	5	5	1	5	5	1
Conclusion of study: 1 = active better than placebo; 2 = active equal to or worse than placebo; 3 = active equal to active; 4 = active better than active; 5 = no conclusion	1	1	1	2	1	1	1

* *Key to references*: as table 5.1.

DISCUSSION: TREATMENT OF ATTACKS

Patient selection (table 5.5)

The vast majority of migraine patients take only symptomatic treatment and have attacks once a month or less. A similar type of patient should ideally be selected for clinical trials of symptomatic medication. Such patients are virtually never seen in hospitals or by specialists, and their impetus to join a controlled trial is probably minimal. Patients who are less representative, i.e. who have more frequent attacks, have therefore virtually always been used. An upper limit of attack frequency must be set as low as considered realistic. We would suggest less than four attacks a month. Such a limit also greatly reduces problems with interval headache (see above).

Some trials have had a limit concerning severity of attacks, patients being allowed to treat only moderate or severe attacks. It has been our experience that one probably cannot expect the patients to do this in a reliable way since most attacks start gradually and patients want to take the treatment early. In acute headache clinics where patients come for treatment of attacks, such a selection of the most severe cases can be done (Tfelt-Hansen *et al.*, 1980, 1982).

Trial design (table 5.6)

All the reviewed trials were double blind and placebo was involved in seven out of 11 papers. It is difficult or impossible from the published results to evaluate the magnitude of the placebo response. In general this is difficult because the migraine attack is self-limiting, and because symptoms are usually not maximal at the time of drug intake. In addition there is a lack of details in the reporting of results. The best way to estimate the placebo response is probably to look at the need for escape medication. In two placebo-controlled studies (Diamond, 1976; Hakkarainen *et al.*, 1979) 50% of the patients got along without escape medication after placebo. These trials did not report how patient information was given and in particular it was not stated whether patients were informed that placebo was included. In a later study of similar drugs where the inclusion of placebo was deliberately and thoroughly explained to the patients, only 17% managed without escape medication after placebo (Tfelt-Hansen and Olesen, 1984). Thus the magnitude of the placebo response in migraineurs can probably be manipulated considerably by the investigators.

Concerning the general design, two different methods have been used. One is to study patients as they come to an acute migraine clinic for the treatment of an individual attack. Under these circumstances patients can be objectively evaluated and it can be assumed that they really have a migraine attack. The disadvantages are problems with recruiting sufficient numbers of

Table 5.5 Statistics

	Reference*										
	a	b	c	d	e	f	g	h	i	j	k
Definition { NIH or WHO											
other non-operational		+							+		+
other operational			+	+	+		+		+	+	+
No. classical/common				17/10	8/12		10/15		19/124	10/12	0/120
Migraine attacks (mean/month)		2				2			2		2
Limits for inclusion			+	+	+	+	+				
Mean duration of migraine disorder (years)								19	19		18
Age limits (years)			+	+		+					
Limits on attack severity or associated symptoms			+	+	+				+		
Sex ratio (M/F)	14/46	16/40	7/33	7/26	0/20	17/133	0/25	0/22	29/114		23/79
Basis population defined: 1 = demographically selected; 2 = general practice; 3 = specialist practice; 4 = migraine clinic; 5 = hospital patient		3				4		4	4		4

** *Key to references:* a, Ryan, 1974; b, Diamond, 1976; c, Somerville, 1976; d, Slettnes and Sjaastad, 1977; e, Hakkarainen et al., 1979; f, Tfelt-Hansen et al., 1980; g, Hakkarainen et al., 1980; h, Hakkarainen and Allonen, 1982; i, Tfelt-Hansen et al., 1982; j, Peatfield et al., 1983; k, Tfelt-Hansen and Olesen, 1984.

Table 5.6 Trial design.

	Reference*										
	a	b	c	d	e	f	g	h	i	j	k
Double blind	+	+	+	+	+	+	+	+	+	+	+
Placebo included	+	+	+	+	+	+		+	+	+	+
Cross-over	+	+	+	+	+		+	+	+		+
Number of test medications	3	3	2	2	4	3	3	4	3	2	3
Single dose or repeated dose in each attack: 1 = single dose; 2 = up to 2 doses; 5 = up to 5 doses	5	5	2	1	1	1	2	1	1	1	1
Number of times each test medication was tested	2	2	1	≥4	2	1	7	2	1	3	1
Entry balance									+		
Patient information described											+
Number of patients included	60	56	34	33	20	150	25	24	150	40	118
Number of patients completed	60	56	28	27	20	140	25	22	143	22	85
Total number of attacks treated	336	336	56	339	160	140	525	176	143	132	283

*Key to references: as table 5.5.

patients, a high workload, and the fact that patients cannot be crossed over since too few tend to come back for a second treatment. The other general approach has been to let patients treat attacks at home according to certain criteria and then fill in a report form after each attack. This is a time-efficient method which allows patients to treat a number of attacks and thus to use the cross-over design. Of course a group comparison would also be possible. This would probably mean better preservation of blindness but at the sacrifice of power, and so the method has not been used. The main disadvantage of home treatment is the uncertainty about what kind of headache the patients actually treat. Probably the placebo response is lower in trials done at home than in a migraine clinic where a placebo response of 70% on nausea could be ascribed to patients being detached from their environment and cared for (Tfelt-Hansen *et al.*, 1980).

The number of test medications including placebo varied from two to four in the reviewed studies. Each compound was taken from one to several times. The aim of repeated intake of the same drug is to reduce variability from attack to attack. The mean result for each subject on each test medication is then used for statistical evaluation. The method seems fairly powerful since positive results have been reported in trials including a small number of patients. One should, however, keep in mind that by treating a small number of patients many times one is still only testing the effect on that particular patient material. The representativeness of small patient numbers is questionable, and we suggest that no less than 30 patients should be included in trials of symptomatic medication.

Evaluation of results (table 5.7)

Duration and severity of attacks, the need for escape medication, effect on head pain and nausea and general parameters such as patients' preference and global evaluation have been used as judgement criteria in previous trials. The choice of judgement criteria depends on the design. Thus trials in a headache clinic where patients come with fully developed attacks have at various times used rating of headache and nausea. Outpatient trials, where drugs are taken at the onset of attack, have mostly used duration and severity of attacks and preference. Regrettably only two studies have reported power calculations. No comparison between the power of the different variables has been published.

In analgesic trials of other conditions the visual analogue scale has proved useful. Calimlin *et al.* (1977) studied the effect of pentazocine, aspirin and placebo on postoperative pain. They studied the discriminative power of various effect parameters and found that a patient's global evaluation of efficacy on an ordinal scale (1 = poor, 5 = excellent) performed much better than various parameters derived from visual analogue scales or verbal pain

Table 5.7 Evaluation of results and statistics.

	Reference*										
	a	b	c	d	e	f	g	h	i	j	k
Duration of attacks	+			+	+		+	+			
Severity of attacks		+		+	+		+	+			
Escape medication		+		+	+	+	+	+	+		+
Effect on head pain				+		+		+	+	+	+
Effect on nausea				+		+					+
Patient's preference	+		+		+			+		+	
Global evaluation	+		+				+				
Systematic prospective recording of side-effects	+	+	+	+	+	+	+	+	+	+	+
Name of test(s)	Wilcoxon, paired t-test	Friedman's ANOVA			Tukey's test, χ-square	Fisher's exact	Friedman's ANOVA	ANOVA, χ-square	Kruskal-Wallis	Wilcoxon, Student's t-test	Monte Carlo
Confidence limits										+	
Power									+	+	
Handling of drop-outs: 1 = excluded; 2 = excluded if unrelated to trial; 3 = regarded as failures; 4 = assigned a relative value			1	1		1		1	1	1	4
Conclusion of study: 1 = active better than placebo; 2 = active equal or worse than placebo; 3 = active equal to active; 4 = active better than active	1.3	1.3	1	1	1.3	1.3	3.4	3.4	2.3	3	1.3

Key to references: as table 5.5.

report scales. A similar approach may be used for each migraine attack scoring it, for example, as very mild, mild, moderate, fairly severe, severe and excruciating. Patients may also use a visual analogue scale to make a global evaluation of the attack. By letting the patient integrate pain intensity and duration, nausea, photophobia, side-effects and other factors important to him or her, we probably get a more reliable estimate than by letting the patient score the different components of the attack and then multiply or add these factors. We strongly recommend that visual analogue scales and global evaluation as well as traditional parameters should be tested prospectively.

Statistics (table 5.7)

In general and in contradistinction to prophylactic drug trials, the use of statistics was reasonably sufficient in these trials probably because of similarity with other analgesic studies. Calculation of confidence limits and power should be used more frequently to enable the readers to evaluate the clinical significance of the results. Level of significance and end-points have not usually been predetermined as they should.

CONCLUSION

We hope that it is obvious to the reader of this chapter that the formulation of a single ideal protocol for a study of migraine prophylaxis or treatment of acute attacks is impossible. The number of patients and their clinical characteristics are bound to vary very much between centres. So are the qualifications and available time of the investigators. The recommendation we make for future migraine trials is to go through the long list of problems discussed in this paper and maybe add a few extra, and then, with a view to resources, expected magnitude of effect of the drug, etc. select the proper solution for the individual study. All questions are not equally important; nor are the answers to the questions equally good. More methodological research is necessary to improve protocols, particularly to improve power. Probably most of such new methodological information will derive from studies of the treatment of acute attacks. We must find out how to rate a single attack in the best possible way before it can become possible to design an optimal headache diary and optimal test parameters in prophylactic drug studies. (See Tables A.1–A.3. on pp. 305–309.)

REFERENCES

Anthony, M., Lord, G. D. A. and Lance, J. W. (1979). Controlled trials of cime-tidine in migraine and cluster headache. *Headache*, **18**, 261-4.

Calimlin, J. F., Wardell, W. M., Phil, D., Davis, H. T., Lasagna, L. and Gil-lies, A. J. (1977). Analgesic efficacy of an orally administered combination of pentazocine and aspirin. With observations on the use and statistical efficiency of GLOBAL subjective efficacy ratings. *Clin. Pharmacol. Ther.*, **21**, 34-43.

Capildeo, R. and Rose, F. C. (1982). Single-dose pizotifen, 1.5 mg nocte: a new approach in the prophylaxis of migraine. *Headache*, **22**, 272-5.

Cohen, J. (1977). *Statistical Power Analysis for the Behavioral Sciences*. Academic Press, New York.

Diamond, S. (1976). Treatment of migraine with isomethoptene, acetaminophen, and dichloralphenazone combination: a double-blind, cross-over trial. *Headache*, **15**, 282-7.

Gelmers, H. J. (1983). Nimodipine, a new calcium antagonist, in the prophylactic treatment of migraine. *Headache*, **23**, 106-9.

Hakkarainen, H. and Allonen, H. (1982). Ergotamine vs. metoclopramide vs. their combination in acute migraine attacks. *Headache*, **22**, 10-12

Hakkarainen, H., Vapaatalo, H., Gothoni, G. and Parantainen, J. (1979). Tolfena-mic acid is as effective as ergotamine during migraine attacks. *Lancet*, **1**, 326-8.

Hakkarainen, H., Quiding, H. and Stockman, O. (1980). Mild analgesics as an alternative to ergotamine in migraine. A comparative trial with acetylsalicylic acid, ergotamine tartrate, and a dextropropoxyphene compound. *J. Clin. Pharmacol.*, **20**, 590-5.

Herrmann, W. M., Horowski, R., Dannehl, K., Kramer, U and Lurati, K. (1977). Clinical effectiveness of lisuride hydrogen maleate: a double-blind trial versus methysergide. *Headache*, **17**, 54-60.

Hübbe, P. (1975). Controlled clinical trials of drugs for use in the prophylaxis of migraine. *Dad. Med. Bull.*, **22**, 92-9.

Kallanranta, T., Hakkarainen, H., Hokkanen, E. and Tuovinen, T. (1977). Clonidine in migraine prophylaxis. *Headache*, **17**, 169-72.

Kangasniemi, P. (1979). Placebo, 1-isopropylnoradrenochrome-5-monosemicarba-zono and pizotifen in migraine prophylaxis. *Headache*, **19**, 219-22.

Lawrence, E. R., Hossain, M. and Littlestone, W. (1977). Sanomigran for migraine prophylaxis; controlled multicenter trial in general practice. *Headache*, **17**, 109-12.

Lindegaard, K. F., Ovrelid, L. and Sjaastad, O. (1980). Naproxen in the prevention of migraine attacks. A double-blind placebo-controlled cross-over study. *Headache*, **20**, 96-8.

Louis, P. (1981). A double-blind placebo-controlled prophylactic study of fluna-rizine (sibelium R) in migraine. *Headache*, **21**, 235-9.

Mørland, T. J., Storli, O. V. and Mogstad, T. E. (1979). Doxepin in the prophylactic treatment of mixed 'vascular' and tension headache. *Headache*, **19**, 382-3.

National Institute of Health *Ad Hoc* Committee on Classification of Headache (1962). Classification of headache. *J. Am. Med. Assoc.*, **179**, 717-18.

Olesen, J., Larsen, B. and Lauritzen, M. (1981a). Focal hyperemia followed by spreading oligemia and impaired activation of rCBF in classic migraine. *Ann. Neurol.*, **9**, 344-52.

Olesen, J., Tfelt-Hansen, P., Henriksen, L. and Larsen, B. (1981b). The common migraine attack may not be initiated by cerebral ischaemia. *Lancet*, **2**, 438-40.

Olesen, J., Krabbe, A. E. and Tfelt-Hansen, P. (1981c). Methodological aspects of prophylactic drug trials in migraine. *Cephalalgia*, **1**, 127–41.

Peatfield, R. C., Petty, R. G. and Rose, F. C. (1983). Double-blind comparison of mefenamic acid and acetaminophen (paracetamol) in migraine. *Cephalalgia*, **3**, 129–34.

Ryan, E. R. (1974). A study of midrin in the symptomatic relief of migraine headache. *Headache*, **14**, 33–42.

Slettnes, O. and Sjaastad, O. (1977). Metoclopramide during attacks of migraine. In Sicuteri, F. (ed.), *Headache: New Vistas*. Biomedical Press, Florence, pp. 201–4.

Somerville, B. W. (1976). Treatment of migraine attacks with an analgesic combination (mersyndol). *Med. J. Aust.*, **1**, 865–6.

Steig, R. L. (1977). Double-blind study of belladonna–ergotamine–phenobarbital for interval treatment of recurrent throbbing headache. *Headache*, **17**, 120–4.

Stensrud, P. and Sjaastad, O. (1979). Clonazepam (rivotril) in migraine prophylaxis. *Headache*, **19**, 333–4.

Stensrud, P. and Sjaastad, O. (1980). Comparative trial of tenormin (atenolol) and inderal (propranolol) in migraine. *Headache*, **20**, 204–7.

Sulman, F. G., Pfeifer, Y. and Superstine, E. (1977). Preventive treatment of migraine with mini-doses of danitracene. *Headache*, **17**, 203–7.

Tfelt-Hansen, P. and Olesen, J. (1984). Effervescent metoclopramide and aspirin (Migravess) versus effervescent aspirin or placebo for migraine attacks. A double-blind study. *Cephalalgia*, **4**, 107–11.

Tfelt-Hansen, P., Olesen, J., Aebelholt-Krabbe, A., Melgaard, B. and Veilis, B. (1980). A double-blind study of metoclopramide in the treatment of migraine attacks. *J. Neurol. Neurosurg. Psychiatr.*, **43**, 369–71.

Tfelt-Hansen, P., Jensen, K., Vendsborg, P., Lauritzen, M. and Olesen, J. (1982). Chlormezanone in the treatment of migraine attacks: a double-blind comparison with diazepam and placebo. *Cephalalgia*, **2**, 205–10.

Tfelt-Hansen, P., Standness, B., Kangasniemi, P., Hakkarainen, H. and Olesen, J. (1984). Timolol versus propranolol versus placebo in common migraine prophylaxis. A double-blind multicenter trial. *Acute Neurol. Scand.*, **69**, 1–8.

World Federation of Neurology, Research Group on Migraine and Headache (1970). Definition of migraine. In Cochrane, A. L. (ed.), *Background to Migraine*, Heinemann, London, pp. 181–2.

6
Methodology of clinical trials in neurology. Evaluation of extracranial arterial disease

J. PHILIP KISTLER and MICHAEL J. G. HARRISON

INTRODUCTION

Trials in cerebrovascular disease, for example of antithrombotic agents, are beset with difficulties. They seek to answer the pragmatic question of whether such a strategy prevents clinical end-points like stroke and death, but they are dependent on a unitary hypothesis about the cause of those end-points. They assume homogeneity of the clinical material, and a uniform pathophysiological mechanism of symptom production.

Clearly in the case of transient ischaemic attacks some are due to non-vascular causes such as sensory epilepsy, hypoglycaemia, subdural haematoma or brain tumour, and in the case of 'strokes' up to 5% are due to tumours presenting acutely. Even when the vascular basis of the episode is correctly assumed, the mechanism may be embolic or haemodynamic. When embolic the source of the embolism may be in the heart, the aorta, the neck vessels or intracranially. The nature of the embolic material varies widely from platelet aggregates to platelet fibrin masses, clotlike material, non-bacterial vegetations, cholesterol crystals, atheromatous debris, and calcific heart-valve fragments.

In so far as a trial tests a hypothesis about disease causation, it is clear that this gross heterogeneity in the case of cerebrovascular disease is going to limit interpretation severely.

What can be done to identify the cerebral and the vascular lesion more accurately when these details are crucial to trial design? In the multicentre trials of antiplatelet agents where the treatment *policy* is under scrutiny, simple measures may suffice. In a trial of new agents or surgical procedures aimed at a specific pathogenic mechanism, a more tightly defined patient group is desirable.

111

THE CEREBRAL LESION

It is important to identify whether clinical end-points are due to infarction, haemorrhage or non-vascular causes, and CT scanning is clearly desirable on entry into trials in which stroke is an end-point, and again when a clinical event occurs. In trials of the acute treatment of stroke victims, the same diagnostic characterisation is clearly needed. In addition the relative roles of oedema and necrosis in the production of morbidity and mortality may be useful information. For example, no trial of anti-oedema therapy has yet been CT scan controlled. Nuclear magnetic resonance (NMR) scanning is likely to be superior to CT scanning in making distinctions between oedema and infarction, and would clearly be desirable in any further trial of anti-oedema treatment.

If attempts are to be made to affect blood flow acutely in the hope of limiting infarct size, then it may be necessary to consider measurement of cerebral blood volume and cerebral oxygen extraction, currently the best indications of true ischaemia. Such studies are limited to those centres with the necessary equipment for PET scanning although regional cerebral blood volume as an indication of a dilated collateral bed is more widely available.

THE VASCULAR LESION

It seems necessary to identify whether the patient's clinical status is due to cardiac or artery-to-artery embolism, whether an embologenic lesion is also haemodynamically significant, and what degree of collateral supply has developed, or is capable of developing. The location and severity of any atherothrombotic lesion at the origin of the internal carotid artery, the 'carotid siphon' or the middle cerebral stem will determine the need for collateral flow around the circle of Willis. The adequacy of such collateral flow can only be determined angiographically.

TRANSIENT ISCHAEMIC ATTACKS

Symptomatic patients with brief attacks attributable to transient ischaemia or minor infarction are known to be at increased risk of major strokes (5–7% per annum). Though the advisability of carotid endarterectomy is hotly debated (Harrison, 1982) and is the subject of a new UK controlled trial, many believe that the procedure is the treatment of choice for patients with TIAs in the carotid territory. There is some suggestion, but no proof, that carotid stenosis of severe degree is more likely to be followed by stroke than when the lesion is minor (Busuttil *et al.*, 1981) and some evidence that complicated ulcerated lesions carry a greater risk of subsequent stroke than shallow, smooth-looking lesions (Moore *et al.*, 1970). We badly need to know if the degree, location and nature of stenotic lesions have a real effect on prognosis since this would influence surgical policy. Surgical trials need to consider separately patients with these differing kinds of carotid lesion. Although the 'tandem' lesion (combined stenosis of the carotid in the siphon and at the bifurcation) has perhaps been overstressed, coincidental stenosis intracranially may influence surgical risk and ideally should be detected preoperatively. Since the presence of bilateral carotid disease adversely affects surgical safety, both carotid systems need to be assessed and patients with bilateral disease need to be analysed separately. In a small number of individuals, TIAs persist after carotid occlusion or are due to intracranial stenosis of the internal carotid or the middle cerebral artery.

There is some evidence that the severity of carotid atheroma (degree of lumen narrowing) affects the prognosis of patients with early features of cerebrovascular disease so trials may need to be stratified according to the severity of the carotid abnormality.

Furthermore, the natural history of a stenotic lesion at the origin of the internal carotid artery or in the carotid siphon will depend greatly on the competence of the circle of Willis above it. For example, the natural history of short-lived stereotyped recurrent transient ischaemic attacks above a tightly stenotic carotid siphon with an incompetent circle of Willis may well be different from the natural history of a single prolonged transient spell (8–12 hours) that might have been embolic. Both spells would be classified as transient ischaemic attacks. Precise documentation of the pathophysiological nature of the transient ischaemic attack is difficult in the single patient, as well as in a group of patients that could be statistically relevant.

Thus in TIA patients admitted to trials there may be a need to provide considerable detail about the nature of any carotid lesion and of haemodynamically significant lesions of the symptomatic and other vessels.

PATIENTS ABOUT TO UNDERGO MAJOR HEART AND AORTO-ILIAC SURGERY

Such individuals are frequently subjected to periods of hypotension with or without cardiac arrhythmia, and face a risk of perioperative stroke. It has been assumed that such events are due to low perfusion pressure in the presence of an asymptomatic neck vessel stenosis. Patients with carotid bruits or with test evidence of carotid disease have therefore been assumed to be especially at risk, and physicians have sought preoperative assessments of the haemodynamic patency of both carotid vessels. In this situation only flow-affecting stenoses are deemed of importance. In practice, several studies now suggest that most strokes during cardiac bypass surgery are embolic in nature, and that patients with bruits or symptomatic stenoses are not at increased risk (Ropper *et al.*, 1983). The exception may be those whose neck vessel lesions have already been symptomatic with TIAs or prior strokes. Further studies in this field need to include assessments of the haemodynamic significance of any demonstrated bruit or stenosis, and if possible measures of collateral potential.

ASYMPTOMATIC BRUITS

Many individuals in the community have a neck bruit. Whereas many are venous or conducted from the thorax, some reflect asymptomatic stenosis of the carotid artery. These patients are important in the longitudinal study of the pathogenesis of evolution of arterial disease, and their sequential study is of great academic interest. Again such a longitudinal study needs to identify the location, nature and severity (residual lumen diameter) of the bruit-causing lesion.

Comment

To reduce the noise in clinical trials, the heterogeneity of the patient group can be reduced by assessment of the cerebral and the vascular lesion. This may be unnecessary when a community-based simple treatment policy is under trial, but, in the case of surgical trials especially, stratification according to the nature of the vascular lesion is desirable. It is also desirable in longitudinal studies of such situations as the asymptomatic bruit against which to audit the results of intervention. The goal is the identification of both the physiological (flow) and anatomical features of arterial lesions. The extent to which published trials have achieved necessary characterisation of their material and the success of non-invasive methods in supplementing or replacing angiography will now be considered.

Review

(1) Natural history of the asymptomatic bruit and atheromatous plaque of the carotid bifurcation: tables 6.1–4.
(2) Risks of stroke in patients with asymptomatic bruit undergoing surgery: tables 6.5–8.
(3) Natural history of carotid bifurcation atheromatous disease and stenosis: tables 6.9–12.
(4) Asymptomatic ulcerative disease without stenosis: tables 6.13 and 14.

Table 6.1   'Asymptomatic bruit and risk of stroke — the Framingham Study' (Wolf *et al.*, 1981).

1. Type of study	Single population, single centre
2. Patient group	Asymptomatic bruit
3. Number of patients identified	5184 subjects, 30–62 years of age
4. Number admitted to study	171: 105 women and 66 men
5. Method of assessment	Carotid auscultation
6. Follow-up period	1–8 years
7. End-points	TIA, stroke, myocardial infarction, death
8. Outcome	Incidence of carotid bruit increased with age (3.5% at 44–54 years to 7.0% at 65–79 years), and greater in diabetics and hypertensives (see conclusions). General mortality increased: 1.7-fold for men, 1.9-fold in women

9. *Authors' conclusions*: TIA and stroke incidence was greater in patients with bruits than those without, yet the nature of the stroke was not necessarily related to an atheromatous plaque at the carotid bifurcation that gave rise to the bruit. Embolic strokes, haemorrhage and lacunar infarction also occurred. Incidence of heart disease was greater in patients with cervical bruits

Comments. Wolf *et al.* have mentioned that the severity of the stenotic lesion, i.e. the tightness of the stenosis, was not assessed in these patients. This may be the single most important factor in identifying those with bruits who are at a greater risk of stroke. Wolf is now conducting a study of the asymptomatic bruit where the tightness of the stenosis is assessed by quantitative angiography and duplex Doppler examination.

Table 6.2 'Risks of stroke in asymptomatic persons with cervical arterial bruits. A population study in Evans County, Georgia' (Heyman *et al.*, 1980).

1. Type of study	Prospective study from Evans County begun 1960
2. Patient group	Asymptomatic cervical arterial bruits
3. Number of patients identified	1620 surviving without heart disease or stroke
4. Number admitted to study	72
5. Method of assessment	Cervical auscultation
6. Follow-up period	2 years
7. End-points	Stroke and TIA
8. Outcome	Prevalence of asymptomatic bruit increased with age, greater in women and in hypertensive subjects

9. *Authors' conclusions*: if asymptomatic bruit was present, the risk of heart disease and death was greater. Incidents of stroke and TIA were not necessarily related to the vessel that had the asymptomatic bruit. Also, since bruits were not assessed using quantitative angiography or duplex Doppler examination, some of the bruits heard might have been a radiated basal murmur or an external carotid bruit

Comments. Three patients studied had strokes in the ipsilateral territory of the carotid artery with the bruit. This signifies a 2% per year stroke rate from an asymptomatic bruit which includes radiated basal heart murmurs and external carotid origin bruits. Would the incidence of ipsilateral stroke be higher in patients with truly tight internal carotid stenosis of 1.5 mm or less residual lumen?

Table 6.3 'Asymptomatic carotid bruit. The long-term outcome of patients having endarterectomy compared with unoperated controls' (Thompson *et al.*, 1978).

1. Type of study	Single-centre retrospective study
2. Patient group	Asymptomatic bruits 'not operated on for one reason or another'. Compared with a group who had undergone carotid endarterectomy
3. Number of patients identified	1286 carotid endarterectomies on 1022 patients
4. Number admitted to study	138 patients in both groups
5. Method of assessment	Angiography
6. Follow-up period	180-month follow-up
7. End-points	Stroke, TIAs
8. Outcome	24/138 (17.4%) patients with asymptomatic bruits had subsequent strokes. 37 patients (26.8%) developed TIAs between 1 and 99 months after detection of bruit

9. *Authors' conclusions*: asymptomatic carotid bruits may be potential stroke hazards, the risk of which can be significantly reduced by appropriately applied endarterectomy

Comments. The study is not a controlled study comparing operated cases and non-operated cases with all patients eligible for surgery. The reasons why some received surgery and others did not is not clearly stated. The severity and location of the stenotic lesion causing the bruit are not clearly stated. The type of the subsequent stroke was not clearly defined.

Table 6.4 'Significance of asymptomatic carotid bruits' (Cooperman *et al.*, 1978).

1. Type of study	Single-centre retrospective study
2. Patient group	Asymptomatic bruit patient group compared with a group of patients with angiographically proven arteriosclerotic plaque at carotid bifurcation and no bruit
3. Number of patients identified	256 patients surgically operated on for arterial occlusive disease of legs
4. Number admitted to study	60 patients, asymptomatic bruits without symptomatic cerebrovascular disease
5. Method of assessment	Auscultation
6. Follow-up period	2–7 years
7. End-points	Stroke only
8. Outcome	Those with a bruit had: 15% stroke rate, 20% TIA, 35% died of other causes during follow-up. Without a bruit: 4% rate, 12% TIA, 16% died of other causes. Asymptomatic: 30% in bruit group, 66% without bruits group

9. *Authors' conclusions*: detection of an asymptomatic carotid bruit is not an innocent finding. It predicts a higher incidence of cerebrovascular complications than that expected on the basis of generalised arteriosclerosis alone

Comments: The authors do not clearly define the tightness of the stenosis that was causing the asymptomatic bruit nor the nature of the associated strokes.

Table 6.5 'Carotid bruit and the risk of stroke in elective surgery' (Ropper *et al.*, 1982).

1. Type of study	Single-centre prospective study
2. Patient group	All patients over 55 years undergoing elective surgery (Tuesday–Friday) at the Massachusetts General Hospital over 9 months
3. Number of patients identified	735 unselected cases preoperatively
4. Number admitted to study	617 postoperative examination (day 1–3); 48 had medical record review
5. Method of assessment	Auscultation of the neck. Bedside/ medical record review
6. Follow-up period	3 days
7. End-points	Stroke only
8. Outcome	104 of 735 patients had cervical bruits (44%). 7% perioperative stroke rate. 4 patients had strokes without bruits, and 1 patient a stroke with bruit

9. *Authors' comments*: no increase in the incidence of stroke with asymptomatic bruits in patients who had surgery

Comments. The authors did not assess the degree of narrowing of the stenotic lesion that produced the bruit or whether it was the result of external carotid stenosis or a radiated basal murmur. Also, many patients on the cardiac surgery service were found to have tightly stenotic lesions at the carotid bifurcation by quantitative phonoangiography and underwent endarterectomy prior to surgery. These patients were excluded from their study.

Table 6.6 'Asymptomatic carotid disease in the cardiovascular surgical patient. Is prophylactic endarterectomy necessary?' (Barnes and Marszalek, 1981).

1. Type of study	Single-centre prospective study
2. Patient group	Admitted for coronary or peripheral vascular (PVD) arterial construction
3. Number of patients identified	314 (273 men + 41 women)
4. Number admitted to study	All
5. Method of assessment	Auscultation/Doppler examination
6. Follow-up period	30 days
7. End-points	TIA, stroke, death
8. Outcome	54 arteries found with more than 50% stenosis (41 patients) = 13.1%; only one-third had cervical bruit. 48 arteries where bruit was heard, 18 (37.5%) associated with 'significant' obstruction by non-invasive screening, 1 perioperative TIA, 1 non-fatal stroke. Perioperative mortality higher in PVD + stenosis or bruit (15.0% and 18.2%) vs. 3.1% and 2.1% without stenosis/bruit

9. *Authors' conclusions*: asymptomatic carotid occlusive disease does not necessarily predispose to perioperative stroke and thus does not necessitate prophylactic carotid endarterectomy prior to coronary or peripheral vascular reconstruction

Comments. The degree of stenosis was not precisely defined. The haemodynamic significance of the lesion producing the bruit was based only on spectral broadening of the Doppler shift signal. Quantitative phonoangiography was needed.

Table 6.7 'Postoperative stroke in cardiac and peripheral vascular disease' (Turnipseed *et al.*, 1980).

1. Type of study	Single-centre prospective study
2. Patient group	Patients with peripheral vascular disease (PVD) or cardiovascular disease (CVD) admitted for elective surgery
3. Number of patients identified	330
4. Number admitted to study	160 patients with PVD and 170 patients with CVD
5. Method of assessment	Cervical auscultation/Doppler imaging combined with spectral analysis
6. Follow-up period	Two-and-a-half years
7. End-points	TIA, stroke
8. Outcome	98 had cervical bruits, 45 of these 'significant stenosis', 17 had 'severe' carotid occlusive disease on ultrasound and no cervical bruit. 16 patients had postoperative 'carotid ischaemia' — 13 strokes and 3 TIAs. 10/16 had no cervical bruits and only 5 had evidence of carotid stenosis

9. *Authors' conclusions*: no direct relationship found between bruit, severity of disease and stroke

Comments. Their conclusions, however, cannot be justified for two reasons. First, the method of non-invasive testing of the severity of carotid stenosis was not described. Doppler imaging and spectral analysis of the Doppler shift signal have not been quantified to the point that the residual lumen diameter of a stenotic lesion at the bifurcation of the common carotid artery can be estimated. At best, these procedures can localise the atheromatous lesion to the common internal or external carotid artery origin and determine the amount of turbulent flow the lesions produce. Secondly, the clinical nature of the deficits were not described except to say focal or diffuse neurological deficits. Therefore, correlations cannot be made between the side of the stenosis and the neurological deficit. In addition, the question of watershed stroke cannot be assessed.

Table 6.8 'Carotid artery stenosis — haemodynamic significance and clinical course' (Busuttil *et al.*, 1981).

1. Type of study	Single-centre prospective study
2. Patient group	TIA, stroke or asymptomatic bruit who had had positive oculoplethysmography
3. Number of patients identified	215 including subgroup of 125 with significant stenosis
4. Number admitted to study	45 patients with asymptomatic bruits (15 had surgery, 30 no surgery)
5. Method of assessment	Auscultation of bruit and OPG
6. Follow-up period	Two-and-a-half years
7. End-points	TIA, stroke or death
8. Outcome	Patients with significant stenosis, 51 (40.8%) endarterectomy and 74 (59.2%) 'no surgery'. Incidence of stroke in non-operated group 12/74 (16.2%) compared with 1/51 (1.9% in operated group. Recurrent TIA = 9/51 (17.6%) compared with 29/74 (39.2%) in 'non-surgery' group. In non-haemodynamically significant carotid stenosis, rise of stroke, death very low. Asymptomatic bruit group: results not statistically significant

9. *Authors' conclusions*: patients with haemodynamically significant stenosis treated non-operatively have a greater risk of death, stroke, TIA, than patients treated with carotid endarterectomy

Comments. The 30 patients followed without operation who had positive OPGs were somehow different from the 15 who had surgery and positive OPGs. We suspect the lesion was much tighter in those who had surgery. In order to have a positive OPG the residual lumen diameter of the carotid stenosis has to be below 2 mm. If the lesion was as tight as 1 mm, then most likely those patients had surgery. The study however suggests that those patients with bruits and a stenotic lesion at the origin of the internal carotid that is tight enough to cause a reduction in the ocular systolic pressure (i.e. <2 mm) are at a greater risk of subsequent stroke. This kind of non invasive quantitative assessment of the carotid bifurcation should be included in any trial of therapy for patients with asymptomatic bruit. The best non-invasive tests are quantitative phonoangiography, duplex Doppler scanning and oculoplethysmography.

Table 6.9 'Unoperated asymptomatic significant internal carotid stenosis: a review of 182 instances' (Humphries *et al.*, 1976).

1. Type of study	Single-centre retrospective study
2. Patient group	Patients with angiographic evidence indicating more than 50% stenosis in one carotid artery and asymptomatic with respect to that artery
3. Number of patients identified	168 patients
4. Number admitted to study	All assessed (clinical record)
5. Method of assessment	Angiography
6. Follow-up period	1–12 years, average 32 months
7. End-points	TIA, stroke, surgery
8. Outcome	182 internal carotid arteries with arteriosclerotic lesion (168 patients). 66% of patients: stenosis 50–70%, 19% had 90% stenosis and 15% greater than 90%. 31% had ulcers also. 26 patients developed TIAs and had endarterectomies, and 'did well'. Of 3 patients with TIAs refusing surgery, all had strokes. 1 patient had a stroke without a TIA warning

9. *Authors' conclusions*: most patients with atheromatous disease in the carotid bifurcation will present with TIAs prior to surgery

Comments. The paper suffers from the small number of patients and also lack of description of the stroke and whether or not it occurred above a very tight stenosis as opposed to the only moderate stenosis: 50–70%. Many investigators agree with the authors' conclusions. Most of the patients in this review had been operated on for the other (symptomatic) carotid artery.

Table 6.10　'Stenosis of the contralateral asymptomatic carotid artery – to operate or not. An update' (Levin *et al.*, 1980).

1. Type of study	Single-centre retrospective study
2. Patient group	Patients who had undergone unilateral endarterectomy and were noted to have asymptomatic atheromatous disease on the other side
3. Number of patients studied	535 operations in 509 patients
4. Number admitted to study	147
5. Method of assessment	Angiography
6. Follow-up period	Up to 20 years
7. End-points	Stroke
8. Outcome	12/137 had stenosis less than 50%, 125 patients 50–90%, and 7 patients more than 90%. 16 patients had TIAs and went on to surgery. 60 patients died, all of non-cardiac disease. None of the 137 patients had stroke during the follow-up period (up to 20 years)

9. *Authors' conclusions*: surgical policy to operate on symptomatic patients only

Comments. Only seven had stenosis of 90%. This is not enough for a survey. 90% stenosis corresponds to residual lumen of 1 mm, but the preciseness of the measurement of percentage of stenosis is not adequate because the denominator is often hard to judge.

Table 6.11 'Asymptomatic contralateral carotid artery stenosis: a five-year follow-up study following carotid endarterectomy' (Podore *et al.*, 1980).

1. Type of study	Single-centre retrospective study
2. Patient group	Patients with greater than 50% stenosis compared with patients with no significant stenosis on the side opposite the symptomatic carotid artery that underwent surgery
3. Number of patients assessed	202
4. Number admitted to study	67 patients with 50% stenosis or over; 50 patients with no stenosis on asymptomatic side
5. Method of assessment	Angiography
6. Follow-up period	5 years
7. End-points	TIA and stroke
8. Outcome	14/67 (21%) became symptomatic, and 11 had stroke without warning. 2/50 control cases symptomatic

9. *Authors' conclusions*: for patients with contralateral carotid artery stenosis the following guideline was suggested: 'undergo staged carotid endarterectomies if the surgeon's stroke and morbidity rate is less than 3%'

Comments. The numbers are too small and the study is retrospective.

Table 6.12 'The natural history of asymptomatic carotid birfurcation plaques', (Durward *et al.*, 1982).

1. Type of study	Single-centre prospective study (see comment)
2. Patient group	Patients with atheromatous lesions of the carotid bifurcation (greater than 50% stenosis, and ulcers)
3. Number of patients studied	324
4. Number admitted to study	73
5. Method of assessment	Angiography
6. Follow-up period	4 years (medical record and telephone review)
7. End-points	TIA, stroke
8. Outcome	50 patients with greater than 50% stenosis: 5 TIA of ipsilateral hemisphere, 1 monocular blindness, 2 developed stroke; 17 patients with stenosis and ulcer: 3 TIAs and no strokes; 6 patients with ulcer only: 1 TIA

9. *Authors' conclusions*: in this series, incidence of stroke in territory of a significant asymptomatic carotid plaque was low (3%). It seems a reasonable approach to consider endarterectomy only if appropriate ischaemic symptoms develop

Comments. Although said to be a prospective study, actually a retrospective review from medical case records. The study suffers from the small number of patients and proper identification of the term TIA. Is TIA a stereotyped short-lived spell lasting 10–15 min or a longer spell of 8–12 up to 24 h, which may not be stereotyped and may be embolic in nature? What is the nature of the short-lived stereotyped TIAs? This point becomes particularly important when assessing patients with asymptomatic ulcers of the carotid artery without stenosis.

Table 6.13 'Natural history of non-stenotic asymptomatic ulcerative lesion at the carotid artery' (Moore *et al.*, 1978).

1. Type of study	Single-centre retrospective study
2. Patient group	Patients with atheromatous ulcers without stenosis
3. Number of patients studied	67 patients with asymptomatic ulcerative lesions
4. Number admitted to study	67 patients and 26 'controls' (who had surgery)
5. Method of assessment	Angiography: A = minimal ulcer; B = large; C = multiloculated large ulcer
6. Follow-up period	72–96 months post-angiography
7. End-points	Stroke
8. Outcome	Group A: 38 patients, group B and C: 29 patients. Annual stroke rate group A = 0.4%; group B and C = 12.5%; 'control group' = 1.47%

9. *Authors' conclusions*: no significant differences in mortality but a highly significant difference in stroke incidence. Annual stroke rate was high in group B and C ulcer patients

Comments. The type and location of strokes were not identified. Furthermore, the nature of the TIAs is not given; were they transient symptoms above the ipsilateral carotid? How many spells occurred? Were they multiple short-lived stereotyped or single prolonged spells? The numbers are small. It is our experience that ulcers alone rarely lead to stroke, i.e. embolic stroke to the middle or anterior cerebral artery or one of their major branches.

Table 6.14 'Prognosis of asymptomatic ulcerating carotid lesions' (Kroener *et al.*, 1980).

1. Type of study	Single-centre retrospective study
2. Patient group	Patients with asymptomatic ulcerative plaques
3. Number of patients studied	79 patients
4. Number admitted to study	76 patients (87 asymptomatic ulcerative plaque)
5. Method of assessment	Angiography (medical record and telephone review)
6. Follow-up period	3–7 years
7. End-points	Stroke, TIA, death
8. Outcome	63 patients 'shallow ulcer group'. 1 patient with stroke, 24 patients in the more severe ulcer groups; none had stroke. 3 TIAs in the shallow ulcer group

9. *Authors' conclusions*: cumulative stroke rate 1% at 7 years. Cumulative mortality was 17% at 3 years and 52% at 7 years. Prophylactive carotid endarterectomy is not justified for asymptomatic carotid bifurcation ulcerations

Comments. The study points out the very low incidence of stroke in patients with a non-stenotic ulceration lesion at the carotid bifurcation.

DISCUSSION

Studies of the natural history of the asymptomatic bruits and the atheromatous plaque at the carotid bifurcation

In all of the studies of the natural history of the asymptomatic bruit, as well as those of the nature of the atheromatous lesion of the bifurcation of the common carotid artery, the pathophysiological nature of the stroke or TIA is not clearly identified. Furthermore, the small number of cases followed, the retrospective nature of most studies, and the lack of precise clinical details of strokes or TIAs limit the conclusions that can be drawn. In all of the studies dealing with asymptomatic bruit the tightness of the stenotic lesion causing the bruit and its location are not identified clearly. In only one study was there an attempt to assess the haemodynamic significance of the bruit, and it was by OPG alone (Busuttil *et al.*, 1981). The evidence suggested from that study is that the tighter the stenosis the more likely the patient with the asymptomatic bruit is to have trouble. In any study of the natural history or therapy of the asymptomatic bruits, patients should have non-invasive assessment of the degree, location and haemodynamic significance of stenosis of the lesion producing the bruit. This is best accomplished by quantitative phonoangiography combined with duplex Doppler examination to identify the source of the bruit and OPG to identify whether it reduces pressure in the distal internal carotid artery. We would suspect that those patients with very tight stenosis, i.e. residual lumen of 1 mm, would be at higher risk for stroke or TIA. Those patients should therefore be the ones to include in a study of the efficacy of medical or surgical therapy.

Evaluation of extracranial carotid arterial disease

Clinical laboratory evaluation of the bifurcation of the common carotid artery may be separated into two parts, the non-invasive vascular examination and the invasive examination (angiography including digital subtraction angiography). In order to understand these and to put them in the proper context, it becomes important to bring to the reader's attention certain facts about the pathophysiology and physical examination of atherosclerotic disease at this location.

Atheroma tends to form in the posterior portion of the origin of the internal carotid artery and distal common carotid artery (Ackerman, 1979). Therefore, the external carotid artery is less often involved and less often gives rise to a bruit. For a stenotic lesion to produce a reduction in flow and a bruit, there has to be a greater than 70% reduction in area, which means a 50% reduction in luminal diameter (De Weese *et al.*, 1970; Burton, 1974; Busuttil *et al.*, 1981). Because it is often difficult to estimate the percentage of luminal diameter reduction, it is useful to think in terms of millimetres of residual lumen diameter. Bruits generally occur when the residual lumen diameter of the carotid bifurcation is 3 mm or less (Fisher, 1951; Duncan *et al.*, 1975; Flanigan *et al.*, 1977). Such bruits are produced by the disturbances in blood flow immediately distal to the stenosis when the jet of blood expands into the post-stenotic vessel. The character of the disturbance or turbulence is determined by the rate of flow proximal to the stenosis and by the residual lumen diameter (Harrison, 1982). This is clinically evident when the pitch of the bruit increases with the tightening of the stenosis. High-pitched bruits with diastolic components are suggestive of a tightly stenotic lesion with less than 1.5 mm residual lumen diameter. Flow distal to the stenotic site is likely to be reduced when the residual lumen diameter is less than 2 mm, and more often when the residual diameter is less than 1.5 mm. When the residual lumen diameter is 1 mm or less, flow is reduced to the point that the bruit intensity falls and the bruit may disappear (Fisher 1951; Flanagan *et al.*, 1977). When flow and pressure are reduced through the carotid bifurcation, collateral flow across the anterior circle of Willis tends to keep the pressure in the ipsilateral middle cerebral artery normal. This further decreases flow in the internal carotid artery and the stenotic lesion becomes in jeopardy of occluding, often asymptomatically. However, with tight stenosis and reduced flow, thrombus formation may occur and give rise to embolic stroke. With occlusion, clot may also propagate the entire length of the internal carotid artery and become lodged in, or embolised to, the middle or anterior cerebral artery. Other aspects of the physical examination include dynamic palpation of the facial pulses, in particular the obliteration of the supraorbital and supratrochlear pulses with intermittent impression of the prearicular artery. This may suggest internal carotid stenosis but is often difficult to do with certainty. The internal carotid artery may be occluded, yet it may still have a palpable pulsation in the high cervical area. A prominent lateral brow pulse may give a more reliable clue to occlusion of the internal carotid artery.

Non-invasive evaluation

Many non-invasive methods have been developed to assess directly or indirectly the degree and location of a stenotic lesion at the carotid bifurcation that produces a bruit (Lees *et al.*, 1970, 1982; Kistler *et al.*, 1981). Because some methods provide more reliable information than others, there has emerged an optimal set of tests (Orgogozo *et al.*, 1978; Wise *et al.*, 1979). Some tests, such as directional supraorbital Doppler examination, ophthalmodynamometry and oculoplethysmography, indirectly assess pressure in the internal carotid artery. These tests are of greatest value when the residual lumen diameter is greater than 2 mm and pressure in the internal carotid artery is not reduced, or when the residual lumen diameter is less than 1 mm and pressure is greatly reduced. Directional supraorbital Doppler examination, an outgrowth of dynamic palpation of the facial pulses, is a reliable indicator of tightly stenotic (1 mm) disease at the origin of the internal carotid artery, but only in experienced hands (Wise *et al.*, 1979). The test is difficult to do reliably. Ophthalmodynamometry, once a preferred bedside diagnostic test, has given way to oculoplethysmography, which measures the intraocular systolic pressure. In most laboratories this is the most reliable 'indirect' non-invasive test.

Non-invasive tests that '*directly*' study the bifurcation of the common carotid artery can be divided into those that utilise ultrasound technology and those that analyse audible sound, i.e. a bruit. Ultrasound technology includes real-time B-mode ultrasound imaging and analysis of the Doppler shift of the returning echo of flowing blood using a range gated pulsed Doppler. Two-dimensional B-mode pulsed ultrasound vascular imaging systems are able to develop an image of the bifurcation of the common carotid artery, but its reliable resolution is limited.

Calcification in atherothrombotic plaque may prevent penetration of the ultrasound beam and soft thrombus may appear similar in density to flowing blood, suggesting patency of an occluded vessel (Kistler *et al.*, 1981). Blood flowing through an atherosclerotic stenotic lesion changes from laminar flow with uniform velocity to streamlined flow at high velocity to turbulent flow with a broad range of velocities. This can be detected with either the CW or range gated pulsed Doppler as broadening of the Doppler-shift frequency range of the returning echoes of flowing blood. Thus, the more spectral broadening of the Doppler shift signal indicates more turbulent flow. This, however, does not give a reliable estimate of the residual lumen diameter of the stenotic lesion.

Duplex ultrasound scanning combines both B-mode imaging of the common carotid artery with range gated pulsed Doppler analysis of the flowing blood at any point in the image. This combination appears to be the current 'state of the art' in ultrasound non-invasive technology.

Quantitative spectral phonoangiography (Lees and Dewey, 1970; Duncan *et al.*, 1975; Kistler *et al.*, 1978, 1981) analyses the frequency intensity components of the audible sound spectrum of the bruit produced by turbulent blood flow. By Fourier analysis of the digitised sound signal, a frequency-intensity power spectrum can be obtained. With turbulent flow that produces a bruit, there is a characteristic frequency beyond which the intensity falls off. This break frequency bears a relationship to the residual lumen diameter of the lesion that produced the bruit and the velocity of flowing blood proximal to the lesion. By assuming a velocity of 500 mg per second, a calculated estimate of the residual lumen diameter of the stenotic vessel can be made. In addition, this test accurately differentiates a bruit rising from the carotid bifurcation from one originating lower in the arterial tree (e.g. from the base of the heart) (Kistler *et al.*, 1978). It tends to be most accurate, approaching the accuracy of angiography, when the bruit arises from a stenotic lesion with a residual lumen diameter between 0.0 and 2.5 mm (Flanigan *et al.*, 1977). This method does not differentiate external from internal carotid bruits. However, compression of the ipsilateral facial and prearicular pulse may cause marked diminution in amplitude of the bruit if it arises from the external carotid artery (Lees and Myers, 1982). In addition, in combination with duplex Doppler examination, the location of the lesion causing the bruit can be more accurately assessed.

For optimum accuracy, many laboratories are putting their emphasis on oculoplethysmography combined with duplex Doppler examination. When a bruit is present, quantitative phonoangiography appears to be the method of choice in analysing its significance. Thus, these three methodologies are emerging as the non-invasive tests of choice. It must be pointed out, however, that severe stenosis with a thread-like lumen may appear as an occluded carotid on non-invasive tests. In this setting there is no substitute for cerebral angiography.

Invasive evaluation

When a TIA or minor stroke suggests that there may be an arterial lesion in the territory of the internal carotid artery, selective cerebral angiography remains the single most important method of assessing the bifurcation of the common carotid artery. It can accurately assess the severity of stenosis and it can demonstrate large ulceration in the plaque and large thrombus formation in the lumen. Most importantly, it can demonstrate lesions in the carotid siphon and stem of the middle cerebral artery that can cause symptoms similar to those caused by a lesion at the origin of the internal carotid artery. In addition, atheromatous disease of the vertebrobasilar circulation can be accurately assessed. Patterns of collateral flow around the circle of Willis and over the hemisphere can be properly assessed by this methodology and are most important in deciding the aetiology of symptoms, as well as therapeutic approaches. Emboli in the branches of the middle cerebral artery may be demonstrated. Because they often fragment and lyse, angiography done 48 hours after an event may not result in a positive diagnosis.

Because of the inherent risk of stroke with cerebral angiography, intravenous digital subtraction angiography has been developed. This methodology can demonstrate occlusion of the internal carotid artery, but will not reliably show severe ulceration. It, like many non-invasive tests, may also suggest occlusion of the internal carotid artery when there is a thread-like lumen. Thus far in the development of this technology subtle important pathological changes in the intracranial arteries cannot reliably be demonstrated.

Digital subtraction angiography is an invasive test and has been known to cause exacerbations in angina and renal insufficiency. Hypotension after a dye load, leading to worsening of an ischaemic deficit, has also been observed in our institution. The procedure requires the patient to hold his breath and not swallow, both of which may be difficult in the elderly. Lastly, the image quality improves with improved cardiac output. Many elderly patients with cardiovascular disease and cerebrovascular disease have poor cardiac outputs.

It is likely that improvement in this technology will circumvent many of these problems. It is also likely that arterialised digital angiography will come into vogue. Here, intracranial arteries may be visualised with a small injection in the aortic arch, which is hopefully safer than selective catheterisation.

In the future, it is likely that nuclear magnetic resonance scanning (NMR) technology and proton NMR imaging will be developed to the point that non-invasive imaging of the common carotid bifurcation will be extremely accurately delineated in three dimensions. In addition, blood flow through the carotid bifurcation will be measured.

CONCLUSION

In the future, any study designed to test the therapeutic efficacy of a drug in prevention of TIAs and stroke will, at the very least, have to be designed as carefully as the Canadian and French aspirin studies (see chapter 7 by Bousser). Careful attention should be paid not only to the quality of symptoms of transient cerebral ischaemia, but also to their frequency and duration in order to assign the symptoms to ischaemia of a particular arterial territory, i.e. carotid, vertebrobasilar, or small vessel. Non-invasive carotid testing including duplex Doppler scanning to assess flow at the bifurcation of the common carotid artery, and OPG to assess pressure in the internal carotid artery should be used to identify those patients with TIA associated with arteriosclerotic stenosis at the origin of the internal carotid artery. If a cervical bruit is present, quantitative phonoangiography will help differentiate a radiated basal murmur and will quantitate the tightness of stenosis at the origin of the internal carotid artery.

Angiography, however, is the only means of identifying siphon stenosis, middle cerebral stem stenosis, or incompetent basilar circulation. This study carries a morbidity which varies from centre to centre. In many centres it is not standard practice to have this study performed in all TIA patients. In most, however, particularly those that are specialising in stroke therapy, angiography is readily available and is the standard practice in patients with bona fide TIAs, particularly in the carotid circulation.

Ideally then, angiography should be performed if serious consideration is to be given to 'surgical versus medical' therapy at the carotid bifurcation and if serious consideration is to be given to middle cerebral stem or carotid siphon stenosis as an aetiology of the transient ischaemia of minor stroke.

CT scanning should also be performed if a TIA or minor stroke has occurred and the patient is to be included in a study. Then, if subsequent stroke occurs, CT scanning should definitely be performed to localise precisely the area of infarction and relate it to the arterial lesion.

Therefore, by clinical history and physical examination and non-invasive testing, as well as by angiography (when available) and CT scanning, patients can be divided into the following groups:

(1) those with suspected carotid bifurcation disease,
(2) those with carotid siphon disease,
(3) those with middle cerebral stem disease,
(4) those with small-vessel disease, or
(5) those with vertebrobasilar disease,

as the cause of their TIA or small stroke.

REFERENCES

Ackerman, R. H. (1979). A perspective on non invasive diagnosis of carotid disease. *Neurology*, **29**, 615–22.

Barnes, R. W. and Marszalek, P. B. (1981). Asymptomatic carotid disease in the cardiovascular surgical patient. Is prophylactic endarterectomy necessary? *Stroke*, **12**, 497–500.

Burton, R. C. (1974). Atheromatous disease of the carotid artery: correlation of angiographic, clinical and surgical findings. *J. Neurosurg.*, **41**, 321–31.

Busuttil, R. W., Baker, J. D., Jameson, R. K. and Muchleder, H. I. (1981). Carotid artery stenosis — haemodynamic significance and clinical course. *J. Am. Med. Assoc.*, **245**, 1438–41.

Cooperman, M., Martin, E. W. and Evans, W. E. (1978). Significance of asymptomatic carotid bruits. *Arch. Surg.*, **113**, 1339–40.

De Weese, J. A., May, A. S., Lipchick, E. O. and Robb, C. S. (1970). Anatomic and haemodynamic correlations in carotid artery stenosis. *Stroke*, **1**, 149–57.

Duncan, G. W., Gruder, J. U., Dewey, C. R. Jr, Myers, G. S. and Lees, R. S. (1975). Evolution of carotid stenosis by phonoangiography. *New Engl. J. Med.*, **293**, 1124–8.

Durward, Q. J., Ferguson, G. G. and Barr, H. W. K. (1982). The natural history of asymptomatic carotid bifurcation plaques. *Stroke*, **13**, 459–64.

Fisher, C. M. (1951). Occlusion of the internal carotid artery. *Arch. Neurol. Psychiatr.*, **69**, 346–77.

Flanigan, D. P., Tullis, J. P., Streeter, V. L., Whitehouse, W. M., Fry, W. J. and Stanley, J. C. (1977). Multiple subcritical arterial stenosis effect on poststenotic pressure and flow. *Ann. Surg.*, **186**, 663–8.

Harrison, M. J. G. (1982). Carotid endarterectomy. In Rice Edwards, J. M. (ed.) *Topical Reviews in Neurology I*, P. S. G. Wright, Bristol, pp. 57–80.

Heyman, A., Wilkinson, W. E., Heyden, S., Helms, M. J., Bartel, A. G., Karp, H. R., Tyroler, H. A. and Hames, C. G. (1980). Risk of stroke in asymptomatic persons with cervical arterial bruits. A population study in Evans County, Georgia. *New Engl. J. Med.*, **302**, 838–41.

Humphries, A. W., Young, J. R., Santilli, P. H., Beven, S. E. G. and deWolfe, D. G. (1976). Unoperated asymptomatic significant internal carotid stenosis: a review of 182 instances. *Surgery*, **80**, 695–8.

Kistler, J. P., Lees, R. S., Friedman, J., Pessin, M., Mohr, J. P., Robertson, G. S. and Ojemann, R. G. (1978). The bruit of carotid stenosis versus radiated basal heart murmurs. Differentiation by phonoangiography. *Circulation*, **57**, 975–81.

Kistler, J. P., Lees, R. S., Miller, A., Crowell, R. M. and Robertson, G. (1981). Correlation of spectral phonoangiography and carotid angiography with gross pathology in carotid stenosis. *New Engl. J. Med.*, **305**, 417–19.

Kroener, J. M., Dorn, P. L., Shoor, P. M., Wickbom, I. G. and Bernstein, E. F. (1980). Diagnosis of asymptomatic ulcerating carotid lesions. *Arch. Surg.*, **115**, 1387–92.

Lees, R. S. and Dewey, C. F. Jr. (1970). Phonoangiography: a new non invasive diagnostic method of studying arterial disease. *Proc. Natl. Acad. Sci. USA*, **67**, 935.

Lees, R. S. and Myers, G. S. (1982). Non invasive evolution of arterial disease. *Adv. Intern. Med.*, **27**, 475–509.

Lees, R., Kistler, J. P. and Sanders, D. (1982). Duplex doppler scanning and spectral bruit analysis offer accurate diagnosis of carotid stenosis. *Circulation*, **66**, I-102–5.

Levin, S. M., Sondaheimer, F. K. and Levin, J. M. (1980). Stenosis of contralateral asymptomatic carotid artery — to operate or not. An update. *Am. J. Surg.*, **140**, 203–5.

Moore, W. S., Boren, C., Malone, J. M., Roon, A. J., Eisenberg, R., Goldstone, J. and Mani, R. (1970). Natural history of non-stenotic asymptomatic ulcerative lesion at the carotid artery. *Arch. Surg.*, **113**, 1352–9.

Moore, W. S., Malone, J. M., Boren, C., Roon, A. J. and Goldstone, J. (1979). Asymptomatic ulcerative lesions of the carotid artery. *Stroke*, **10**, 96.

Orgogozo, J. M., Enjalbert, O., Beloussoff, T. and Loiseau, P. (1978). L'examen doppler en pathologie carotidienne: semeiologie, resultats et revue de la litterature. *Rev. Med.*, **19**, 1021–34.

Podore, P. C., De Weese, J. A., May, A. G. and Robb, C. G. (1980). Asymptomatic contralateral carotid artery stenosis: a five-year follow-up study following carotid endarterectomy. *Surgery*, **88**, 748–52.

Ropper, A. H., Wechsler, L. R. and Wilson, L. S. (1982). Carotid bruit and the risk of stroke in elective surgery. *New Engl. J. Med.*, **307**, 1388–91.

Thompson, J., Patman, R. D. and Talkington, C. D. (1978). Asymptomatic carotid bruit. The long-term outcome of patients having endarterectomy compared with unoperated controls. *Ann. Surg.*, **188**, 308–16.

Turnipseed, W. D., Berkoff, H. A. and Belzerm, F. O. (1980). Postoperative stroke in cardiac and peripheral vascular disease. *Ann. Surg.*, **192**, 365–8.

Wise, G., Parker, J. and Burkholder, J. (1979). Supraorbital doppler studies of carotid bruits and arteriography in unilateral ocular or cerebral ischaemic disorders. *Neurology*, **29**, 34–7.

Wolf, P. A., Kindall, P. S. and McNamara, T. (1981). Asymptomatic bruit and risk of stroke — the Framingham Study. *J. Am. Med. Assoc.*, **245**, 1442–5.

7

Trials of secondary prevention after transient ischaemic attacks.
Part I: Analysis of previous clinical trials

M. G. BOUSSER

INTRODUCTION

In order to define precisely the basis of this review, I should like to emphasise that this critique of previous clinical trials will deal with:

(1) *Secondary prevention,* thus eliminating studies of primary prevention such as Blakely and Bent's trial of sulfinpyrazone (1975) or Heikinheimo and Jarvinen's trial of aspirin (1971). Despite its importance, the control of risk factors will not be discussed here because it concerns mainly primary prevention, although there is some evidence that careful correction or control of risk factors — particularly arterial hypertension — is helpful in secondary prevention (Leonberg and Elliott, 1981).
(2) *Secondary prevention of stroke* (including death and myocardial infarction), thus discarding studies limited to the recurrence of TIA (Evans, 1973; Herskovits *et al.*, 1981).
(3) *Secondary prevention of ischaemic strokes due to 'atherosclerosis',* thus excluding other causes of ischaemia (which admittedly is not always easy) such as embolic infarction from cardiac source, cerebral arteritis, blood disorders, etc. The issue of the use of anticoagulants in cerebral embolism of cardiac origin will not be discussed here. In summary, it could be said that (see Easton and Sherman, 1980), in patients without rheumatic heart disease or myocardial infarction, anticoagulants decrease the incidence of cerebral emboli, but that, in patients with 'idiopathic' atrial fibrillation, the effect of anticoagulation is still unknown since there is not a single randomised study devoted to this condition.

(4) *Secondary prevention after TIA and stroke*. Some studies deal only with
TIA *stricto sensu*, but the majority include TIA, reversible ischaemic
neurological deficits (RIND), minor strokes and even non-disabling
major strokes. The rationale for this is that:
  (a) there is no fundamental difference in the pathogenesis of strokes
  and long-lasting TIA; and
  (b) patients who have made a good recovery after a stroke are no less in
  need of secondary prevention than those with TIA. It should be said
  that there is still no general agreement on the definition of all these
  categories of ischaemic event, even for TIA, usually lasting less than
  24 hours but in some studies less than 1 hour (Acheson *et al.*, 1969,
  1972).
(5) *Prospective randomised clinical trials*, thus excluding individual cases,
retrospective studies, and non-randomised studies. This is particularly
important for carotid surgery for which there are numerous non-
randomised series, most of which have suggested (on the basis of
unacceptable evidence) that surgery was an effective therapeutic procedure. This also applies to about half of the anticoagulant trials which
were not randomised (see the review by Genton *et al.*, 1977), and which
indicated a reduced incidence of stroke in patients treated by anticoagulants.
(6) *Prospective randomised trials of carotid endarterectomy, anticoagulants
and antiplatelet drugs*. Other treatments such as vasodilators and venesection will not be discussed here.

One should bear in mind that some of these studies — particularly those
with anticoagulants — were carried out 20 years ago, before the CT-scan
era, and will be judged here against standards and methodologies which
have improved in recent years. My purpose is not to denigrate work done in
the past, but to provide information on previous studies which might be of
value for future clinical trials.

CAROTID ENDARTERECTOMY

Surgery of vertebral or subclavian arteries will not be discussed here since
there is not a single randomised clinical trial devoted to this surgery.
    Carotid endarterectomy is now routinely performed and many series with
a combined total of several thousands of patients have been reported in the
literature. Very regrettably, only one was a randomised clinical trial (Fields
et al., 1970) (figure 7.1).
    In this trial, 24 medical centres recruited 316 patients with carotid stenosis
who had experienced TIA or minor stroke: 169 patients were randomly
allocated to carotid endarterectomy and 147 to 'the best available medical

treatment'. The mean follow-up period was 42 months. This trial *did not show an overall benefit for surgery* since there were 20 strokes in the surgical group (12%) and 19 in the medical (13%). However, if the strokes as an immediate result of surgery are removed from the analysis, the rates of stroke and/or death are significantly less ($p<0.05$) in the surgical group (4%) than in the medical group (12%), suggesting that if patients survive surgery without stroke, then the risk of subsequent strokes is reduced. Most surgeons argue that surgical morbidity and mortality are now far less than they were in the American trial where mortality ranged from 2 to 36% depending on the centre (which is probably true in highly specialised centres but certainly not in routine surgical practice). It has been calculated that if surgery is to reduce the overall risk of stroke, the stroke and/or death rate due to the operation itself must be something less than 3–4%. Among other points, this study showed a reduction of continuing carotid TIA in the surgery group (although not statistically significant), and subgroup analysis suggested that patients with isolated unilateral carotid stenosis fared best whatever the treatment, but the numbers were very small (figure 7.1).

Some criticisms have been made of this study, as follows:

● not every patient had experienced carotid distribution events before randomisation;
● no attempt was made to consider separately strokes arising in the cerebral hemisphere ipsilateral to the operated arteries;
● the study compared surgery with the 'best available medical treatment' versus 'the best available medical treatment plus surgery';
● finally, the sample size was rather small (although it is larger than in most studies performed with anticoagulants and antiplatelet drugs!).

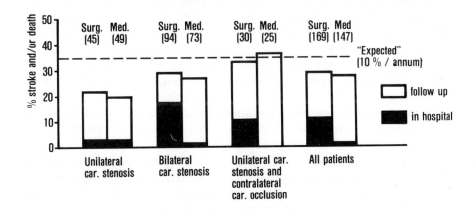

Figure 7.1 American joint study (Fields *et al.*, 1970).

For all these reasons, it has been felt that there is a very real need for a further randomised trial of sufficient size to determine whether carotid endarterectomy, using modern surgical and anaesthetic techniques, confers any long-term benefit, and if so of what degree, in patients with carotid symptomatic stenosis who have experienced a minor carotid event. Such a study is now in progress in the UK, France and Holland.

ANTICOAGULANTS

Trials of anticoagulants in patients with progressing strokes, and studies to assess the influence of anticoagulants on immediate mortality in patients with completed strokes will not be discussed here.

There are 11 randomised controlled clinical trials evaluating anticoagulants in the secondary prevention of 'atherothrombotic' cerebral ischaemic events: four in patients with TIA, six in patients with completed stroke and one in patients with either TIA or completed stroke. These studies are summarised in table 7.1. It can be seen that there is no statistical difference in stroke or death between those treated and the controls, and that there is a trend for increased bleeding in those treated with anticoagulants.

There is no need to go into the details of these studies because they are all unsatisfactory from the methodological point of view. In all of them the sample size was far too small to have a reasonable chance of detecting anything except an enormous difference between the two groups, and there was not even a trend in favour of anticoagulants. There were numerous other difficulties:

● most studies were not double blind;
● follow-up was usually too short and sometimes different in the two groups, with more frequent visits in the treated than in the controls;
● it is not always clear whether strokes occurring after treatment was withdrawn were analysed;
● the adequacy of anticoagulant treatment was not always indicated;
● in some studies, strokes due to cerebral haemorrhage were left out of the analysis;
● elderly patients and patients with hypertension were excluded in some studies, but included in others with an unusually high mortality.

These controlled trials are so imperfect that it is absolutely impossible to draw any conclusion on the efficacy or inefficacy of anticoagulants, although, reviewing the same data, some experts (Sandok *et al.*, 1978) have concluded that anticoagulants are beneficial. We think that, at the moment, it is not possible to make a rational decision to use or not to use anticoagulants after a TIA or stroke (due to atherosclerosis). The only

Table 7.1 Anticoagulants in the secondary prevention of atherothrombotic brain infarction: randomised clinical trials.

Study	Entry episode	Double blind	Number of subjects — Treated	Number of subjects — Control	Average follow-up (months)	Results* Lethal strokes T	Lethal strokes C	Ischaemic strokes T	Ischaemic strokes C	All deaths T	All deaths C	Bleeding T	Bleeding C
Baker (1961)	TIA	No	22	15	11	0	0	1	0	1	0	31	5
Baker et al. (1962)	TIA	No	24	20	20	0	1	1	4	5	2	11	1
Pearce et al. (1965)	TIA	+	17	20	11	0	1	5	2	0	3	0	0
Baker et al. (1966)	TIA	No	30	30	40	0	1	6	4	9	5	3	2
Baker (1961)	CS	No	56	62	11	6	2	12	4	12	7	31	5
Baker et al. (1962)	CS	No	72	60	11	6	5	9	6	18	15	31	2
Hill et al. (1962) phase I†	CS	No	71	71	10	4	0	22	4	8	1	5	0
phase II			65	65	30	5	1		19	12	4	12	0
Howard et al. (1963)	CS	+	15	15	12			20	22	3	3	3	3
McDowell and McDevitt (1965)	CS	?	92	99	38	4	7	5	10	53	57	32	14
Enger and Boyesen (1965)	CS	+	51	49	23	1	3			6	6	10	0
Bradshaw and Brennan (1975)	TIA/CS	No	24	25	18	0	1	1	3	1	4	0	0

*T = Treated; C = controls.
†In phase II, the trial was modified by withdrawing the patients with hypertension.

solution would be another randomised trial but with up-to-date methodology and a large number of patients.

However, because anticoagulants are difficult to handle, particularly in the elderly and in patients with hypertension, and because they carry a risk of haemorrhagic complications, we believe it is probably correct to concentrate on antiplatelet drugs at the present time.

COMPARISON BETWEEN ANTICOAGULANTS AND ANTIPLATELET DRUGS

There are two studies comparing anticoagulants and antiplatelet drugs in the secondary prevention of atherothrombotic brain infarction, but neither is satisfactory from the methodological point of view.

In Buren and Ygge's study (1982), the sample size was too small (125 patients), there was no proper randomisation, the doses of aspirin and dipyridamole were not indicated, and the modalities of anticoagulant treatment were not given. Therefore, as the authors stated themselves: 'no firm conclusion can be drawn about the value of treatments reported here'.

In another Swedish study (Olsson *et al.*, 1980), 156 patients with TIA or RIND were all treated by anticoagulants for 2 months and then randomised into two groups: coumadin (68) or aspirin 1 g + dipyridamole 150 mg (67). At 2 years' follow-up there were significantly less ($p<0.001$) cerebral ischaemic events in the anticoagulant group but significantly more bleedings. This study does not permit one to draw conclusions about the relative efficacy of anticoagulant and antiplatelet drugs since all patients were initially treated by anticoagulants. It simply suggests that, in the long run, anticoagulants may be more powerful but also more dangerous than antiplatelet drugs.

ANTIPLATELET DRUGS

Of the numerous drugs that alter platelet behaviour, only five have been evaluated in the secondary prevention of atherothrombotic brain infarction, and 11 randomised trials have so far been published (table 7.2.).

Dipyridamole

An early study (Acheson *et al.*, 1969) did not demonstrate any benefit for dipyridamole alone but the sample size was small and the follow-up short. The same criticisms apply to the only study devoted to clofibrate (Acheson *et al.*, 1972).

Table 7.2 Secondary prevention of atherothrombotic brain infarction by antiplatelet drugs: randomised trials

Drug	Study	Double blind	Entry episode	Dose	Number of subjects — Treated	Number of subjects — Placebo	Follow-up (months)	Results — Events	Results — Significance
Dipyridamole	Acheson et al. (1969)	+	TIA/CS TIA/CS	400 mg 800 mg	77 62	76 66	14 11	TIA + CS TIA + CS	NS NS
Clofibrate	Acheson et al. (1972)	+	TIA/CS hyper-cholesterolaemia	1.2 g	47	48	60	TIA + CS	NS
Aspirin	Fields et al. (1977)	+	TIA	1.3 g	88	90	24	TIA, CS + death	$p < 0.01$, NS
Aspirin	Reuther and Dorndorf (1978)	+	TIA/RIND	1.5 g	29	29	24	TIA + CS	NS
Aspirin	Fields et al. (1978)	+	TIA + carotid surgery	1.3 g	65	60	24	TIA + CS + death	NS
Aspirin	CCSG (1978)*	+	TIA/RIND	1.3g	144 + 146*	156 + 139*	26	TIA CS + death	$p < 0.05$ $p < 0.05$
Aspirin	Guiraud (1982)†	No	TIA/RIND	1 g	147	Hydergine 155	36	CS + death	NS
Aspirin	Candelise et al. (1982)	+	TIA	1 g	63	Sulfinpyrazone 61	11.2	TIA + CS + death + MI	NS
Aspirin	Bousser et al. (1983)**	+	CS 84%; TIA 16%	1 g	198 + 202**	204	36	CS	$p < 0.05$
Aspirin	Sorensen et al. (1983)	+	TIA/RIND	1 g	101	102	25	TIA + death	NS
Flurbiprofene	Dehen (1983)‡	No	CS	100 mg	191	192 'controls'	36	CS	$p < 0.02$

*Four treatment groups: aspirin (144); aspirin + sulfinpyrazone (146); sulfinpyrazone (156); placebo (139).
†Three treatment groups: dihydroergocornine (138); dihydroergocornine 4.5 mg per day + aspirin (147); dihydroergocornine + dipyridamole (150 mg) + aspirin (138); dihydroergocornine (155).
**Three treatment groups: aspirin (198); aspirin + dipyridamole 225 mg/day (202); placebo (204).
‡The control group was not a placebo group but received the 'usual treatment in such a condition'
Note: CS = completed stroke; TIA = transient ischaemic attack(s); RIND = reversible ischaemic neurological deficit.

Dipyridamole in combination with aspirin was studied in two French trials (Guiraud-Chaumeil *et al.*, 1982; Bousser *et al.*, 1983), but no benefit was shown for this combination over aspirin alone. A North American study is currently testing this combination again versus aspirin in patients with TIA (Persantine–aspirin trial; American–Canadian Cooperative Study Group, 1983).

Sulfinpyrazone

An early study dealing mainly with primary prevention (Blakely and Bent, 1975) suggested that sulfinpyrazone produced a reduction in mortality (particularly from vascular causes) in those patients who had a history of prior stroke. However, this result was obtained by subgroup analysis and was not confirmed in the Canadian CCSG (1978) study. An Italian study (Candelise *et al.*, 1982) did not show any difference between sulfinpyrazone and aspirin, but the sample size (128) was far too small to detect anything except a very large difference, even if there was one.

Flurbiprofene

Flurbiprofene is a non-steroidal anti-inflammatory drug which has been recently studied in a French trial (Dehen, 1983). There was a significant ($p<0.02$) decrease in stroke incidence in the treated group compared with controls. There are several problems with this study among which are the following.

(1) It was not blind and there was no blind evaluation of the clinical events.
(2) There was no placebo group but controls received 'the usual treatment in such a condition' (details are not given).
(3) Most of the risk factors were more prominent (but not significantly so) in the control group.

Thus, although flurbiprofene is a very active antiplatelet drug *in vitro*, its *in vivo* efficacy in the secondary prevention of stroke needs to be confirmed in other, better-designed studies.

Aspirin

Aspirin (ASA) has been the most widely studied antiplatelet drug in secondary stroke prevention. The Italian study (Candelise *et al.*, 1982) comparing ASA and sulfinpyrazone will not be discussed again (see above). The French Toulouse study (Guiraud-Chaumeil *et al.*, 1982) included 440 patients with TIA or RIND in carotid or vertebrobasilar territories. There were three treatment groups: dihydroergocornine (DHE) alone, DHE + ASA 900 mg, and DHE + ASA 1 g + dipyridamole (150 mg). At 3 years' follow-up there was no statistical difference in stroke and death between the three groups. However, the combination of stroke recurrence and vascular death was 12.7% in the ASA group compared with 25% in the DHE group. The major problem with this study is that it was not blind.

All other studies were double-blind randomised studies with a placebo group (Fields *et al.*, 1970, 1978; CCSG, 1978; Reuther and Dorndorf, 1978; Bousser *et al.*, 1983; Sorensen *et al.*, 1983). These studies will be divided into two groups according to the sample size. In the four studies of the first group (Fields, 1970, 1978; Reuther and Dorndorf, 1978; Sorensen *et al.*, 1983), the sample size was relatively small (203 patients or less); entry episodes were TIA and/or RIND referrable mostly to the carotid territory (except in the study by Sorensen *et al.*, 1983). In these four studies there was no statistically significant difference between ASA and placebo as far as stroke incidence and death were concerned.

Various criticisms have been made of each of these studies. However, the main difficulty, strongly emphasised by Dyken (1983b), is that the numbers of patients are too small to avoid a type II error. This means that, although no statistical difference was observed, there might very well be a real difference, and one should therefore not conclude from these studies that aspirin is ineffective.

In the second group are two multicentre studies with a much larger sample size: the Canadian study (CCSG, 1978), and the French AICLA study (Bousser *et al.*, 1983).

The Canadian study was designed to have a sample size large enough to detect a 50% reduction in the risk of stroke with a type I (α) error of 0.05 and a type II (β) error of 0.20. The 585 patients with carotid and vertebrobasilar TIA (62%) or stroke with mild to moderate residual deficit (32%) were randomly assigned to four treatment groups:

- Group 1: ASA 1.3 g;
- Group 2: ASA 1.3 g + sulfinpyrazone 800 mg;
- Group 3: sulfinpyrazone 800 mg;
- Group 4: placebo.

When the two groups treated with aspirin were compared with the two not treated with aspirin, a statistical difference was noted. After 26 months of average follow-up, TIA, stroke and death were decreased by 19%, and stroke and death by 31% ($p<0.05$). Subgroup analyses revealed that these differences were limited to men, who had a 48% reduction in stroke and death ($p<0.005$). Although this study was better than all the previous ones, it has been vigorously attacked (Whisnant, 1978; Kurtzke, 1979).

The main criticisms have been that:

(1) when the end-points were limited to stroke alone, whether fatal or not, the risk reduction attributable to aspirin was no longer significant;
(2) the beneficial effect of aspirin might have been due to a positive interaction between ASA and sulfinpyrazone;
(3) the differences by sex might have been due to chance, since it was observed only by retrospective subgroup analysis.

Although it is essential to study stroke and death, it remains difficult to understand why in this study there was no significant reduction in the first stroke occurring after inclusion in the trial. There was indeed a positive interaction between ASA and sulfinpyrazone but it was not statistically significant. Because of the well-known difficulties in subgroup analysis (Lee *et al.*, 1980), the sex difference observed in response to aspirin, though impressive in this trial, clearly needs further confirmation.

The French AICLA study (Bousser *et al.*, 1983) was designed to have a sample size large enough to detect a 50% risk reduction in cerebral infarction with a type I error of 0.05 and a type II error of 0.10. The 604 patients were randomly assigned to three treatment groups.

● Group 1: ASA 1 g;
● Group 2: ASA + dipyridamole 225 mg (ASA + D);
● Group 3: placebo.

The main difference in baseline characteristics compared with the Canadian study was that the majority of patients (84%) had a completed stroke and only 16% had TIA. As in the Canadian study, ischaemic events were referrable either to the carotid or vertebrobasilar circulation, and angiography was not mandatory. With the exception of patients who withdrew from the study, each patient was followed for 3 years. Another important difference was that the only major end-point was cerebral infarction, whether fatal or not. The cumulative rates for cerebral infarction were 18% in the placebo group, 10.5% in the ASA group and 10.5% in the ASA + dipyridamole group. There was no difference between ASA and ASA + dipyridamole groups. A significant difference with a risk reduction of 41% was present between ASA and placebo group ($p<0.05$) and between the placebo group and the two ASA-treated groups taken together ($p<0.02$) (ASA and ASA + dipyridamole). Myocardial infarction was significantly less frequent in the two treated groups ($p<0.05$). Subgroup analysis failed to show a significant sex difference in the efficacy of aspirin.

One of the main criticisms of the French study was that withdrawn patients were not counted in the analysis. In fact, they were counted until the date of withdrawal but it was not thought necessary, in an explanatory approach, to take into account events occurring after cessation of trial medication. Another important point was that all strokes including cerebral haemorrhages and all deaths should have been counted. This has been done since and the results are as follows.

(1) There is no significant difference between the three groups for the two following end-points:
   (a) cerebral infarction + all deaths (figure 7.2);
   (b) cerebral infarction + vascular deaths.
(2) By contrast there is a significant difference ($p<0.05$) for the two following end-points:
   (a) stroke + myocardial infarction + all deaths;
   (b) all strokes (infarction + haemorrhage);
   with cumulative rates of 19% in the placebo group, 12% in the ASA group and 10.5% in the ASA + dipyridamole group (figure 7.3).

The results of this study thus showed a beneficial effect of aspirin (1 g) in the secondary prevention of stroke, so confirming and extending the favourable results obtained in the Canadian study.

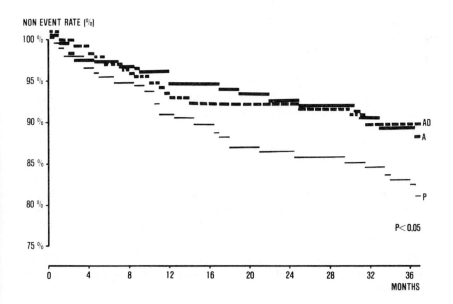

Figure 7.2   Cerebral infarcts and death, all causes.

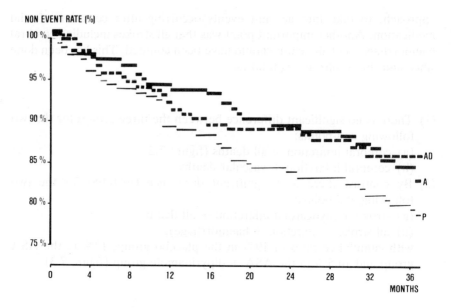

Figure 7.3   All strokes.

CONCLUSION

Although there is a great deal of controversy, one might conclude from these studies of secondary stroke prevention that:

(1) The benefit of carotid endarterectomy is not established since the only randomised clinical trial did not show an overall benefit for surgery.
(2) The benefit of anticoagulants is not established since it is impossible to draw any conclusion from the 11 controlled trials so far performed, because of their poor methodology.
(3) Among antiplatelet drugs there is at this time no evidence that any other antiplatelet or a combination of agents is superior to aspirin (results of ongoing studies might prove otherwise). Results of the two largest studies done so far are concordant in showing a 30 to 40% decrease in stroke occurrence in patients with TIA or strokes. As Dyken (1983a) stated: 'It is obvious that there is much more evidence for the value of therapy with aspirin in cerebrovascular disease than there is for any other specific therapy that has ever been reported'. The beneficial effect of aspirin was obtained with a daily dose of about 1 g; therefore one should be cautious about using lower doses until adequate studies have established their efficacy. Such a study comparing 300 mg and 1 g is

currently in progress in the United Kingdom (UK-TIA Study Group, 1979).

The results of the ongoing studies are awaited expectantly to confirm the beneficial effect of aspirin, to obtain data on the optimal dose, to re-examine the possible sex difference in response to aspirin, and to evaluate other antiplatelet drugs such as ticlopidine or combinations of antiplatelet drugs.

REFERENCES

Acheson, J., Danta, G. and Hutchinson, E. C. (1969). Controlled trial of dipyridamole in cerebral vascular disease. *Brit. Med. J.*, **1**, 614–15.

Acheson, J., Danta, G. and Hutchinson, E. C. (1972). Controlled trials of clofibrate in cerebral disease. *Atherosclerosis*, **15**, 177–83.

American –Canadian Cooperative Study Group (1983). Persantine–aspirin trial in cerebral ischemia. *Stroke*, **14**, 99–103.

Baker, R. N. (1961). An evaluation of anticoagulant therapy in the treatment of cerebrovascular disease. *Neurology*, **11**, 132–8.

Baker, R. N., Broward, J. A., Fang, H. C., Fisher, C. M., Groch, S. N., Heyman, A., Karp, H. R., McDevitt, E., Scheinberg, P., Schwartz, W. and Toole, J. F. (1962). Anticoagulant therapy in cerebral infarction. Report on cooperative study. *Neurology*, **12**, 823–35.

Baker, R. N., Schwartz, W. S. and Rose, A. S. (1966). Transient ischaemic strokes: a report of a study of anticoagulant therapy. *Neurology*, **16**, 841–7.

Blakely, J. A. and Bent, M. (1975). Platelets, drugs and longevity in a geriatric population. In Hirsh, J., Cade, J. F. and Gallus, A. S. (eds), *Platelets, Drugs and Thrombosis*. Karger, Basel, pp. 284–91.

Bousser, M. G., Eschwege, E., Haguenau, M., Lefauconnier, J. M., Thibult, N., Touboul, D. and Touboul, P. J. (1983). 'AICLA' controlled trial of aspirin and dipyridamole in the secondary prevention of atherothrombotic cerebral ischemia. *Stroke*, **14**, 5–14.

Bradshaw, P. and Brennan, S. (1975). Trial of long-term anticoagulant therapy in the treatment of small stroke associated with a normal carotid arteriogram. *J. Neurol. Neurosurg. Psychiatr.*, **38**, 642–47.

Buren, A. and Ygge, J. (1982). Treatment program and comparison between anticoagulants and platelet aggregation inhibitors after transient ischemic attacks. *Stroke*, **12**, 578–80.

Canadian Cooperative Study Group (1978). A randomized trial of aspirin and sulfinpyrazone in threatened stroke. *New Engl. J. Med.*, **299**, 53–9.

Candelise, L., Lanli, G., Perrone, P., Bracchi, M. and Brambilla, G. (1982). A randomized trial of aspirin and sulfinpyrazone in patients with TIA. *Stroke*, **13**, 175–9.

Dehen, H. (1983). Essai contrôlé du Flurbiprofène (anti-agrégant plaquettaire) dans la prévention secondaire des infarctus cérébraux de l'athérosclérose. *Presse Med.*, **12**, 521.

Dyken, M. L. (1983a). Anticoagulant and platelet antiaggregating therapy in stroke and threatened stroke. Neurologic clinics. In Barnett, H. J. M. (ed.), *Cerebrovascular Diseases*. W. B. Saunders, Philadelphia, pp. 223–42.

Dyken, M. L. (1983b). Editorial. Transient ischemic attacks and aspirin, stroke and death; negative studies and type II error. *Stroke,* **14**, 2–4.

Easton, J. D. and Sherman, D. G. (1980). Management of cerebral embolism of cardiac origin. *Stroke,* **11**, 433–42.

Enger, E. and Boyesen, S. (1965). Long-term anticoagulant therapy in patients with cerebral infarction: a controlled clinical study. *Acta Med. Scand. Suppl.,* **438**, 1–61.

Evans, G. (1973). Effect of platelet suppressive agents on the incidence of amaurosis fugax and transient cerebral ischemia. In McDowell, F. H. and Brennan, R. W. (eds). *Cerebral Vascular Disease. Eighth Conference.* Grune & Stratton, New York, pp. 297–9.

Fields, W. S., Maslenikov, V., Meyer, J. S., Hass, W. K., Remington, R. D. and Macdonald, M. (1970). Joint study of extracranial arterial occlusion. V. Progress report of prognosis following surgery or non-surgical treatment for transient cerebral ischaemic attacks and cervical carotid artery lesions. *J. Am. Med. Assoc.* **211**, 1993–2003.

Fields, W. S., Lemak, N. A., Frankowski, R. F. and Hardy, R. J. (1977, 1978). Controlled trial of aspirin in cerebral ischemia. I: *Stroke,* **8**, 301–14; II *Stroke,* **9**, 309–19.

Genton, E., Barnett, H. J. M., Fields, W. S., Gent, M. and Hoak, J. C. (1977). Cerebral ischemia XIV. The role of thrombosis and of antithrombotic therapy. *Stroke,* **8**, 150–75.

Guiraud-Chaumeil, B., Rascol, A., David, J., Boneu, B., Clanet, M. and Bierme, R. (1982) Prévention des récidives des accidents vasculaires cérébraux ischémiques par les anti-agrégants plaquettaires. Résultats d'un essai thérapeutique contrôlé de 3 ans. *Rev. Neurol. (Paris),* **138**, 367–85.

Heikinheimo, R. and Jarvinen, K. (1971). Acetylsalicylic and arteriosclerotic–thromboembolic diseases in the aged. *J. Am. Geriat. Soc.,* **19**, 403–5.

Herskovits, E., Vazques, A., Famulari, A., Smud, R., Tamaroff, L., Fraiman, H., Gonzalez, A. M., Vila, J. and Matera, V. (1981). Randomised trial of pentoxifylline versus acetylsalicylic acid plus dipyridamole in preventing transient ischaemic attacks. *Lancet,* **I**, 966–8

Hill, A. B., Marshall, J. and Shaw, D. A. (1962). Cerebro-vascular disease. Trial of long-term anticoagulant therapy. *Brit. Med. J.,* **2**, 1003–6.

Howard, F. A., Cohen, P. and Hickler, R. B. (1963). Survival following stroke. *J. Am. Med. Assoc.,* **183**, 921–5.

Kurtzke, J. F. (1979). A critique of the Canadian T.I.A. study. *Ann. Neurol,* **5**, 597–9.

Lee, K. L., McNeer, J. F., Starmer, C. F., Harris, P. J. and Rosati, R. A. (1980). Clinical judgment and statistics. Lessons from a simulated randomized trial in coronary artery disease. *Circulation,* **61**, 508–15.

Leonberg, S. C. and Elliott, F. A. (1981). Prevention of recurrent stroke. *Stroke,* **12**, 731–5.

McDowell, F. and McDevitt, E. (1965). Treatment of the completed stroke with long-term anticoagulant. In Millikan, C. H., Siekert, R. G. and Whisnant, J. P. (eds), *Cerebral Vascular Diseases.* Grune & Stratton, New York, pp. 185–99.

Olsson, J. E., Brechter, C., Backlund, H., Krook, B., Muller, R., Nitelius, E., Olsson, O. and Tornberg, A. (1980). Anticoagulant vs antiplatelet therapy as prophylactic against cerebral infarction in transient ischaemic attacks. *Stroke,* **11**, 4–9.

Pearce, J. M. S., Gubbay, S. S. and Walton, J. M. (1965). Long-term anticoagulant therapy in transient cerebral ischaemic attacks. *Lancet,* **1**, 6–9.

Reuther, R. and Dorndorf, W. (1978). Aspirin in patients with cerebral ischaemia and normal angiograms or non-surgical lesions. Results of a double-blind trial. In Breddin, K., Dorndorf, W., Loew, D. and Marx, R. (eds), *Acetylsalicylic Acid in Cerebral Ischemia and Coronary Heart Disease.* F. K. Schattauer Verlag, Stuttgart, pp. 97–106.

Sandok, B. A., Furlan, A. J., Whisnant, J. P. and Sundt, T. M. (1978). Guidelines for the management of transient ischemic attacks. *Mayo Clin. Proc.,* **53**, 665–74.

Sorensen, P. S., Pedersen, H., Marquarsden, J., Petersson, H., Heltberg, A., Simonsen, N., Munck, O. and Andersen, L. A. (1983). Acetyl salicylic acid in the prevention of stroke in patients with reversible ischemic attacks. A Danish cooperative study. *Stroke,* **14**, 15–22.

UK-TIA Study Group (1979). Design and protocol of the UK-TIA Aspirin Study. In Tognoni, G. and Garattini, S. (eds), *Drug Treatment and Prevention in Cerebrovascular Disorders.* Elsevier North Holland, Amsterdam, pp. 387–94.

Whisnant, J. P. (1978). The Canadian trial of aspirin and sulfinpyrazone in threatened stroke. *New Engl. J. Med.,* **299**, 953.

8

Trials of secondary prevention after transient ischaemic attacks.
Part II: Towards better clinical trials

CHARLES P. WARLOW

INTRODUCTION

It is not difficult to design a clinical trial which is sufficiently unbiased and large to determine reliably whether some particular treatment reduces the long-term risk of stroke and myocardial infarction (MI) after a transient ischaemic attack (TIA), since the methodological and analytical techniques are well known (Peto *et al.*, 1976; Peto, 1982, 1983). It is, however, far more difficult to recruit enough patients in a reasonable time, maintain them on tenacious follow-up, maximise compliance with treatment, keep control of the organisation and the data, and contain costs. In this review, while attempting to cover all the components currently thought to be necessary in a clinical trial, I shall concentrate on the more controversial and difficult areas.

RANDOMISED TREATMENT ALLOCATION

It is almost impossible to evaluate treatment accurately without a randomised comparison against the 'standard' treatment of the day unless it has an extraordinarily major effect on the risk of stroke or myocardial infarction. Although desirable, this is unlikely. Non-random comparisons, based on either historical or concurrent controls, may very well come up with the right — or wrong — answer, but are extremely vulnerable to a number of systematic errors (McPherson, 1984). Moreover, they cannot be as convincing as randomised comparisons even if attempts are made to allow for any imbalance of important prognostic variables, such as age and hypertension, between treated and untreated groups of patients. There will inevitably be

153

unknown and yet to be discovered prognostic variables which influence the outcome, particularly if one remembers the extraordinary variation in the reported 'natural' history of TIA (Warlow, 1982). Even within one institution (Christie, 1979) or with tightly controlled treatment protocols (Pocock, 1977), there can be surprisingly large and inexplicable differences in outcome between groups of similar patients treated in apparently the same way, but at different times. There is also the possibility, usually unevaluated, that patients with the best prognosis receive the most favoured treatment, so making the effects of that treatment appear beneficial (Ravid *et al.*, 1980). In short, non-randomised comparisons are potentially extremely misleading and tend to overestimate true treatment effects, or find them where none exists (Sacks *et al.*, 1982); 'the argument for randomisation is not that no truths can emerge without it, but that without it moderate biases can easily emerge' (Peto, 1983).

Telephone randomisation

In large, or even small, multicentre trials, randomisation by telephone to a central trials office is an enormous advantage. The office will know at once when a patient is entered into the trial and from that moment all end-points must be accounted for and kept in the analysis. The office will also be able to calculate the expected dates of follow-up and when notification (entry) and follow-up forms are to be expected. It is impossible for a distant collaborator to 'cheat' by, for example, rejecting a patient after an envelope with the treatment allocation is opened. Allocation by day of the week, date of birth, or by alternating patients is hardly random and easily manipulated by a biased clinician. Using the telephone may also allow particularly simple trials to collect *all* the relevant notification data *before* allocating treatment. This eliminates the difficult and tedious task of extracting such data from distant and recalcitrant collaborators who may be irritatingly slow at completing written notification forms, particularly if the forms are at all complicated.

Unequal treatment allocation

It has been traditional to randomise patients so that equal numbers receive each treatment. This is not strictly necessary since the power of the analysis is very little reduced even if the treatments are allocated in as extreme a ratio as 7:3 (Peto *et al.*, 1976). This can be an advantage if, on past experience or theoretical grounds, one treatment is thought to be more effective than the other. By randomly allocating more than half the patients to the favoured treatment one may (perhaps irrationally) make collaborators more willing to participate by reducing their ethical doubts about doing the trial at all. This is particularly useful if the trial is challenging what has become an accepted therapeutic dogma without any good evidence, for example the value of carotid endarterectomy after TIA, or of anticoagulation in patients in atrial fibrillation.

Sample size

The sample must be large enough to control random errors, and its size depends on:

(a) the natural history of TIA (uncertain but might involve an annual risk of stroke and/or death of about 10%: Warlow, 1982; Wiebers and Whisnant, 1982);
(b) the effect of treatment which, by definition, is not known but to be clinically relevant would need to reduce the above risk by perhaps 25% (about 15 000 patients under the age of 75 are likely to present to their general practitioner with TIA every year in England and Wales; a reduction of 25% in a 10% per annum risk of stroke and/or death would 'save' about 1500 patients from stroke and/or death by the end of 5 years, and several thousand low-risk patients would perhaps have received the treatment unnecessarily);
(c) the patient accession rate given the requirement that the duration and funding of the trial have finite limits and any projected accession rate tends to be an overestimate;
(d) the requirement for a formally statistically significant treatment effect ($p<0.05$, or preferably <0.01);
(e) a reasonable power, perhaps 80% or more.

Any sample size calculation will be something of a guess, but if we have 500 patients in the control group recruited over 4 years and followed for another year, about 150 may be expected to have a stroke or die. If this risk were reduced by 25%, then, in an equal number of treated patients, there would be 112 with a stroke or dead at 5 years. This difference would be statistically significant ($p<0.01$) and the chance of the trial giving this result or better would be about 50%. Unfortunately, the chance of that trial giving a less convincing result is also about 50%, a probability that can only be substantially reduced by entering many more patients, or continuing follow-up much longer.

In general, therefore, trials in this area require several hundred or even a few thousand patients to have much hope of success in a reasonable period of time. Indeed, it is probably important to aim for a fairly quick answer since a potentially useful treatment may not be available outside the trial; nihilistic doctors may be denying a potentially useful but available treatment to non-trial patients while the trial grinds on its way; and enthusiastic doctors may be giving a potentially harmful treatment to non-trial patients while hoping for the practice to catch up with the theory. Furthermore, the theoretical basis for the trial treatment may change (e.g. the current controversy about the dose of aspirin), or the interest in and relevance of the trial question may disappear with increasing knowledge from other sources. Finally, a drug may outrun its patent, which would cause considerable distress to its makers. The disadvantage of a large short-term trial as compared with a smaller but long-term trial with the same number of end-points (and equal power) is that a side-effect appearing only in the long-term may very well be missed. This might be avoidable if the patients are 'flagged' for death (and even cancer) with central government records in countries where this can be done (see below).

These arithmetic imperatives lead to the inevitable conclusion that trials in TIA patients have to be organised on a multicentre basis even though TIAs are a common condition. This requires considerable attention to eligibility and exclusion criteria, documentation (see below), and liaison between centres. However, there are advantages to multicentre trials: they improve our ability to make agreed and therefore generalisable definitions, they improve communications and reduce conflicts between neurologists working in different centres and countries, and they improve the knowledge of the collaborators less familiar with the disease in question by exposure to those who specialise in it. There is no need to exclude centres randomising a rather small number of patients since, contrary to some reports (Sylvester *et al.*, 1981), I have found that small centres can be excellent in completing documentation accurately and keeping patients on follow-up. Indeed, small centres may have the advantage of *not* being particularly interested in TIA and not, therefore, running any other trials or experiments which might compete with the multicentre trial. Large centres are more attractive in a multicentre trial (provided they can keep to the trial discipline), and non-teaching centres need to be actively encouraged to collaborate since very often they deal with many more patients than more prestigious institutions.

If, at the end of a trial, or at an interim analysis, it seems that more end-points will be needed to show a significant treatment effect (which is so often more modest than first anticipated), then one probably should not feel obliged to stop the trial at the originally predetermined time. More end-points will accrue fairly rapidly if the patients can just be followed for another year or two, and this may well be easier and cheaper than continuing to randomise more patients *and* continue follow-up. However, this strategy does beg the question as to how best to treat the new TIA patients who are no longer entering the trial, particularly if the interim analysis had not been revealed to the collaborators. Naturally *p* values will need to be more extreme to take account of any interim analyses that are done (McPherson, 1974).

ONE TRIAL, OR MORE?

However large and well designed, a single trial whatever the result will still be criticised on the general philosophy that it is only one experiment, and before accepting the result as the truth, the experiment should be repeated. Exactly this problem has arisen following the publication of the Extra-cranial to Intra-cranial Bypass Surgery Trial (EC/IC Bypass Study Group, 1985). Indeed, large randomised trials seem to attract an extraordinary amount of criticism (some of it well based and much of it unsound) which can only really be countered by having more than one trial giving the same general conclusion. However, if one trial is completed and shows that a treatment seems to work, it then becomes ethically difficult to withhold that treatment from a group of patients in a further trial to confirm the result of the first. It is also tedious to be doing confirmatory rather than innovatory trials. A way round this problem would be for investigators, pharmaceutical companies and national medical research agencies to try to arrange for two or three trials of a particular treatment to start at about the same time. Competition between trial collaborators as to who finishes first might even increase a flagging accession rate.

ELIGIBILITY AND INELIGIBILITY

In theory, the results of a trial are only applicable to patients who entered that trial, but in practice the results have to be generalised to future similar patients in the trial centres and elsewhere. It is, therefore, crucial that the trial patients are very carefully described and that any future patients given the trial treatment (if it is found to be effective) are reasonably similar although they cannot be exactly the same.

A particular problem with TIA is that, although the definition is clinical and widely accepted, the 24-h division between TIA and stroke is arbitrary and has no pathophysiological basis. A TIA can be defined as an acute loss of focal cerebral or ocular function with symptoms lasting less than 24 h, and which, after adequate investigation, is presumed to be due to embolic or thrombotic vascular disease (Warlow and Morris, 1982). It is also important to be quite clear in excluding patients who have certain symptoms in isolation (e.g. vertigo, drop attacks) which although they occur in vertebro-basilar ischaemia also occur frequently in other non-vascular conditions. The assumption is widely held in the literature, and in practice, that the long-term management of patients whose focal vascular episodes recover in minutes, hours or days is the same. Thus if a trial treatment prevents stroke after TIA, it will almost inevitably be given — in the future — to mild-stroke as well as TIA patients. This may or may not be the correct thing to do but it is theoretically possible that an antihaemostatic drug such as aspirin may carry more risk after stroke than after TIA (because some strokes are due to primary intracerebral haemorrhage, or because of the possibility of exacerbating haemorrhagic infarction), or that carotid endarterectomy may carry a greater risk of stroke or death in a stroke patient compared with a TIA patient. There seem to be two possible strategies to deal with this: first, taking a purist line and only treating future TIA patients with the treatment found to be effective in the trial while running separate trials (consecutively or concurrently) on stroke patients; or, secondly, including mild-stroke patients in a 'TIA' trial (which in fact is what most people have done) and if necessary looking at them as a separate subgroup. Whatever the strategy, there will be a post-trial tendency for doctors to generalise and give an effective treatment to a rather wider category of patients than had been entered into any previous trial. In many ways this may be scientifically sensible and ethically necessary although the quantitative benefit of the treatment may be less, or more, than in the sort of patient originally entered into the trial.

In general, I favour being overinclusive rather than overexclusive with trial entry criteria and then, if necessary, describing the results in predefined subgroups although I am uncomfortably aware of the chance effects which can ruin subgroup analysis (Lee *et al.*, 1980; Peto, 1982). Naturally, if this strategy is to be used, enough data must be collected at randomisation to allow the identification of appropriate subgroups and their size needs to be large.

A rather special problem of the generalisability of trial results occurs when the treatment is surgical, since surgical (and anaesthetic) skill does vary between institutions and this variation must in part be responsible for the differences in surgical morbidity and mortality over and above the explanation that selection criteria for surgery also differ between centres. Thus, it is fallacious to assume that the morbidity and mortality following surgery in a published trial can be generalised to one's own institution. One must determine the risk of surgery in one's *own* institution, add this to the outcome after successful surgery, which can be determined from the randomised trials of surgery, and then compare this overall outcome with the predicted outcome without surgery, which can also be determined from the randomised trials of surgical treatment. This can only be done if the trial patients are well described and similar to one's own patients.

Finally, it is important to remember that all published and ongoing trials in TIA are largely concerned with *long-term* management rather than acute treatment because of the logistic difficulty of identifying and randomising patients quickly after their last TIA.

Excluded patients

If one is tending to be overinclusive and wants the trial patients to be broadly representative of real and future patients (which seems sensible), then exclusions must be kept to a minimum, i.e. patients who refuse to be randomised, or where trial treatment is contraindicated, or follow-up impractical or in the presence of some other serious disorder which is likely to be fatal in a matter of months.

I doubt if it is worth spending much or any time checking the validity of each patient who is randomised since the collaborators ought to be well trained and disciplined enough to agree and stick to the entry definition of TIA, mild stroke, etc. Indeed, how would one deal with patients found to be ineligible *after* randomisation other than by keeping them in an 'intention to treat' analysis (see below)? If, as we all do, the trial collaborators inadvertently include some unsuspected cases of migraine or hysteria, this will not much matter in the analysis since these patients will be unlikely to have a stroke or die, and provided they are randomly distributed in equal proportions between the treatment groups, not much harm will be done. But, if the trial treatment is exceptionally risky, then inadvertent inclusion of good-prognosis patients with the wrong diagnosis would be more serious. However, I suspect that patients who get into a well-run clinical trial are on average diagnosed far more accurately than those who end up, in routine clinical practice, getting the same treatment if it turns out to be effective. An exception is those few patients who are found to have an intracranial tumour or some other 'non-vascular' serious condition. This will usually become obvious fairly quickly, and I believe it is legitimate to stop the trial treatment and withdraw the patient from the analysis provided this is done 'blind' to treatment allocation, and there is no likelihood of differential withdrawal rates between treatment groups. If in any doubt, these patients can at least be kept on follow-up and included in one analysis, if not in the main analysis itself. The problem of withdrawals from trial medication or analysis is considered in detail later.

Accounting for excluded patients

There is a school of thought that the number of patients screened, but not randomised, should be reported so that the degree of selection for the trial can be assessed against one's own clinical practice (Hampton, 1981). I think this is relatively unimportant, and moreover it is a slight nuisance in a multicentre study since it may be very difficult to persuade trial collaborators to keep the appropriate records, particularly when one is pressing them for much more important data on the patients who *do* actually get into the trial. If the randomised patients are accurately described, they can then be compared with anyone's clinical practice without knowing about the larger group from which they were selected. In practice most of the selection for a trial occurs long before the moment the patient is seen by a collaborator and can therefore be 'counted'. In the UK a patient with a TIA must bother to report it to his general practitioner, the general practitioner has to recognise it for what it is, he then has to decide to refer the patient to hospital, the patient has to be referred to a hospital involved in the trial, and finally the patient has to find his way to one of the collaborators working in that hospital. Only *after* this point can any selection for the trial be accurately assessed, and it is likely to be a very small part of the overall selection process. For example, about 25 000 patients first report to their general practitioners with TIA every year in England and Wales (Oxford-shire Community Stroke Project, unpublished data) and yet only about 500 are entered into the UK-TIA Aspirin Trial. Clearly a lot of selection is going on but very little of it is to do with the collaborating neurologists. If resources are limited, it is far more important to describe properly who does get randomised, and not waste time trying to count who does not get randomised.

END-POINTS: WHAT DO WE EXPECT TREATMENT TO ACHIEVE?

Recurrent TIA is not a satisfactory end-point for analysis because:

(1) a treatment which stops TIA may not necessarily reduce the risk of a more substantial thrombo-embolic event such as stroke;
(2) a treatment which stops TIA might do so only at the price of unaccept-able side-effects and it may even *increase* the risk of stroke (e.g. an antihaemostatic drug which stops TIA might cause cerebral haemorr-hage); and
(3) TIA themselves are by definition transient, leaving the patient symp-tomless (if anxious), and in practice rather few patients have very many or very frequent attacks.

The most relevant objective, and therefore end-point for analysis, is the reduction in the risk of stroke which in a TIA patient is about ten times that in a non-TIA patient (Whisnant *et al.*, 1973). For the patient, it does not matter too much whether a stroke of a given severity is occlusive or haemorrhagic as long as the *overall* stroke risk is reduced and it is, therefore, essential that *all* strokes are analysed whether they are occlusive or haemorrhagic. Naturally, it is of interest to know, from the explanatory and theoretical points of view, the cause of any stroke, and for this reason CT scanning is useful if it is available. Of some potential concern is the possibility that a treatment which reduces the risk of stroke might make any stroke that does occur more severe. It is not inconceivable, for example, that the haemostatic defect caused by aspirin or anticoagulants might actually worsen cerebral infarction by potentiating any tendency for the infarct to become haemorrhagic. This is a difficult notion to deal with since, as well as any quantitative reduction in stroke risk, we may need to be concerned with the severity of stroke in treated and untreated patients. It is, of course, easy to examine stroke mortality as well as stroke incidence but this may not be a sensitive enough measure of stroke severity. Unfortunately there is no easy way to measure stroke severity. Indeed, how does one compare global aphasia, hemiplegia, urinary incontinence, and thalamic pain? All these problems are 'severe' but their impact will depend on the individual patient. In the UK-TIA Aspirin Trial we decided to count, in the main analysis, only those strokes causing symptoms for more than a week (so-called 'major' stroke), but it might, in retrospect, have been sensible to subdivide these strokes further in terms of disability. How this could have been done, and whether it could be done without undue effort in a large multicentre study, is questionable. However, very recently we have decided to attempt some measure of stroke severity by using the Rankin Disability Scale.

Another relevant end-point, at least in antihaemostatic drug trials, is myocardial infarction and 'vascular' deaths which are mostly related to the complications of atheroma (e.g. sudden death, ruptured aortic aneurysm, etc.). To date only one trial has examined the effect of treatment on MI (Bousser *et al.*, 1983). This is a pity since after TIA as many major events are likely to be due to MI and vascular — usually 'sudden' — death as to stroke (table 8.1). It is, therefore, very reasonable to include MI as an end-point by itself, or in a 'basket' of end-points with stroke.

Finally, total mortality — or all vascular deaths which is almost the same thing (table 8.1) — must be accounted for, particularly because mortality is high in TIA patients, with an excess risk of about three times (Heyden *et al.*, 1980). Furthermore, the most relevant issue for the patient is the probability of survival free of stroke, survival free of MI, or survival free of either stroke or MI. Failure to account for non-stroke deaths leads to an unrealistic analysis, particularly since a trial treatment such as carotid surgery may actually cause non-stroke death (e.g. acute MI during anaesthesia). I agree with Sackett (1978) who writes 'dead patients cannot have strokes, and to confine an analysis to fatal and non-fatal strokes could produce the situation in which the drug which decimates the ranks of potential stroke victims by killing them from other causes will spuriously appear efficacious', and with Peto (1982) who writes 'counts of recurrences alone which do not also include patients who died without recurrence may be misleading if there is any possibility that some of the deaths without recurrence might have been caused by, or prevented by, one or other treatment'.

In conclusion, all strokes, MIs and deaths should be analysed, and this requires all patients to be followed up, preferably continuing to take trial medication, but, even if they are withdrawn from trial medication, until death even if a non-fatal stroke or MI occurs. These non-fatal events are not, therefore, really 'end-points' but 'major analysable events'. For an individual patient the trial does not 'end' until he is dead or the trial is stopped.

Table 8.1 The outcome after TIA. (Unpublished data from the UK-TIA Aspirin Trial, August 1983; these data are based on approximately 3600 patient-years of follow-up, and the mean age of the patients is 59 years.)

First major stroke*	
Fatal	20
Non-fatal	80
Total	100
First myocardial infarct	
Fatal	11
Non-fatal	28
Total	39
Other vascular deaths†	61
Total vascular deaths	92
Non-vascular deaths	19
Total deaths	111
Total patients with MI, stroke, death	219

*Symptoms lasting more than one week.
†31 'sudden'; 4 ruptured aortic aneurysm; 3 pulmonary embolism; 23 vascular but uncertain cause.

BLIND OR NON-BLIND EVALUATION OF END-POINTS

Apart from all-cause mortality, the reporting and evaluation of end-points should be done double blind if this can be arranged. This is self-evident when end-points are variably reported by patients and open to diagnostic bias by clinicians; in this context TIAs, if they are going to be used as an end-point, must be assessed blind.

One might think that more major events such as stroke or MI could be reasonably evaluated without a double-blind technique. This is not so because there is no reliable 'gold standard' for the diagnosis of all cases, particularly mild cases which can so easily be misclassified as TIA for stroke, or angina for MI. A mild stroke, for example, might not be reported by the patient or even neurologist if either had knowledge of the treatment and were biased in favour of it.

Chest pain might be more likely to lead to an ECG, and hence the diagnosis of MI, if a physician is biased against the treatment the patient is having. There are *always* grey areas between a definite (and yet mild) stroke and TIA, and between a definite (and yet mild) MI and angina. In ordinary clinical practice this sort of distinction is irrelevant since it does not influence management, but in a clinical trial a distinction *must* be made and the event analysed or discarded. Even at post mortem, diagnostic bias can arise in the case of a patient who is found dead and who has 'coronary atheroma', but no evidence of myocardial infarction. This can very easily be counted as a 'myocardial infarction' even though there are thousands of live patients with coronary arteries in a similar state.

Blindness is scientifically desirable to avoid diagnostic bias but sometimes it is almost impossible to arrange, and almost always it is expensive. In trials of surgical treatment, blindness for the patient might in theory be possible but is ethically unacceptable since a general anaesthetic and skin incision would be required in the 'no-surgery' group. Some patients might even die under the general anaesthetic, since TIA patients are elderly and often have ischaemic heart disease, and the analysis would then be biased against the 'surgery' group. Although the patient may be biased in what symptoms he reports and what he ignores, it would at least be feasible for the collaborating neurologist to be 'blind' to the treatment allocation even though it would be very difficult for him to avoid noticing the surgical scar. In practice, the best that can be done is for an independent audit committee to review the evidence for any end-point without knowledge of treatment allocation. Even then one has to consider the possibility of a non-blind collaborating neurologist over- or under-reporting a possible end-point depending on his view of the treatment.

For drug trials blindness is usually possible unless the active treatment has obvious effects unrelated to the outcome under consideration. This applies, for example, to the bradycardia caused by beta-blockers. In the TIA context it would be possible, but difficult, to give anticoagulants without the knowledge of the assessing neurologist. It is quite easy to make antiplatelet drug trials blind, but at a cost since instead of merely asking half the patients to take a drug openly (usually at the expense of the health service, a medical insurance scheme, or a pharmaceutical company), the cost of the drug and the placebo has to be borne by the trial budget. Moreover, if calendar packaging is thought to be desirable to increase compliance, and I believe it is, then this will increase costs dramatically. For example, in the UK-TIA Aspirin Trial the cost of the drugs and their packaging will be about £400 000 which is more than 50% of the total cost of the trial. If this trial had been 'open', the cost to the British Medical Research Council would be less than it is since most of the patients would be old enough to receive 'free' aspirin under the National Health Service, and the rest would pay only a modest prescription charge. Not surprisingly it is difficult, it not impossible, to persuade a pharmaceutical company to invest large sums of money in a trial, or even supply the medication, unless the drug is still protected by patent. Thus commercial rather than scientific pressures may dictate which trials get done, since in this field, where potential profits from a successful drug are enormous, it may be far easier to get a trial funded by a pharmaceutical company than by a national research or charitable agency.

FOLLOW-UP

The frequency of follow-up visits should be determined by the need for the collaborator to be made aware of and evaluate all important end-points; to notice and evaluate any side-effects of treatment; and to maintain compliance with trial medication. In surgery trials the last point is irrelevant as long-term treatment compliance is not an issue and even the second point is of little relevance since treatment side-effects occur early (i.e. surgical mortality and morbidity which is usually defined as any event related to surgery and starting within 30 days of the operation). In a surgery trial, therefore, annual follow-up is probably adequate to detect stroke and MI, particularly if resources are stretched, and it is usually quite easy to obtain records of these events retrospectively if they occur without the trial collaborator's earlier knowledge. In the United States this is not so easy, and to keep track of even surgical trial patients 3- or 4-monthly follow-up visits are probably desirable. Marking the outside of hospital and general practitioner records of trial patients helps in the early notification of major events to a collaborator.

In a drug trial, follow-up every 3 or 4 months is required so that compliance with medication can be reinforced and any side-effect detected. It may need to be more frequent if some blood test is necessary when a new drug is on trial. Particularly frequent blood tests may be required if a drug has been reported to cause leukopenia or hepatic damage (e.g. Ticlopidine) or if dosage control is necessary (e.g. anticoagulation). Exact monitoring of compliance is expensive and probably unnecessary, particularly if one is using a 'pragmatic' rather than 'explanatory' analysis (see below). Pill counts are somewhat naive since patients will soon discover what is happening and it is probably better to detect a trial drug or its metabolite in the plasma or, preferably, urine (because it is easier and cheaper) by some sort of qualitative test. Quantitative tests are usually more complicated and more expensive. Compliance can presumably be maximised by reasonably frequent follow-up, an enthusiastic and persuasive physician, simple treatment regimes (one pill daily being ideal), and calendar packaging which has been used for the oral contraceptive for many years.

Patients who stop trial medication, either known or unknown to the trial collaborator, must still be followed and included in an 'intention-to-treat' analysis (see below). This can be tiresome if there is a high incidence of early side-effects with consequent withdrawal from trial medication. In fact this has been such a nuisance in the UK-TIA Aspirin Trial that every effort is made to stop neurologists randomising patients who are likely to develop indigestion on aspirin. None the less, the withdrawal rate — mostly because of side-effects — is so high in the first 4 months that one might argue that in a trial like this there should be a run-in period on active medication for all, followed by randomisation of only those patients able to tolerate the drug.

However, such a design would miss any influence of treatment in the first few weeks of the natural history of TIA.

In some countries it is possible to ensure that follow-up is complete until death or emigration by 'flagging' patients with central government records (e.g. the Office of Population Censuses and Surveys in England and Wales). In the event of death (or emigration), the trial office is informed and a copy of the death certificate is made available. This has the added advantage that a *fatal* long-term side-effect might be identified even after the trial is complete. For example, if exposure to daily aspirin for a few years were substantially to increase the risk of gastric carcinoma several years later, it would be very difficult to detect without such a system.

It may also be a good idea to ask the collaborators to record on the follow-up forms all events requiring medical attention. This need not necessarily be coded at the time, but at least it is available for retrospective coding and analysis if an interesting idea turns up from some other source. For example, if we had done this in the UK-TIA Aspirin Trial we would have been able to look at the question of whether aspirin protects against cataract.

ANALYSIS

There are well-known and acceptable methods, based on life-table techniques, for the analysis of long-term clinical trials, and they are reliable if the patients are randomised, the end-points well defined, and the sample size appropriate (Peto *et al.*, 1976). There is agreement that the overwhelming advantages of randomisation are lost if patients are changed from one treatment group to the other and yet not analysed in their original treatment group; thus in a trial of surgery there will be some patients randomised to surgery who do not receive it for some reason (e.g. prior death), and some randomised to no-surgery who end up having it (e.g. for very frequent TIA). Provided this does not happen too often, the analysis will be little affected, as was the case in the European Coronary Surgery Trial (European Coronary Surgery Study Group, 1980). It is also agreed that comparing patients who complied with trial medication with those who did not is likely to lead to large errors (Coronary Drug Project Research Group, 1980).

There is a certain amount of doubt as to how far subgroup analysis is permissible since this can suggest large treatment differences where none exists (Lee *et al.*, 1980; Peto, 1982). In general, if the overall results of the trial are negative, subgroup analysis is very risky. Even if the overall trial results are positive, treatment effects in subgroups can appear surprisingly large, and even statistically apparently significant when in fact no treatment differences exist. It is, therefore, probably best to view unexpected subgroup effects chiefly as hypothesis generating and not as hypothesis proving, and to accept subgroup effects only if there is some strong *a priori* reason to do so or if several trials come up with the same result. An example of how difficult this situation can be is the apparently very positive interaction between aspirin and male sex in one trial (Canadian Cooperative Study Group, 1978) whereas, in the two more recent trials, females on aspirin fared better than males on aspirin (Bousser *et al*; 1983; Sørensen *et al.*, 1983). It seems unlikely that there is a *qualitative* interaction between aspirin and sex (such that aspirin is 'good' for males and 'bad' for females), but far more likely that any interaction is *quantitative* (such that aspirin reduces the risk of stroke in males and females but to a differing extent). Qualitative and quantitative interactions are discussed further by Peto (1982).

The dangers of interim analysis have been stressed and accepted by most trialists (McPherson, 1982). This, however, leads one into the knotty problem of how to apply stopping rules to maximise scientific validity while minimising any ethical difficulty in allowing the trial to run on longer than necessary. In the UK-TIA Aspirin Trial we are not planning to stop until one of the treatment arms has an outcome better or worse than three standard deviations from that expected on the null hypothesis that all three treatment arms have the same outcome. Some critics regards this rule as too extreme but at least we are taking a conservative position and are highly unlikely to make a type I error.

If, by ill chance, the treatment groups in a randomised trial are badly matched for prognostic variables affecting the end-points, it is possible to adjust for this retrospectively in the analysis. Indeed, adjustment is often worth making even if any mismatching is not statistically significant since this will allow a more accurate estimate of the true treatment effect. In very large randomised trials, mismatching is highly unlikely to occur but oddly enough just such a problem did occur in the largest trial of aspirin in the secondary prevention of myocardial infarction (Aspirin Myocardial Infarction Study Research Group, 1980). Naturally there is nothing that can be done about any mismatch in unknown prognostic variables, nor about any which become appreciated during the trial (from non-trial evidence) unless they happen to have been measured at randomisation. Since adjustment techniques are not accepted by all statisticians, it is sensible to publish the analysis with and without adjustment for prognostic variables and, if possible, to have a large enough study to make the problem minimal. One can plan to stratify for prognostic variables prospectively at randomisation but this may be hopelessly complex if more than three or four are used, and sometimes is even counterproductive if the sample size is small (Friedman *et al.*, 1981). However, the use of minimisation and a microcomputer may solve this particular problem. Our policy in the UK-TIA Aspirin and Multicentre Carotid Surgery Trials is to stratify only by centre at time of randomisation.

The most important debate in the analysis of these trials is how to analyse patients who stop trial medication which is inevitable even if one avoids randomising inappropriate patients (e.g. vagrants, or patients with duodenal ulcers in a trial of aspirin). If such patients are withdrawn from the analysis of end-points from the moment of stopping trial medication, then bias might result if the withdrawn patients on one treatment are systematically different with respect to prognosis from those on the other treatment. Any such difference may be extremely hard to quantify. One obvious example would be that if a patient developed very frequent severe TIA he might be withdrawn from trial medication and anticoagulated or might undergo carotid surgery. If such co-intervention were ineffective and if the patient went on to have a stroke, then that stroke would not be analysed in an 'on treatment' analysis even though its origin was clearly in the increasingly frequent TIA which had actually occurred 'on treatment'. This particular problem can be avoided by analysing all events which occur up to 6 months from stopping trial medication as was done in the Canadian trial of aspirin (Canadian Cooperative Study Group, 1978). However, more subtle biases are possible and almost certainly do occur, so biasing the trial results towards or away from the null hypothesis.

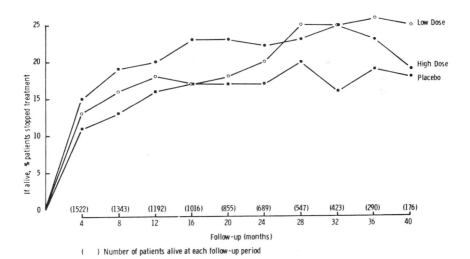

Figure 8.1 Unpublished data from the UK-TIA Aspirin Trial to show the proportion of patients who stopped treatment during the trial. (High dose = 600 mg b.d. and low dose = 300 mg daily.)

One solution to this problem is to make sure that all the patients randomised to a particular treatment (medication, surgery, or whatever) do actually receive it, and, if the treatment is a drug, that the patients take it to the end of the trial or prior death. In such a Utopian situation the 'on treatment' and 'intention to treat' analysis would be identical. In practice this does not happen but the ideal can be approached by avoiding randomising patients who are likely to get side-effects, or abscond from trial medication or follow-up. To me the more pragmatic 'intention to treat' analysis is preferable to the more explanatory 'on treatment' analysis, but I think it is important to report both (cf. the Australian trial in mild hypertension, Management Committee, 1980). The 'on treatment' analysis may well give a more extreme p value, although in the Canadian trial of aspirin it did not. Provided the two analyses point to the same conclusion, even if one is not formally statistically significant, then probably that conclusion is correct. Thus it follows that every patient must be followed until the end of the trial or prior death and every effort made to record all strokes, MIs, and deaths. This issue is further discussed by Sackett and Gent (1979) and May *et al.* (1981).

During a TIA trial it is probably as well to monitor the use of other drugs and co-interventions which might influence the end-point frequency, although usually there is no particular reason why most of them should not be given equally to each treatment group. For example, beta-blockers might influence MI incidence but would probably be given to each group equally unless the trial treatment influenced angina. The control of hypertension is unlikely to be systematically different between the treatment groups in a randomised trial, particularly if it is blind, but since hypertension is the most important treatable risk factor for stroke it should be monitored to look for any differences between treatment groups. Obviously one can make this sort of monitoring more and more complex, and thus more and more expensive, but probably only for marginal gain. The decision to monitor a co-intervention or prognostic variable during follow-up should depend on whether imbalance between treatment groups is likely, whether imbalance will make much difference to the outcome, and whether the collaborating neurologists are willing to provide the data.

Finally, more use should be made of 2×2 factorial designs as in the Canadian trial of aspirin and sulfinpyrazone (Canadian Cooperative Study Group, 1978). For the same number of patients, to compare 'treatment A' with placebo it is possible simultaneously to compare 'treatment A' with 'no treatment A' and 'treatment B' with 'no treatment B'. In addition, but with 50% of the sample size, such a design allows one to compare 'treatment A' alone, with 'treatment B' alone, with both together and with placebo. If treatments A and B interact, some of the advantages of the design will be lost but at least this very design will be the best way to detect any interaction if it exists. This design is not applicable if the two treatments are likely to be dangerous when given together (e.g. aspirin and anticoagulants), but is ideal for two treatments likely to act through different mechanisms such as carotid endarterectomy and an antihaemostatic drug.

DOCUMENTATION

However large, well designed and well defined the entry criteria and end-points, a randomised trial will fail if the patients and end-points are not documented reasonably accurately. These difficulties increase with increasing trial size and are magnified by increasing the number of trial centres which is so very necessary, even in quite common disorders like TIA.

Telephone randomisation (see above) is extraordinarily helpful since the trial office has an up-to-date file of all patients and can generate (by computer) lists of patients, alphabetically or chronologically at convenience, in the whole trial, in any one centre, or for any one individual collaborator. It is then an easy matter to compare centres with each other for various performance criteria, and to try to help or bully all centres into providing missing information or finding 'lost' patients. Each collaborator can be sent computerised lists of his patients, their treatment codes, dates of the next follow-up, and details of missing information.

In the UK, where notification and follow-up forms are usually completed by the collaborating neurologists (or more unreliably by their junior colleagues), it is very difficult to expect clinicians to handle long and complicated forms, and certainly not forms in a format ready for computer card punching (see tables A.4 and A.5, pp. 310–315). In North America, where large trials seem to be more often staffed by research nurses in each collaborating centre, this does not seem to be such a problem and the documentation is far more extensive than on my side of the Atlantic. The advantages of short simple forms, and ours are *very* short and simple, is that the trial need not depend on expensive research nurses and overall costs can be kept within reason. At randomisation it is not necessary to collect more than the patient's name, centre and date of birth along with any known prognostic variables and the nature of the qualifying event(s). At follow-up one needs to know only whether an end-point has been experienced, whether side-effects have been noted, whether potentially biasing co-interventions have been used, and the degree of compliance with drug treatment. Further information on end-points or interesting side-effects can then be collected retrospectively at leisure from hospital, general practitioner or post-mortem records and put together for a clinical audit committee. Information in excess of this minimum is tiresome and expensive to collect, attempts to do so may irritate the collaborators and thus prejudice adequate patient recruitment, and often it never gets analysed because it is as dull as it is incomplete.

FEASIBILITY

The final question is whether it is possible to organise large and usually multicentre, blind, randomised trials in well-defined yet representative TIA patients with clear and relevant end-points. The analysis is not difficult provided the problem of withdrawn patients is considered. Even if the trial is feasible, can it be done at reasonable cost? In my view to get a trial off the ground there are several criteria which must *all* be fulfilled:

(1) The therapeutic question must be clinically important enough to require an answer. If it is not, no one will agree to collaborate and even if they do they will soon lose interest and stop randomising patients.
(2) There must be a clinician organising the trial who has a long enough tenure (and is young enough) to see the trial through to the end, and who is prepared to devote time to it. It is probably helpful for the same person to randomise patients in the trial so as to experience the stresses and strains of following trial patients and filling in the documentation while attempting to do routine clinical practice at the same time.
(3) A full-time trial administrator is required who is probably not medically qualified since the skills needed are not clinical but in organisation, liaison and data management. There must be adequate secretarial and clerical support and this requirement will increase as the trial gets larger, as will the need for more space.
(4) A statistician who will devote time to the trial and whose grasp of clinical reality matches his or her understanding of statistical necessity. There must also be adequate computer and programmer support.

Other things may well be important and these include, in no particular order of preference:

(1) Annual, or if necessary more frequent, visits by the clinical co-ordinator and/or trial administrator to each centre to encourage collaboration, collect missing data, solve logistical problems, etc.
(2) An annual meeting of all the collaborators in a central and congenial place to discuss the ongoing results (even though the main treatment comparison may be concealed until the end), problems, end-points, grievances, and such like. This meeting should be scientifically interesting, educational and stimulating, and by it *esprit de corps* will be fostered. It is also an opportunity to have a break, meet old friends, and make new ones. We always try to give prizes to the 'best' performers, e.g. the collaborator with the lowest number of withdrawn patients or greatest proportion of complete forms.
(3) An easily accessible trials office. This should have a telephone independent of any hospital switchboard if the trial is multicentre, and an answer

phone is highly desirable. The office must be able to respond quickly and effectively to questions from the outlying centres.

(4) Medical, nursing, or secretarial help for those centres which are randomising, and therefore having to follow, large numbers of patients. This should ensure that entering a patient is not a chore but is no more, and maybe even less, work than is usually involved for a TIA patient in routine practice.

(5) Regular newsletters from the trial office to the collaborators to keep them in touch with developments and to disseminate information and instructions.

(6) Regular printouts of patients with follow-up dates sent to each collaborator.

(7) Simple but adequate documentation.

(8) Publication of the results as a group without any star billing for the main investigators.

(9) Most collaborators should be involved in the initial discussions on treatment options and protocol design. It may be undesirable to impose a protocol on collaborators, particularly if it has been written by a committee of people who are not themselves putting people into the trial.

Given these criteria it is inevitable that successful trials will be moderately expensive, particularly if one remembers the cost of computing, telephone, postage, printing, photocopying, travel expenses for the patients if necessary, compliance testing, and the medication and its packaging. However, the costs need not be as great as in some recent and current trials if one is prepared to make some compromises and use simple documentation. The UK-TIA Aspirin Trial and the North American Ticlopidine trial are about the same size and yet the former is costing about $1.1 million and the latter about $22 million. It is difficult to reconcile these two figures, and the difference cannot be attributed entirely to the more extensive collection of side-effect data which is necessary for Ticlopidine.

If trials become outrageously expensive, then national research agencies may be unwilling to fund them and the investigators will have to turn to the pharmaceutical industry which itself is becoming increasingly concerned at the expense of testing even patented compounds. There is then a danger that drugs will be tested only if they are of commercial interest, and this interest may not necessarily coincide with clinical or scientific interest. One wonders whether the proliferation of drug trials compared with the paucity of surgical trials is at least something to do with the availability of funds from the pharmaceutical industry for the former, and not entirely because surgeons have an ingrained resistance to the proper evaluation of their treatments. Of course, in a country like the UK, the cost of a trial to a government agency may be very worth while if the result shows no effect for a treatment which another government agency would have had to pay for if it became widely used. On the other hand, an effective low-cost treatment which reduces the risk of stroke could save a large sum of money which would otherwise have to be devoted to the care of the disabled.

CONCLUSION

There is no shortage of patients for TIA trials and the methodological and analytical techniques are well known, mostly uncontroversial, and — with computers — easily applied. The main difficulties are in working together to collect enough patients in a reasonable time in a well-organised and inexpensive fashion.

REFERENCES

Aspirin Myocardial Infarction Study Research Group (1980). A randomised, controlled trial of aspirin in persons recovered from myocardial infarction. *J. Am. Med. Assoc.*, **243**, 661–9.

Bousser, M. G., Eschwege, E., Haguenau, M., Lefauconnier, J. M., Thibult, N., Touboul, D. and Touboul, P. J. (1983). "AICLA" controlled trial of aspirin and dipyridamole in the secondary prevention of athero-thrombotic cerebral ischae-mia. *Stroke,* **14**, 5–14.

Canadian Cooperative Study Group (1978). A randomised trial of aspirin + sulphinpyrazone in threatened stroke. *New Engl. J. Med.,* **299**, 53–9.

Christie, D. (1979). Before-and-after comparisons: a cautionary tale. *Brit. Med. J.,* **4**, 1629.

Coronary Drug Project Research Group (1980). Influence of adherence to treatment and response of cholesterol on mortality in the coronary drug project. *New Engl. J. Med.,* **303**, 1038–41.

EC/IC Bypass Study Group (1985). Failure of EC/IC arterial bypass to reduce the risk of ischaemic stroke. Result of an international randomised trial. *New Engl. J. Med.,* **313**, 1191–1200.

European Coronary Surgery Study Group (1980). Prospective randomised study of coronary artery bypass surgery in stable angina pectoris. *Lancet,* **2**, 491–5.

Friedman, L. M., Furberg, C. D. and De Mets, D. L. (1981). *Fundamental of Clinical Trials*, John Wright, Boston.

Hampton, J. R. (1981). Presentation and analysis of the results of clinical trials in cardiovascular disease. *Brit. Med. J.,* **282**, 1371–3.

Heyden, S., Heiss, G., Heyman, A., Tyroler, A. H., Hames, C. G., Pazzschke, W. and Manegold, C. (1980). Cardiovascular mortality in transient ischaemic attacks. *Stroke,* **11**, 252–5.

Lee, K. L., McNeer, J. F., Starmer, C. F., Harris, P. J. and Rosati, R. A. (1980). Clinical judgment and statistics. Lessons from a simulated randomised trial in coronary artery disease. *Circulation,* **61**, 508–15.

McPherson, K. (1974). Statistics: the problem of examining accumulating data more than once. *New Engl. J. Med.,* **290**, 501–2.

McPherson, K. (1982). On choosing the number of interim analyses in clinical trials. *Statistics in Medicine*, **1**, 25–36.

McPherson, K. (1984). The evaluation of treatment. In Warlow, C. and Garfield, J. (eds), *Dilemmas in the Management of the Neurological Patient*. Churchill Livingstone, Edinburgh, pp. 277–85.

Management Committee (1980). The Australian therapeutic trial in mild hypertension. *Lancet*, **1**, 1261–7.

May, G. S., De Mets, D. L., Friedman, L. M., Furberg, C. and Passamani, E. (1981). The randomised clinical trial: bias in analysis. *Circulation*, **64**, 669–73.

Peto, R. (1982). Statistical aspects of cancer trials. In Halnan, K. E. (ed.), *Treatment of Cancer*, Chapman & Hall, London.

Peto, R. (1983). What treatments for rheumatoid arthritis can best be assessed by large, simple, long-term trials? *Brit. J. Rheumatol.*, **22** (Suppl.), 3–8.

Peto, R., Pike, M. C., Armitage, P., Breslow, N. E., Cox, D. R., Howard, S. V., Mantel, N., McPherson, K., Peto, J. and Smith, P. G. (1976). Design and analysis of randomised clinical trials requiring prolonged observation of each patient. 1. Introduction and design. *Brit. J. Cancer*, **34**, 585–612.

Peto, R., Pike, M. C., Armitage, P., Breslow, N. E., Cox, D. R., Howard, S. V., Mantel, N., McPherson, K., Peto, J. and Smith, P. G. (1977). Design and analysis of randomised clinical trials requiring prolonged observation of each patient. 2. Analysis and examples. *Brit. J. Cancer*, **35**, 1–39.

Pocock, S. J. (1977). Randomised clinical trials. *Brit. Med. J.*, **1**, 1661.

Ravid, M., Kleiman, N., Shapira, J., Lischner, M. and Feigl, D. (1980). Anticoagulant therapy in acute myocardial infarction: demonstration of a selection bias in a retrospective survey. *Thrombosis Research*, **18**, 753–7.

Sackett, D. L. (1978). The Canadian trial of aspirin and sulphinpyrazone in threatened stroke. *New Engl. J. Med.*, **299**, 955.

Sackett, D. L. and Gent, M. (1979). Controversy in counting and attributing events in clinical trials. *New Engl. J. Med.*, **301**, 1410–12.

Sacks, H., Chalmers, T. C. and Smith, H. (1982). Randomised versus historical controls for clinical trials. *Am. J. Med.*, **72**, 233–40.

Sørensen, P. S., Pedersen, H., Marquardsen, J., Petersson, H., Heltberg, A., Simonsen, N., Munck, O. and Andersen, L. A. (1983). Acetylsalicylic acid in the prevention of stroke in patients with reversible ischaemic attacks. *Stroke*, **14**, 15–22.

Sylvester, R. J., Pinedo, H. M., De Pauw, M., Staquet, M. J., Boyse, M. E., Renard, J. and Bonadonna, G. (1981). Quality of institutional participation in multicentre clinical trials. *New Engl. J. Med.*, **305**, 852–5.

Warlow, C. P. (1982). Transient ischaemic attacks. In Matthews, W. B. and Glaser, G. H. (eds), *Recent Advances in Clinical Neurology — 3*. Churchill Livingstone, Edinburgh.

Warlow, C. and Morris, P. J. (1982). *Transient Ischaemic Attacks*. Marcel Dekker, New York and Basel, p. ix

Whisnant, J. P., Matsumoto, N. and Elveback, L. R. (1973). Transient cerebral ischaemic attacks in a community. Rochester, Minnesota — 1955 through 1969. *Mayo Clin. proc.*, **48**, 194–8.

Wiebers, D. O. and Whisnant, J. P. (1982). Epidemiology. In Warlow, C. and Morris, P. J. (eds), *Transient Ischaemic Attacks*. Marcel Dekker, New York and Basel, pp. 1–19.

9
Methodology of clinical trials in stroke. Part I: Analysis of previous clinical trials

R. CAPILDEO and J. M. ORGOGOZO

INTRODUCTION

Since 1972, there have been at least 21 acute stroke trials reported in the English literature. Most of the trials have reported negative results, and even those trials reporting a positive result have not been confirmed by further investigators. This has led to a feeling of therapeutic nihilism in the acute treatment of the stroke patient which has led some authors to question whether stroke patients should even be admitted to hospital (Mulley and Arie, 1978). Dexamethasone and glycerol have been most commonly used. In animal experiments, both agents seemed promising, particularly if given *before* the ischaemic insult or immediately afterwards, within 1 hour. This experimental situation is totally artificial and does not relate to the human situation. It is exceptionally rare for a stroke patient to be admitted to hospital within 4 hours. In Europe and in the United States of America, 80% of stroke patients are admitted within 24 hours whereas the equivalent figure in the United Kingdom is about 40%.

It is generally accepted that these stroke trials have indicated a lack of efficacy of the therapeutic agent being tested. For example, in a review by Anderson and Crawford (1979) on corticosteroids in ischaemic stroke the authors conclude that 'most clinical evidence suggests that corticosteroids are not of benefit in ischaemic cerebral infarction'. Even more forcefully, after yet another negative study with steroids (this time using high-dose dexamethasone), Norris and Hachinski (1986) go still further: 'High dose steroid therapy was ineffective in ischaemic stroke and the data suggests that further evaluation by a larger multicentre trial is not justified.' Is this a fair conclusion?

In 1975 a leader in the *Lancet* reviewing the use of glycerol in acute cerebral infarction stated that: 'Further trials will be required in which

175

particular effort should be made to distinguish more precisely the type of lesion responsible for the stroke.' This statement is still true. Even in the very few studies so far reported in which CT scanning has been employed, investigators have still included brainstem strokes with hemisphere strokes (Strand *et al.*, 1984; Norris and Hachinski, 1986).

In reviewing previous acute stroke trials, what lessons can we learn from past experience when trying to design new acute stroke trials (see Chapter 10 by Orgogozo and Capildeo)?

METHOD OF REVIEW

The approach to this review has been to analyse each trial in turn according to 12 parameters:

(1) *Type of study*. This refers to whether the trial is 'open, single blind, double blind, randomised control, against placebo, etc.'.

(2) *Patient group*. 'Stroke', like 'anaemia', is not a specific disease entity. It can be defined but the definition does not separate out the different types of strokes (Capildeo *et al.*, 1977). However, having defined 'stroke', we must ask: 'Where is the lesion and what is the lesion?', i.e. the anatomical and pathological substrate; how the diagnosis was confirmed; what is the possible aetiology; severity of disability on admission and on subsequent assessment, etc. This information can be summarised and forms the basis of a new classification proposed by Capildeo *et al.* (1978).

(3) *Criteria of selection*. This depends upon definition of the patient group and the choice of investigations to confirm diagnosis in order to obtain a homogeneous patient group. The single most important investigation should be CT scanning and preferably serial CT scanning.

(4) *Number of patients assessed*. This figure indicates the degree of selection; for example, if 50 patients are assessed and all 50 patients are admitted to the trial, then no selection has taken place and the result of the trial is immediately open to doubt. If 55 patients are assessed and 50 patients are included, then the selection criteria may not be strict enough. If 500 patients are assessed and only 50 patients are included in the trial, then overselection will have taken place. Even if the result is 'positive', the question will be raised, 'But what about the other 450 patients? They are more like the patients we treat!'

(5) *Number admitted to trial*. Although authors may state the number of patients admitted to the trial, the analysis is invariably on fewer patients because of 'protocol violation', withdrawals, e.g. through complications of therapy, related or non-related concurrent illnesses,

etc. Ideally, the group of patients who do not complete the study should also be described accurately.

(6) *Time limit*. This refers to the period allowed in each trial between onset of stroke and initiation of therapy. It depends not only upon the agent and its supposed mode of action but also on those factors which may mean delay before patients are assessed or admitted to the trial.

(7) *Treatment groups*. This depends upon trial design. Even a large study, by having several treatment groups, may be inconclusive.

(8) *Judgement criteria*. Assessment methods are notoriously difficult to devise and carry out, hence the generalisation that there are 'as many methods available for assessing strokes as there are assessors'. Measurement of immediate outcome in terms of neurological recovery is quite different from assessment of functional recovery. Mortality and length of survival are far less important measures than type and degree of recovery in relation to quality of life. The final outcome in terms of discharge as well as the duration in hospital are some of the other parameters that have to be considered (see Chapter 10 by Orgogozo and Capildeo).

(9) *Duration of treatment*. This is a reflection in part on the type of medication being evaluated. It could explain (if all other parameters were comparable) why, although on the same medication, one treatment regime succeeds when another does not.

(10) *Duration of follow-up*. This can vary widely in different trials. It is important to know whether early successes are maintained or whether there are late complications.

(11) *Complications*. These should be clearly described not only in the treated group but also in the control group.

(12) *Authors' conclusions*. It is worth reviewing the authors' conclusions after analysing their paper according to the parameters suggested here. Many readers assume the summary to be 'fair comment' without further analysis.

In view of the small number of patients involved in these different studies (see tables 9.1–9.21), the merit of the authors' method for statistical analysis has not been included.

Table 9.1 'Double-blind study of the effects of dexamethasone on acute stroke' (Patten *et al.*, 1972).

1. Type of study	Double blind, dexamethasone versus placebo
2. Patient group	Acute stroke
3. Criteria of selection	Clinical (LP, EEG, isotope scan)
4. Number of patients assessed	38
5. Number admitted to trial	31
6. Time limit	Less than 24 h
7. Treatment groups	17 placebo/14 dexamethasone (16 mg daily for 10 days then 12 mg tapering over 7 days)
8. Judgement criteria	Global
9. Duration of treatment	17 days
10. Duration of follow-up	17 days
11. Complications	None reported

12. *Authors' conclusions*: steroid group improved their functional status during the treatment period an average of 12%, those on placebo got worse by 12%; severely affected patients (15) improved 23%, placebo worse by 14%; '. . . that dexamethasone can be a useful adjunct to the therapy of the patient with a severe stroke'.

Comments. This trial is frequently quoted but it can be criticised on the following seven points: (2) Patient group was not defined. (4) Number of patients assessed is too few. (5) Number admitted to trial is too small. (6) Treatment groups are not comparable — 3 cases of cerebral haemorrhage in the placebo group and 2 cases of brainstem infarction in the steroid group. (8) Global assessment method only used. (10) Duration of follow-up is too short. (12) Authors' conclusions are not tenable.

Table 9.2 'Double-blind evaluation of glycerol therapy in acute cerebral infarction' (Mathew *et al.*, 1972).

1. Type of study	Double blind, glycerol versus placebo
2. Patient group	Acute cerebral infarction
3. Criteria of selection	Clinical (LP, EEG, isotope scan)
4. Number of patients assessed	62
5. Number admitted to trial	54 cerebral infarction, 8 cerebral haemorrhage
6. Time limit	Less than 4 days
7. Treatment groups	25 placebo/29 glycerol (i.v. infusion 50 g glycerol in 500 ml 5% glucose in 25% physiological saline in 24 h)
8. Judgement criteria	Global
9. Duration of treatment	4–6 days
10. Duration of follow-up	14 days
11. Complications	None reported

12. *Authors' conclusions*: 'Patients with cerebral infarction treated with glycerol showed significant improvement in neurological status compared to patients treated with placebo.' 6 days' treatment with glycerol seemed better than 4 days. No benefit to patients with spontaneous intracerebral haemorrhage.

Comments. The following seven points can be criticised. (4) Number of patients assessed is too few. (5) All patients assessed were included in the trial. Adding 8 cerebral haemorrhage cases confuses the picture. (6) Time limit for inclusion is too long. (7) Placebo group received 5% glucose in 25% physiological saline. (8) Global assessment method only used. (1) Duration of follow-up is too short. (12) Authors' conclusions cannot be justified.

Table 9.3 'Dexamethasone as treatment in cerebrovascular disease. 1. A controlled study in intracerebral haemorrhage' (Tellez and Bauer, 1973).

1. Type of study	Double blind, dexamethasone versus placebo
2. Patient group	Cerebral haemorrhage
3. Criteria of selection	Clinical/CSF more than 200 RBCs
4. Number of patients assessed	42
5. Number admitted to trial	40
6. Time limit	Within 48 h
7. Treatment groups	21 placebo/19 dexamethasone (12 mg i.v. at onset; 4 mg i.m. 6-hourly, 3 days, then reducing, 120 mg given over 10 days)
8. Judgement criteria	Individual parameters/global
9. Duration of treatment	10 days
10. Duration of follow-up	14 days
11. Complications	GI bleeding: 2 patients in placebo-treated and 2 patients in dexamethasone-treated group

12. *Authors' conclusions*: Several parameters of the neurological examination showed an improved quality of survival in the dexamethasone treated group, but this was found only at certain days in the study. No overall statistically significant difference was found between the two therapies.'

Comments. The authors provide a lot of background data. The following four points can be criticised. (4) Number of patients assessed is too few. (5) Number admitted to trial is too small. (7) Treatment groups were not directly comparable — the control group was 'less ill'. (1) Duration of follow-up is too short.

Note. For 'level of consciousness' parameters, mean change from initial values for days 4, 6, 8, 10 and 14 gave statistically significantly better results with dexamethasone than with placebo.

Table 9.4 'Dexamethasone as treatment in cerebrovascular disease. 2. A controlled study in acute cerebral infarction' (Bauer and Tellez 1973).

1. Type of study	Double blind, dexamethasone versus placebo
2. Patient group	Acute cerebral infarction/brainstem infarction
3. Criteria of selection	Clinical/CSF findings
4. Number of patients assessed	54
5. Number admitted to trial	54
6. Time limit	Within 48 h
7. Treatment groups	26 placebo (includes 4 brainstem) 28 dexamethasone (as in table 9.3, 120 mg over 10 days)
8. Judgement criteria	Individual parameters/global
9. Duration of treatment	14 days
10. Duration of follow-up	14 days
11. Complications	GI bleeding: 2 in placebo-treated group only

12. *Authors' conclusions*: 'When comparison of patients with similar levels of consciousness was made, there was no significant difference between those patients receiving dexamethasone and those receiving placebo.'

Comments. Study was conducted in two parts. Part 1: 17 placebo and 20 dexamethasone-treated patients. Part 2 contained 9 placebo and 8 dexamethasone-treated patients. Part 2 was conducted because patient groups in Part 1 were dissimilar in terms of initial severity. This was not eliminated by the addition of Part 2. Analysis was based on Part 1 and Part 2 combined. The following four points can be criticised. (4) Number of patients assessed is too few. (5) All patients assessed were included in the trial. (7) Treatment groups were not comparable in terms of severity. (10) Duration of follow-up is too short.

Table 9.5 'Management of completed strokes with dextran 40. A community hospital failure' (Spudis *et al.*, 1973).

1. Type of study	Open study, randomised
2. Patient group	'So-called completed stroke'
3. Criteria of selection	Clinical/CSF findings
4. Number of patients assessed	167
5. Number admitted to trial	59
6. Time limit	Less than 24 h
7. Treatment groups	29 controls/30 dextran (500 cc low molecular weight, in 10% glucose water: 1 h, loading dose: 1000 cc each 24 h for 3 days)
8. Judgement criteria	Individual parameters
9. Duration of treatment	3 days
10. Duration of follow-up	3 weeks
11. Complications	1 dextran-treated patient, severe flushing and apnoea 5–8 min after dextran given (eliminated from study)

12. *Authors' conclusions*: 'A greater percentage of dextran-treated patients improved with respect to consciousness and strength in upper and lower extremities, but showed less restoration of language than untreated patients. The differences in the two groups were not significant.'

Comments. The study covers a 3-year period. Assessment on admission 1 week and 3 weeks by each author in turn: inter-author reliability 'was felt to be good'; no data presented to confirm this. Patient groups smaller than anticipated: of 78 patients rejected, 36 improved spontaneously, 12 had cardiac arrhythmia, etc. The trial can be criticised on the following four points: (1) It is an open study. (2) The patient group is not accurately defined. (8) Assessments done by different observers at different times. (9) Duration of follow-up is too short.

Table 9.6 'High-dosage dexamethasone in treatment of strokes in the elderly' (Wright, 1974).

1. Type of study	Open study
2. Patient group	'Stroke in the elderly' (age: 61 to 94 years; average 77 years)
3. Criteria of selection	Clinical
4. Number of patients assessed	247
5. Number admitted to trial	61
6. Time limit	Less than 7 days
7. Treatment groups	186 controls/61 dexamethasone (30 cases 4 mg q.d.s. for 3 days; 31 cases, for 7 days)
8. Judgement criteria	Discharges/long-stay hospitals/deaths
9. Duration of treatment	3–7 days
10. Duration of follow-up	3 months
11. Complications	None

12. *Author's conclusions*: in the dosage and duration used on early elderly stroke cases admitted to hospital 'one cannot expect to achieve any significant beneficial difference in the ultimate outcome'.

Comments. The study covers a 4-year period. This trial can be criticised on the following seven points: (1) It is an open study. (2) The patient group is not accurately defined. (6) The time limit for inclusion is too long. (7) The treatment groups are not strictly comparable since dexamethasone-treated patients (admitted under the author) on one ward were compared with those from other wards. (8) Assessments were made only in terms of disposal or death. (9) Duration of treatment may have been too short. (1) Duration of follow-up is too short.

Table 9.7 'Controlled trial of glycerol versus dexamethasone in the treatment of cerebral oedema in acute cerebral infarction' (Gilsanz *et al.*, 1975).

1. Type of study	Controlled, randomised
2. Patient group	Acute cerebral infarction
3. Criteria of selection	Clinical (LP/isotope scan)
4. Number of patients assessed	Not specified
5. Number admitted to trial	68 (61 cerebral infarction, 7 cerebral haemorrhage)
6. Time limit	Within 36 h
7. Treatment groups	30 glycerol (10% glycerol in saline i.v. 500 ml in 24 h)/31 dexamethasone (4 mg 6-hourly i.m. 6 days). Modified from Mathew *et al.* (table 9.2)
8. Judgement criteria	Global
9. Duration of treatment	6 days
10. Duration of follow-up	15 days
11. Complications	GI haemorrhage: 1 case receiving dexamethasone; 2 cases of local thrombophlebitis and 1 of haemoglobinuria with renal failure and death, in glycerol-treated group.

12. *Authors' conclusions*: 'Improvement was significantly greater in the glycerol group after 8 and 15 days. No improvement was noted using either glycerol or dexamethasone in 7 patients with spontaneous intracerebral haemorrhage.'

Comments. The seven intracerebral haemorrhage cases confuse the study. They were excluded from the analysis but not the summary. This trial can be criticised on the following points: (1) It is an open study. (4) Number of patients assessed is not specified. (8) Global assessment method only used. (10) Duration of follow-up is too short. (12) Authors' conclusions are untenable.

Table 9.8 'Combined dexamethasone and low-molecular-weight dextran in acute cerebral infarction: double-blind study' (Kaste *et al.*, 1976).

1. Type of study	Double blind, dexamethasone and dextran 40 against placebo
2. Patient group	Acute cerebral infarction
3. Criteria of selection	Clinical/CSF findings (isotope scan)
4. Number of patients assessed	Not specified
5. Number admitted to trial	40
6. Time limit	24–48 h
7. Treatment groups	20 placebo/20 active (dexamethasone, 10 mg i.m. at onset, 5 mg 6-hourly for 7 days, tapering to zero over 7 days, total 215 mg; dextran 40, 500 ml i.v. 1–2 h, 500 ml/12 h for 72 h)
8. Judgement criteria	Global
9. Duration of treatment	14 days
10. Duration of follow-up	29 days
11. Complications	1 patient in active treatment group, psychotic episode at 3 days

12. *Authors' conclusions*: 'There were no differences in mortality or in improvement of the neurological or mobility scores between the 2 groups.'

Comments. Patients were admitted after 24 h (to exclude transient ischaemic attacks). This trial can be criticised on the following five points: (4) Number of patients assessed is not specified. (5) Number of patients admitted is too small. (7) Placebo group received 9% saline in place of dexamethasone and 10% glucose in place of dextran 40. (8) Global assessment method only used. (10) Duration of follow-up is too short.

Table 9.9 'Controlled trial of intravenous aminophylline in acute cerebral infarction' (Geismar *et al.*, 1976).

1. Type of study	Double blind, aminophylline versus placebo
2. Patient group	Acute cerebral infarction
3. Criteria of selection	Clinical (LP)
4. Number of patients assessed	Not specified
5. Number admitted to trial	79
6. Time limit	Less than 4 days
7. Treatment groups	39 placebo/40 aminophylline (10 ml 2% solution in saline, on admission, 3 h and 6 h)
8. Judgement criteria	Global
9. Duration of treatment	Less than 24 h
10. Duration of follow-up	3 weeks
11. Complications	None

12. *Authors' conclusions*: 'Intravenous aminophylline in patients with ischaemic strokes can bring about an immediate symptomatic relief, but without appreciably influencing the ultimate recovery.'

Comments. The assessor did not witness administration of treatments. This trial can be criticised on the following five points: (4) Number of patients assessed is not specified. (5) Time limit for inclusion is too long. (8) Global assessment method only used. (9) Duration of treatment is too short. (10) Duration of follow-up is too short.

Table 9.10 'Double-blind trial of glycerol therapy in early stroke' (Larsson *et al.*, 1976)

1. Type of study	Double blind, intravenous glycerol and intravenous dextrose
2. Patient group	'Early stroke'
3. Criteria of selection	Clinical
4. Number of patients assessed	Not specified
5. Number admitted to trial	27
6. Time limit	Less than 6 h
7. Treatment groups	15 dextrose/12 glycerol (500 ml over 6 h, on consecutive days, either 10% dextrose or 10% glycerol in 5% dextrose)
8. Judgement criteria	Global
9. Duration of treatment	6 days
10. Duration of follow-up	10 days
11. Complications	None reported

12. *Authors' conclusions*: 'There was no difference in mortality or in improvement in neurological score between the 2 groups.'

Comments. This was an attempt to treat stroke patients as soon as possible. This trial can be criticised on the following six points: (2) Patient group was not defined as accurately as possible even after treatment was started. At post mortem, 5 patients were found to have massive cerebral haemorrhage and 2 patients had acute myocardial infarction. A further 2 patients had gross blood-staining of the CSF. (4) Number of patients assessed is not specified. (5) Number of patients admitted to the trial is too few, particularly since patient group is heterogeneous. (8) Global assessment method only used. (10) Duration of follow-up is too short. (12) Authors' conclusions are untenable.

Table 9.11 'A blind-controlled trial of dextran 40 in the treatment of ischaemic stroke' (Matthews *et al.*, 1976).

1. Type of study	'Blind controlled', dextran 40 versus placebo
2. Patient group	'Ischaemic stroke'
3. Criteria of selection	Clinical/CSF findings
4. Number of patients assessed	Not specified
5. Number admitted to trial	100
6. Time limit	Less than 48 h
7. Treatment groups	48 placebo/52 dextran 40 (includes 7 brainstem strokes in each group)
8. Judgement criteria	Individual parameters
9. Duration of treatment	3 days
10. Duration of follow-up	6 months
11. Complications	None reported

12. *Authors' conclusions*: 'In the treated group mortality in the acute stage in patients with severe strokes was significantly reduced but survivors were severely disabled and 6 months later no significant benefit could be detected. In less severe strokes no effect of treatment was found.'

Comments. This trial was important in that it showed that the duration of follow-up should be for at least 6 months. It can be criticised on the following 4 points. (1) The study was probably 'single blind'. (4) Number of patients assessed was not specified. (7) The inclusion of 14 brainstem strokes confuses the overall picture. (9) Duration of treatment is probably too short.

Table 9.12 'Steroid therapy in acute cerebral infarction' (Norris 1976).

1. Type of study	Double blind, dexamethasone versus placebo
2. Patient group	Acute cerebral infarction
3. Criteria of selection	Clinical (LP, isotope scan)
4. Number of patients assessed	Not specified
5. Number admitted to trial	53 completed
6. Time limit	Less than 24 h
7. Treatment groups	27 placebo/26 dexamethasone (8 mg bolus, 4 mg 6-hourly, then decreased, total dose 140 mg)
8. Judgement criteria	Global assessment
9. Duration of treatment	12 days
10. Duration of follow-up	29 days
11. Complications	GI bleeding: 3 patients in dexamethasone group and 1 in placebo group. 'Serious exacerbations of mild diabetes'; 4 patients with serious infections (2 died pneumonia, 1 staphylococcal septicaemia, 1 brain abscess) in steroid group. None in placebo group.

12. *Author's conclusions*: '41 patients survived for longer than 28 days and patients treated with steroid fared slightly worse than those treated with placebo at the end of this time.'

Comments. This trial can be criticised on the following points: (4) Number of patients assessed is not specified, only the number completing the trial. (7) Method of giving dexamethasone not indicated. (8) Global assessment method only employed. (10) Duration of follow-up is too short. (11) More details should have been given concerning side-effects in the steriod group, 7 out of 26 cases specified and an unspecified number of 'severe exacerbations of mild diabetes'. (12) In the author's comment '. . . Bauer and Tellez and Tellez and Bauer noted an increased incidence of gastrointestinal haemorrhage similar to this present series. . .'. However, see Tables 9.3 and 9.4 for facts.

Table 9.13 'New approach to treatment of recent stroke' (Admani, 1978).

1. Type of study	Double blind, naftidrofuryl vs placebo
2. Patient group	'Acute stroke'
3. Criteria of selection	Clinical
4. Number of patients assessed	Not specified
5. Number admitted to trial	91
6. Time limit	1–10 days
7. Treatment groups	44 placebo/47 naftidrofuryl (200 mg t.d.s. for 4 weeks, 100 mg t.d.s. for 8 weeks)
8. Judgement criteria	Global
9. Duration of treatment	12 weeks
10. Duration of follow-up	12 weeks
11. Complications	Minor side-effects in 5 of the naftidrofuryl-treated patients and 1 of controls (not specified)

12. *Author's conclusions*: 'Both treatment groups greatly improved over the 12 weeks but the naftidrofuryl-treated patients made greater neurological progress, . . . spent only half as long in hospital as the controls, and deaths attributable to stroke were significantly fewer.'

Comments. This trial can be criticised on the following points. (2) The patient group is not accurately defined. (4) Number of patients assessed is not specified. (6) The time limit is far too broad. (8) Global assessment method only used. (10) Duration of follow-up is too short. (11) Complications are not specified. (12) Author's conclusion is untenable (see Steiner *et al.*, 1979).

Table 9.14 'Intravenous glycerol in cerebral infarction: a controlled 4-month trial' (Fawer *et al.*, 1978).

1. Type of study	Double blind, glycerol vs placebo
2. Patient group	Cerebral infarction
3. Criteria of selection	Clinical/CSF findings (EEG, isotope scan)
4. Number of patients assessed	64
5. Number admitted to trial	51
6. Time limit	Less than 48 h
7. Treatment groups	25 placebo/26 glycerol (25 g in 5% glucose and 9% saline, i.v., b.d.)
8. Judgement criteria	Individual parameters
9. Duration of treatment	6 days
10. Duration of follow-up	4 months
11. Complications	None

12. *Authors' conclusions*: 'Glycerol significantly improved global performances and motor and sensory functions in patients with moderate disability, but its effect on global performances was transient. Patients with severe disability were not improved at all.'

Comments. Although these authors have studied more than 50 patients, in a double-blind, randomised trial comparing treatment against placebo, assessing individual parameters and following patients for 4 months, they were unable to control 'the use of anticoagulants and agents which reduce platelet aggregation'. With these patients excluded, the data could not be analysed. Although stating that 'these patients were evenly distributed in the control and the glycerol groups', no details are offered to support this. It is not therefore possible to say if glycerol was better than placebo since the other drugs used might have affected the outcome. Note also authors' conclusions.

Table 9.15 'Dexamethasone in acute stroke' (Mulley *et al.*, 1978).

1. Type of study	Double blind, dexamethasone versus placebo
2. Patient group	Acute stroke
3. Criteria of selection	Clinical/CSF findings
4. Number of patients assessed	256
5. Number admitted to trial	118
6. Time limit	Less than 48 h
7. Treatment groups	57 placebo/61 dexamethasone (4.2 mg 6 hourly i.m., 10 days, 8-hourly day 11, 12-hourly day 12 and 13, single dose day 14)
8. Judgement criteria	Various parameters (mortality, morbidity, etc.)
9. Duration of treatment	14 days
10. Duration of follow-up	12 months
11. Complications	1 patient on dexamethasone developed tuberculosis

12. *Authors' conclusions*: 'At one year there was no significant difference in the number of survivors or in the quality of life between the 2 groups. The results suggest that there is no indication for the routine administration of dexamethasone to a heterogeneous group of patients with stroke.'

Comments. The main criticism, in an otherwise well-executed trial, was that (2) the patient group was not adequately defined. The authors' conclusion that 'dexamethasone is not indicated for a heterogeneous group of patients with stroke' is probably true. The trial should have been directed towards identifying patient groups that might benefit from dexamethasone. Hence it is a vital prerequisite to define the patient group as accurately as possible from the outset. The trial gives excellent background data and discusses patients assessed and not included and withdrawals from the trial.

Table 9.16 'Is there a real treatment for stroke? Clinical and statistical comparison of different treatments in 300 patients' (Santambrogio *et al.*, 1978).

1. Type of study	Randomised, comparative
2. Patient group	Stroke
3. Criteria of selection	Clinical
4. Number of patients assessed	300
5. Number admitted to trial	166
6. Time limit	Less than 24 h
7. Treatment groups	33 hydergine/34 dexamethasone/28 mannitol/32 placebo
8. Judgement criteria	Global
9. Duration of treatment	10 days
10. Duration of follow-up	10 days
11. Complications	Not stated

12. *Authors' conclusions*: 'No statistically significant difference emerged among any of the treatment groups and the reference group in terms of objective therapeutic results.'

Comments. The trial can be criticised on the following six points: (1) It is an open study. (2) The patient group is not accurately defined. It included '241 diagnosed as ischaemic stroke, 189 in the carotid artery territory, 40 in the vertebrobasilar territory'. In 12 classification was uncertain. (7) Despite the large number of patients assessed, the effect of having 3 treatment groups and 1 placebo control group is that small numbers of patients are being compared and (not surprisingly) no significant difference has been found. (8) Global assessment method only used. (10) Duration of follow-up is too short. (12) The trial did not achieve what it set out to achieve, and the conclusion is untenable.

Table 9.17 'The effect of ornithine alpha-ketoglutorate in stroke' (Woollard *et al.*, 1978).

1. Type of study	Double blind, ornithine alpha-ketoglutorate (OAKG) versus placebo
2. Patient group	Acute stroke
3. Criteria of selection	Clinical
4. Number of patients assessed	50
5. Number admitted to trial	45
6. Time limit	Within 96 h
7. Treatment groups	23 placebo/22 OAKG (25 g OAKG in 5000 ml, 5% dextrose i.v. infusion)
8. Judgement criteria	Global/individual parameters
9. Duration of treatment	5 days
10. Duration of follow-up	10 days
11. Complications	None

12. *Authors' conclusions*: 'Significant improvement was found in patients treated with OAKG when examined on the fifth day of therapy as compared to their control cases . . . at 10 days, no differences.'

Comments. The trial can be criticised on the following six points: (2) The patient group is not accurately defined. (4) Number of patients assessed is too few. (5) Number of patients admitted to trial is too small. (6) Time limit for inclusion is too long. (9) Duration of treatment is probably too short. (10) Duration of follow-up is too short.

Table 9.18 'Association of glycerol to dexamethasone in treatment of stroke patients' (Albizzati *et al.*, 1979).

1. Type of study	Randomised, 2 treatment groups: hypertonic glycerol + dexamethasone versus dexamethasone. Open study
2. Patient group	All types of stroke
3. Criteria of selection	Clinical (some EEG, CT scan)
4. Number of patients assessed	123
5. Number admitted to trial	93
6. Time limit	24 h
7. Treatment groups	46 (G & D) group, 47 dexamethasone
8. Judgement criteria	Neurological score/coma scale/disability
9. Duration of treatment	7 days
10. Duration of follow-up	30 days
11. Complications	Non-reported

12. *Authors' conclusions*: no difference between 2 treatments on survival rates and quality of survival at 7 and 30 days post-stroke.

Comments. Patients recruited over 6- or 7-month period. Number who had EEG or CT scan not specified. The following three points can be criticised: (1) Open study. (2) All types of stroke patients included. Although a lot of statistics employed, 'raw data' not given. Since 'all types of strokes' included, (5) numbers were too small.

Table 9.19 'Lack of effect of theophylline on the outcome of acute cerebral infarction' (Britton *et al.*, 1980).

1. Type of study	Double blind, aminophylline versus placebo
2. Patient group	Acute cerebral infarction
3. Criteria of selection	Clinical/CSF
4. Number of patients assessed	Not specified
5. Number admitted to trial	46
6. Time limit	50% within 24 h, range 18-114 h
7. Treatment groups	22 treated, 24 placebo. Treatment = bolus dose/infusion
8. Judgement criteria	2 neurological scores (after Mathew *et al.*, 1972; Geismar *et al.*, 1976)
9. Duration of treatment	3 days
10. Duration of follow-up	Until hospital discharge (average 3 weeks)
11. Complications	No serious side-effects

12. *Authors' conclusions*: No significant difference in outcome between the 2 groups

Comments. The following points can be criticised: (2) Patient group not really confirmed by (3). (4) Number of patients assessed not specified, and (5) number admitted was too small. (8) Results are given on global neurological scores.

Table 9.20   'A randomised controlled trial of haemodilution therapy in acute ischaemic stroke' (Strand *et al.*, 1984).

1. Type of study	Randomised, controlled 'blind' assessor. Haemodilution group (venesection + dextron 40) versus non-treated controls
2. Patient group	Acute ischaemic stroke
3. Criteria of selection	Clinical, CSF (CT scan later)
4. Number of patients assessed	109
5. Number admitted to trial	102
6. Time limit	Within 48 h
7. Treatment groups	52 treated, 50 controls
8. Judgement criteria	Neurological score (after Mathew *et al.*, 1976)
9. Duration of treatment	6 days
10. Duration of follow-up	3 months
11. Complications	2 patients receiving haemodilution: anaphylactoid reactions.

12. *Authors' conclusions*: 85% treated group improved in neurological scoring over first 10 days, compared with 64% in control group ($p < 0.025$); unable to walk at 3 months = 8% in treated group and 31% of control; hospitalisation at 3 months = 13% versus 39% in control ($p < 0.01$).

Comments. The following three points can be criticised: (1) Control group was 'no-treatment group'. (2) Patient group contained hemisphere and brainstem strokes. (3) Although CT scanning used, insufficient information on numbers scanned at 0–3 days or 'up to 3 weeks'. Haemodilution achieved by venesection and dextron 40 administration.

Table 9.21 'High-dose steroid treatment in cerebral infarction' (Norris and Hachinski, 1986).

1. Type of study	Double blind, dexamethasone versus placcbo
2. Patient group	Acute cerebral infarction
3. Criteria of selection	Clinical/CT scanning
4. Number of patients assessed	270
5. Number admitted to trial	113 (13 subsequently withdrawn)
6. Time limit	Up to 48 h
7. Treatment groups	54 patients dexamethasone = total 480 mg over 12 days. 59 control
8. Judgement criteria	Toronto stroke scoring system
9. Duration of treatment	12 days
10. Duration of follow-up	21 days
11. Complications	Diabetes (4 cases) in treated group. 4 cases infection placebo (0 in steroid group) and GI bleeding similar 3:2. 13 patients withdrawn = 7 steroid and 6 placebo

12. *Authors' conclusions*: high-dose steroid therapy was ineffective in ischaemic stroke and the data suggest further evaluation by a larger multicentre trial is not justified

Comments. The following points can be criticised: (2) Although 'cerebral infarction' specified, 4 patients with brainstem strokes included. (3) Although CT scanning was used, no details given. (1) Authors argue that this is an acute study — therefore outcome, e.g. at one year, not relevant. (12) Conclusions are 'debatable'. Authors appear to have shown less coning in patients who died having received steroid therapy (7 cases) compared with the controls (12 cases).

DISCUSSION

Defining the patient group

Of the 21 studies reviewed, only 12 attempted to define the patient group. The studies of Matthews *et al.* (1976) and Strand *et al.* (1984) were on 'ischaemic stroke' although in the latter study CT scanning was used. Tellez and Bauer (1973) reported on a controlled trial in intracerebral haemorrhage, the only trial reported on this subject. The other 10 trials defined their patients as having had an 'acute cerebral infarction'.

It is important to note that eight trials made no attempt to define their patient group. All stroke patients were included, i.e. the infarction or haemorrhage cases, the lesion being either in the left or right hemisphere or in the brainstem. The trial by Patten *et al.* (1972) clearly demonstrates this type of bias (Capildeo and Rose, 1979). It would be equally illogical to do a trial on 'brain tumours' pretending that all types of brain tumour are the same with a similar natural history and prognosis and would respond similarly to treatment.

How was the patient group defined?

In nine trials, stroke was defined primarily on clinical grounds. Therefore cerebral infarction could not have been distinguished from cerebral haemorrhage or even cerebral tumour with any degree of certainty.

In seven trials, cerebrospinal fluid examination was carried out to confirm the diagnosis, and in the other five studies, technetium scans were also performed.

Although two trials (Strand *et al.*, 1984; Norris and Hachinski, 1986) use CT scanning to define their patient group, little detail is given as to when CT scanning was actually performed. Although the trialists excluded cerebral haemorrhage, brainstem strokes were included. No analysis was made of those patients who had a 'normal' CT scan despite clinical evidence of stroke as opposed to patients who had definite areas of infarction in the brain within the presumed territory affected according to the pattern of neurological deficit. In particular the study by Norris and Hachinski (1986) did not comment on the appearance on the CT scan of cerebral swelling since this study was specifically looking at the effect of high-dose dexamethasone as an anti-oedema agent in the acute phase following stroke. In this trial, patients who died were investigated at post-mortem for evidence of coning, and there appeared a significant difference in that coning seemed to be twice as common in placebo-treated patients as opposed to the dexamethasone-treated patients although the total number of deaths in the two groups was the same.

Number of patients assessed

What is the correct ratio of 'number of patients assessed to number of patients included in the trial'? This cannot be answered simply. It really does depend upon the patient group being studied, i.e. we come back to the definition of the patient group. If the trial is on acute cerebral infarction, which compromises approximately 80% of all stroke cases, in order to get 80 cases in the trial it may be necessary to screen 200–240 cases on the premiss that there will be 160–180 cases of cerebral infarction and that less than 50% will be eligible for the trial. If the trial is on acute cerebral haemorrhage, which comprises approximately 20% of all stroke cases, in order to get 80 cases in the trial it may be necessary to screen four times the number required for acute cerebral infarction, i.e. 800–960 cases. These numbers suggest that future stroke trials should be multicentre despite the additional problems that these types of study cause.

In a trial reported by Wright (1974), 61 patients were selected from 247 patients screened. In the study by Norris and Hachinski (1986), 270 patients were assessed and 113 were included in the trial. Because of complications 13 patients were subsequently withdrawn, leaving 100 patients for eventual analysis.

Most trials do not give the possible number of patients, i.e. the number of patients with presumed stroke admitted during the trial period. This number is important because it indicates that a degree of selection has been made. Again, if these patients could be followed up in the same way as those patients in the trial, it certainly would enhance the study.

Trial design

Of the trials reviewed, 14 were double blind against placebo. The trial by Matthews *et al.* (1976) was called a 'blind-controlled trial against placebo' by the authors, possibly meaning a single-blind study. One trial was uncontrolled (Wright, 1974) and five were randomised trials with either open controls or controls not receiving treatment. Since there is 'no proven therapy' for the treatment of acute stroke, trials should be double blind, comparing the active agent against placebo.

Ten trials have used dexamethasone. The study by Gilsanz *et al.* (1975) compared dexamethasone against glycerol and reported a favourable result for glycerol. The trial by Albizzati *et al.* (1979) compared glycerol and dexamethasone against dexamethasone. This apparently was a negative study. Patten *et al.* (1972) was the only trial reporting a favourable response to dexamethasone, but this study has already been criticised on methodological grounds. Santambrogio *et al.* (1978) compared a placebo group against three treatment groups: dexamethasone, hydergine and mannitol. This was an open, randomised trial and hence seriously liable to bias. The trial by Kaste *et al.* (1976) combined dexamethasone with dextran 40 against placebo, treatment being started after 24 hours 'to exclude transient ischaemic attacks'.

Four trials have assessed glycerol against placebo. It can be argued that the intravenous use of glucose or dextrose as placebo in three studies

(Mathew *et al.*, 1972; Larsson *et al.*, 1976; Fawer *et al.*, 1978) may have affected the outcome. The results were not conclusive. The trial by Larsson *et al.* (1976) is exceptional in that treatment was attempted within 6 hours of the onset of stroke.

Three trials have assessed dextran 40 (Spudis *et al.*, 1973; Kaste *et al.*, 1976; Matthews *et al.*, 1976) and one study has used dextran 40 as part of haemodilution therapy (Strand *et al.*, 1984). The study by Matthews *et al.* (1976) showed a lower mortality in the acute stage in patients with severe stroke treated with dextran 40 but survivors were severely disabled at 6 months with no significant benefit found. In less severe strokes no benefit was found. This study would seem to indicate that follow-up after acute stroke should be for at least 6 months. The study from Strand *et al.* (1984) was a positive result in favour of the patients' receiving haemodilution therapy. Although an overall neurological scoring system was used to indicate improvement in the treatment group, at 3 months treated patients were significantly better in terms of walking and far fewer patients were hospitalised at 3 months in the treated compared with the control groups (13% as against 39%).

Other agents that have been tried include aminophylline (Geismar *et al.*, 1976; Britton *et al.*, 1980), naftidrofuryl (Admani, 1978; Steiner, 1987), hydergine and mannitol (Santambrogio *et al.*, 1978) and ornithine ketoglutarate (Woollard *et al.*, 1978). The study by Admani (1978) has been severely criticised on methodological grounds (Steiner *et al.*, 1979).

The major problem in design revolves around the time limit for admission to the trial and for the initiation of treatment. This clearly depends upon the action of the agent being used, i.e. whether treatment must be given as soon as possible or whether delayed treatment may still be efficacious. Of the 21 trials reviewed, only the trial by Larsson *et al.* (1976) initiated treatment within 6 hours. Admani (1978) included patients up to 10 days after the ictus. Seven studies included patients admitted within 24 hours only and three studies included patients after 24 hours to exclude a transient ischaemic attack, since this is defined as 'an acute disturbance of cerebral function of vascular origin causing disability lasting less than 24 hours'. This suggests that one must wait until 24 hours have elapsed before initiating treatment to see whether the disability completely resolves. There is seldom a need to do this in practice. Treatment can be initiated as soon as possible and patients recovering within 24 hours will have to be excluded from subsequent analysis of the acute stroke trial, i.e. secondary exclusion. However, providing there are comparable groups from the outset, the rate of early recovery between active and placebo-treated patient groups can still be compared and might provide valuable information concerning initiation of early treatment. Seventeen trials initiated treatment within 48 hours and four included patients after 48 hours.

Randomisation cannot be expected to be able to match patients adequately, as can be seen by the trial reported by Bauer and Tellez (1973) where patient groups were never comparable even when the number of patients was extended from 37 to 54 trial patients. A self-randomisation plan has been described by Nordle and Brantmark (1977) and adapted for acute stroke trials by Capildeo and Rose (1978). It may be necessary in the future to match patients according to CT scan appearances.

Duration of treatment

This depends upon the actions of the therapeutic agent being tested. Seven of the trials gave treatment for only 7 days. Regimes varied widely between trials.

Judgement criteria

There is little agreement in any of the trials as to how best to assess the patient's progress. Our main objective is to measure disability in the survivors, in terms of the activities of daily living. The problems of assessment are considerable (Capildeo and Rose, 1979). Fourteen of the trials used a global assessment, basically a total score made up of a series of subsets, each subset being the invention of each trialist. This method is statistically unsound since it assumes that each parameter has equal weighting. Even for those methods that include some form of weighting system, it must be noted that, although it may have been validated in one particular centre, so far these systems have not been completely reproducible in other centres.

It can be argued that individual parameters should be evaluated independently. There is a greater chance that over time a difference could be shown that is due entirely to chance if a large number of different parameters are assessed, hence the need to decide on the important parameters to assess; providing the number is small, these parameters should be assessed and evaluated independently.

One trial measured outcome in terms of disposal, i.e. discharges, deaths, referral to a long-stay institution (Wright, 1974). The length of assessment and follow-up is important, particularly if the conclusion of Matthews *et al.* (1976) is confirmed. Norris and Hachinski (1986) argue that outcome at 1 year is influenced by a lot of other factors independent of the acute stroke illness, for example heart disease, and therefore may not be relevant in a study which is aimed at looking at acute therapy. Most trials assess patients for only 4 weeks. There is very little information as to how long trials took to complete. The trial carried out by Spudis *et al.* (1973) took 3 years; Admani (1978) took 16 months; Mulley *et al.* (1978) took 13 months and Albizzati *et al.* (1979) managed to recruit 93 patients in 6 or 7 months.

SUMMARY

So far, no multicentre trial has been reported. Although CT scanning has been available for 10 years, very few trials have been reported using CT scanning to define the patient group and also for stratification when it comes to the randomisation of patients. No working party has been set up to standardise methods for assessing the acute stroke patient. A new classification of stroke may help towards this aim (Capildeo *et al.*, 1977, 1978). There needs to be a basic agreement as to the major problems in designing acute stroke trials, and it is hoped that there may be moves towards this in the near future.

Of the trials included in this analysis, only four have attempted to:

(1) define the patient group;
(2) perform a double-blind controlled study comparing active agent against placebo;
(3) initiate treatment within 48 hours;
(4) include over 50 patients in the study.

Three of the trials have been previously criticised (Bauer and Tellez, 1973; Matthews *et al.*, 1976; Norris, 1976). The best trial to date happens to be the latest study from Norris and Hachinski, and it is hoped that this study will stimulate other workers in the field.

Since there are pathological problems with all the trials previously reviewed, it follows that no claim can be made as to the efficacy or lack of it of any therapeutic regime that has been tried to date. That is, it is not a question of 'no therapy in acute stroke'; it is that the trials themselves have not been designed to provide an answer.

REFERENCES

Admani, A. K. (1978). New approach to treatment of recent stroke. *Brit. Med. J.*, **2**, 1678–9.
Albizzati, M. G., Candelise, L., Capitani, E., Colombo, A. and Spinnler, H. (1979). Association of glycerol to dexamethasone in treatment of stroke patients. *Acta Neurol. Scand.*, **60**, 77–84.
Anderson, D. C. and Crawford, R. G. (1979). Current concepts of cerebrovascular disease. Stroke: corticosteroids in ischaemic stroke. *Stroke*, **10**, 68–71.
Bauer, R. B. and Tellez, H. (1973). Dexamethasone as treatment in cerebrovascular disease. 2. A controlled study in acute cerebral infarction. *Stroke*, **4**, 547–55.
Britton, M., Faire, V. de, Helmers, C., Miah, K. and Rane, A. (1980). Lack of effect of theophylline on the outcome of acute cerebral infarction. *Acta Neurol. Scand.*, **62**, 116–23.

Capildeo, R. and Rose, F. C. (1978). The design of an acute stroke trial. In Jukes, A. M. (ed.), *Baclofen: Spasticity and Cerebral Pathology*. Cambridge Medical Publications, Northampton, pp. 85–94.

Capildeo, R. and Rose, F. C. (1979). The assessment of neurological disability. In Greenhalgh, R. M. and Rose, F. C. (eds), *Progress in Stroke Research 1*. Pitman Medical, Tunbridge Wells, pp. 106–16.

Capildeo, R., Haberman, S. and Rose, F. C. (1977). New classification of stroke: preliminary communication. *Brit. Med. J.*, **2**, 1578–80.

Capildeo, R., Haberman, S. and Rose, F. C. (1978). New classification of stroke. *Quart. J. Med.*, **47**, 177–96.

Fawer, R., Justafre, J. C., Berger, J. P. and Schelling, J. L. (1978). Intravenous glycerol in cerebral infarction: a controlled 4-month trial. *Stroke*, **9**, 484–6.

Geismar, P., Marquardsen, J. and Sylvest, J. (1976). Controlled trial of intravenous aminophylline in acute cerebral infarction. *Acta Neurol. Scand.*, **54**, 173–80.

Gilsanz, V., Rebollar, J. L, Buencuerpo, J. and Chantres, M. T. (1975). Controlled trial of glycerol versus dexamethasone in the treatment of cerebral oedema in acute cerebral infarction. *Lancet*, **1**, 1049–51.

Kaste, M., Fogelholm, R. and Waltimo, O. (1976). Combined dexamethasone and low-molecular-weight dextran in acute brain infarction: double-blind study. *Brit. Med. J.*, **2**, 1409–10.

Lancet Leader (1975). Glycerol in acute cerebral infarction. *Lancet*, **2**, 1246–7.

Larsson, O., Marinovich, W. and Barber, K. (1976). Double-blind trial of glycerol therapy in early stroke. *Lancet*, **1**, 832–4.

Mathew, N. T., Meyer, J. S., Rivera, V. M., Charney, J. A. and Hartmann, A. (1972). Double-blind evaluation of glycerol therapy in acute cerebral infarction. *Lancet*, **2**, 1327–9.

Matthews, W. B., Oxbury, J. M., Grainger, K. M. R. and Greenhall, R. C. D. (1976). A blind-controlled trial of dextran 40 in the treatment of ischaemic stroke. *Brain*, **99**, 196–206.

Mulley, G. and Arie, T. (1978). Treating stroke: home or hospital? *Brit. Med. J.*, **2**, 1321–2.

Mulley, G., Wilcox, R. G. and Mitchell, J. R. A. (1978). Dexamethasone in acute stroke. *Brit. Med. J.*, **2**, 994–6.

Nordle, O. and Brantmark, B. (1977). A self-adjusting randomisation plan for allocation of patients into two treatment groups. *Clin. Pharmacol. Therap.*, **22**, 825–8.

Norris, J. W. (1976). Steroid therapy in acute cerebral infarction. *Arch. Neurol.*, **33**, 69–71.

Norris, J. W. and Hachinski, V. C. (1986). High-dose steroid treatment in cerebral infarction. *Brit. Med. J.*, **1**, 21–3.

Patten, B. M., Mendell, J., Bruun, B., Curtin, W. and Carter, S. (1972). Double-blind study of the effects of dexamethasone on acute stroke. *Neurology (Minneap.)*, **22**, 377–83.

Rose, F. C. and Capildeo, R. (1981). *Stroke: The Facts*. Oxford University Press, Oxford.

Santambrogio, S., Martinotti, R., Sardella, F., Porro, F. and Randazzo, A. (1978). Is there a real treatment for stroke? Clinical and statistical comparison of different treatments in 300 patients. *Stroke*, **9**, 130–2.

Spudis, E. V., de la Torre, E. and Pikola, L. (1973). Management of completed strokes with dextran 40. A community hospital failure. *Stroke*, **4**, 895–7.

Steiner, T. (1987). To be published.

Steiner, T., Capildeo, R. and Rose, F. C. (1979). New approach to the treatment of recent stroke. *Brit. Med. J.,* **1**, 412.

Strand, T., Asplund, K., Eriksson, S., Hägg, E., Lithner, F. and Webster, P. O. (1984). A randomised controlled trial of haemodilution therapy in acute ischaemic stroke. *Stroke,* **15**, 980–9.

Tellez, H. and Bauer, R. B. (1973). Dexamethasone as treatment in cerebro-vascular disease. 1. A controlled study in intracerebral haemorrhage. *Stroke,* **4**, 541–56.

Woollard, M. L., Pearson, R. M., Dorf, G., Griffith, D. and James, I. M. (1978). Controlled trial of ornithine alpha ketoglutarate in patients with stroke. *Stroke,* **9**, 218–22.

Wright, W. B. (1974). High-dosage dexamethasone in the treatment of strokes in the elderly. *Gerontology-Clinics,* **16**, 88–91.

10
Methodology of clinical trials in stroke. Part II: Future trials — Recommendations

J. M. ORGOGOZO and R. CAPILDEO

INTRODUCTION

Chapter 9 has shown the methodological shortcomings encountered in most of the published trials on drug therapy following acute stroke. Clearly, better designed trials are necessary, but are they possible?

One basic problem shared with the drug trials in dementia (see chapter 14) is the lack at the present time of any treatment likely to dramatically affect the course of stroke. The challenge is to try to distinguish between a small effect and no effect at all, an uneasy task when dealing with such a heterogeneous disease as stroke.

Another thorny issue is the definition of what is meant by improvement in a disease where the natural history is towards spontaneous improvement. Early mortality occurs only in the more severe cases, and often preventing these patients from dying will leave them with such a degree of handicap that it is hardly possible to speak of a 'therapeutic benefit' (Matthews et al., 1976).

On the other hand, it would not be realistic to aim at a *restitutio ad integrum* in completed strokes since, by definition, neurological disability lasts more than 24 hours, implying some degree of irreversible brain damage. In between is the modest objective of improving as much as possible the extent and/or the speed of recovery, i.e. adding to the largely unpredictable natural process a presumably moderate effect of the drug under trial.

The practical consequences of these difficulties on the methodology of acute stroke trials are the subject of this chapter and we shall discuss some solutions that we are currently testing within the framework of an international multicentre trial on acute cerebral hemisphere infarction.

207

AIM OF THE STUDY

First, it is important to state if the drug (or other treatment) under trial is supposed to act through a specific or a non-specific effect (Kurtzke, 1982).

Non-specific treatment goals

Non-specific treatment goals include:

(1) the improvement of wakefulness;
(2) the prevention of complications such as deep vein thrombosis and pulmonary embolism, or cardiac and respiratory insufficiency;
(3) the prevention or treatment of secondary depression;
(4) the management of sequelae, i.e. the residual impairment of motor or other function after the acute stage of stroke.

Such non-specific aims are sometimes easier to achieve since either the selection criteria (such as depression) or the end-points (such as pulmonary embolism) are relatively well defined and *independent of the precise type of stroke involved.*

Specific treatment goals

Specific treatment goals will aim at one or several of the following effects:

(1) preventing the spread of brain oedema;
(2) reducing the size of the 'penumbra' around an area of infarction;
(3) improving the metabolism and function of remote areas involved by 'diaschisis';
(4) improving the rate of early recovery;
(5) preventing deterioration (due to extension of the arterial thrombosis or to continued haemorrhage);
(6) preventing early recurrence (e.g. repeated embolism or rebleeding).

Among those objectives some (e.g.(5)) are pragmatic and merely descriptive; others are based on physiopathological concepts. Others (e.g. (5) and (6)) are a mixture of both.

It is obviously necessary to specify why a given treatment is being submitted to a trial, in order to select the appropriate patients and choose the appropriate criteria to observe the expected effects. Patients with lacunes are unlikely to be satisfactory cases for the study of an antioedematous agent, whereas patients with an early shift of the midline structures seen on CT scanning from an hemisphere infarction will be suitable. It may seem obvious that one should not expect antithrombotic agents to be of any value in cases of intracranial haemorrhage, but some trials carried out before the advent of CT scanning included such cases.

If there is a general rule to propose, then it is to choose between a scientific trial, based on well-defined physiopathological concepts, and a more pragmatic trial designed to observe a clinical benefit in a wider selection of cases. In the first instance the result will be valid only for the model chosen, whereas in the second it will be of value to any general practitioner first seeing a stroke patient.

Side-effects and complications

Side-effects and complications of treatment are of special importance in stroke since in this group of diseases it is easier to make matters worse rather than aid recovery. For example, steroids have been shown to be detrimental in at least one study (Norris, 1976); and vasoactive drugs have been accused of 'stealing' blood away from the ischaemic area (Olesen and Paulson, 1971) and may cause a drop in blood pressure through peripheral vasodilatation, thereby reducing blood supply to the ischaemic brain (Astrup *et al.*, 1981). Other presumably important factors for outcome include respiratory function, which is depressed by barbiturates although previously recommended for stroke (Smith, 1977). Blood viscosity, as determined by haematocrit, if increased appears to aggravate brain infarction. This can be induced by diuretics and osmotic agents (Harrison *et al.*, 1981). Hyperglycaemia may increase the size of an infarction (Plum, 1983).

Some additional and well-known prognostic variables in the acute phase of stroke are cardiac dysrhythmias, high blood pressure, renal failure and coagulation abnormalities. The possible effects of treatment on all these variables should be looked for in order to correct any abnormality which may worsen the clinical picture, or at least to understand why a promising treatment may in fact be unsafe. Even if the treatment has no effect on these variables, they should be recorded and reported in order to make sure that an uneven distribution of any of them is not interfering with the result of the trial.

TYPE OF STUDY

In chapter 3 the reason for clinical trials to be double blind has already been discussed. This is also required in acute stroke trials, but as always there are exceptions to this golden rule. An obvious example is surgery. A sham operation cannot be used for ethical reasons, and the compromise is an open evaluation using an assessor independent of the surgeon. The same may be true if the active treatment demands a high level of monitoring, such as barbiturates in cases of coma, or requires mechanical ventilation

(Christensen *et al.*, 1973). Other kinds of treatment have side-effects which make patients receiving active treatment recognisable (e.g. bradycardia with beta-blockers) or which need laboratory control (e.g. anticoagulants). In these cases a single-blind or even an open trial is unavoidable. The result is that only major objective end-points like death or recurrence of stroke can be analysed with confidence, if recorded by an independent observer.

The first choice is usually a double-blind study comparing treatment under trial against something else — but what else? Placebo is the correct choice since no convincingly active treatment is available in stroke (Yatsu, 1982).

Randomisation is now a part of clinical trials which also applies in stroke. The real problem is stratification. Among variables which can affect the prognosis are: age; sex; side, size and nature of the lesion; severity of motor disturbance; sensory signs; hemianopia; deviation of gaze; associated conditions such as hypertension; and most of all impairment of consciousness (Oxbury *et al.*, 1975; Miller and Miyamoto, 1979; Sheikh *et al.*, 1983). It is not possible to take into account so many stratification factors otherwise the number of cases in each cell of the stratification table will be far too small. Our choice has been to stratify only for the level of consciousness and for the extent of motor impairment in a clinical model chosen to minimise the effects of the other factors (see below). This means that the study must be large enough to ensure comparability between groups, i.e. that a multicentre trial is mandatory.

PATIENT GROUP

In order to give a precise and thorough description of each possible type of stroke, the nature of the lesion, its size, its location (and side, if in the cerebral hemisphere), the associated arterial lesion, the mechanism(s) of that lesion, the aetiological and risk factors involved and the other vascular or neurological problems which may be present should be stated. Here lies probably the major difficulty of clinical trials in acute stroke:

(1) the different conditions presenting as stroke may be differently, or even adversely, influenced by treatment (e.g. anticoagulants in cerebral thrombosis or haemorrhage);
(2) the number of subcategories is such that a balance between the treatment groups is most unlikely in reasonably sized trials;
(3) restricting the study to only one category of stroke will yield a result valid only for that category.

Faced with the cost and complexity of organising a very large multicentre trial, as compared with the unlikeliness of getting a positive answer after such an enterprise with the available drugs, one is forced to accept a compromise. In a current trial (Anagnostou, C. N., Capildeo, R., Rose, F. C., Dartigues, F., Juge, O., Lefort, D., Orgogozo, J. M., Pere, J. J., Steiner, T. J., Yotis, A.) we have chosen the following model.

Patients with rapidly progressing and recent (not less than 24 and not more than 72 hours) neurological deficit of moderate degree which is clinically related to an ischaemic process involving the middle cerebral artery territory: this early inclusion will allow the earliest possible treatment but the diagnosis should later be confirmed by CT scan (between the third and eighth day post-stroke), and lacunes will be excluded.
Sex: males and females
Side of the insult: right and left
Age: 55 to 75 years
Level of consciousness: patients with disturbance of consciousness such as deep coma or stupor (Plum and Posner, 1980) are excluded from the trial
Severity of neurological deficit: patients with either paresis of face and arm or hemiplegia are included
Stratification of the patients: they are stratified according to the level of consciousness (normal versus obtunded) and to the extent of the deficit (face–arm paresis versus hemiplegia). The randomisation of the trial substances is done according to the corresponding four subgroups. For reasons of convenience each trial centre will have its own randomisation list

Other such restrictive but explicit models can be chosen, e.g. hemispheric haemorrhages, brainstem infarctions, lacunar infarctions, etc. The elements of choice should take into account *feasibility* (with too rare a condition the study will never end) and whether the model is *representative* (a trial done on male aphasics under 50 with cardiac embolism will yield conclusions valid only for that category of patients). We feel that if a beneficial effect is observed in the patient group as defined above, it may be reasonable to generalise the conclusion to other types of brain infarction but possibly not to lacunar infarction and not to brain haemorrhage.

CRITERIA OF SELECTION

The specificity of the clinical diagnosis of stroke is good (Von Arbin *et al.*, 1980), but as soon as one wants to specify the nature, location, mechanism, etc. of the lesion (see preceding paragraph) the clinical information is not sufficient. So, if the trial is to be made on a specific subgroup of strokes, the diagnosis must be proven. This previously difficult problem is partly solved by CT scanning but the question of timing of the CT scan remains crucial:

(1) A study on completed stroke supposes, by definition (Joint Committee for Stroke Resources, 1975), that some deficit will persist after 24 hours. Therefore, one should either wait for 24 hours before including the patient, or exclude secondary patients who recover completely within 24 hours if the treatment is started early. Both approaches would miss a treatment capable of cure within 24 hours — theoretically possible but unlikely!

(2) If done before 48 hours, the CT scan will show all cases of intracerebral haemorrhage but it will fail to demonstrate the location and extent of most cases of cerebral infarction (Constant *et al.*, 1977). To document a brain infarction by CT scanning, it is necessary to wait 2 or 3 days after the onset (Tubman *et al.*, 1981). To wait until this time to establish the diagnosis is too late to start a treatment for acute stroke. An acceptable solution is initially to include patients using clinical criteria, so that treatment begins soon enough, and then to allow secondary exclusions when, for example, CT scanning fails to demonstrate the presumed site and nature of the lesion.

Stroke is the result of arterial disease, and the extent of the arterial lesion (disease) can only be shown by angiography. If this procedure is included in the protocol, a number of patients will be excluded because of the risks associated with the technique whereas others may be submitted to further unnecessary risks. Our recommendation is not to include cerebral angiography as a selection criterion, but if it must be done in an individual patient for diagnostic reasons, any complication should be charged against the treatment group of that patient since it cannot be ruled out that the treatment has influenced this event.

NUMBERS OF PATIENTS ASSESSED AND ADMITTED

As explained in chapter 3, these numbers are useful:

(1) to assess the representativity of the study; and
(2) to monitor whether any participating centre is introducing bias into the study by selecting a category of patient according to additional criteria.

They also illustrate how apparently liberal inclusion criteria can dramatically affect the rate of inclusion, a phenomenon popularly known as 'Lasagna's law'. Figure 10.1 illustrates this fact as observed in our ongoing stroke trial: indeed this inclusion rate of 7% makes one understand why such studies are difficult to complete and need the co-operation of several very active centres.

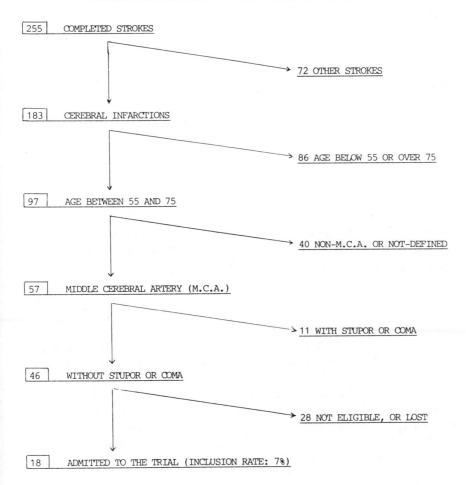

Figure 10.1 Ratio of admitted/observed cases in a clinical trial on acute stroke at the Department of Neurology-Neurosurgery, Bordeaux, July–December, 1982.

Another number to specify is that of the patients lost for follow-up. To achieve this, the best way is for patients to remain hospitalised during the first few weeks but after that everything must be done to review patients on the target dates (see below), and this includes home visits.

METHODS OF ASSESSMENT

Most stroke patients seen in the hospital do improve (Walker *et al.*, 1981) and therefore the best that can be expected from a treatment is to increase the rate and/or speed of recovery. First, let us consider some other criteria of outcome.

Death

This is a well-defined and objective criterion, which should probably be included in all trials on stroke. It could even be the sole or main criterion in trials on severe strokes (i.e. with alteration of consciousness), or when the treatment is aimed at one of the mechanisms most often responsible for early deaths after stroke, such as brain oedema or bronchopneumonia (Silver *et al.*, 1984). As stated previously, there is some concern about the real benefit of preventing early deaths and leaving massive residual deficits with a high probability of delayed deaths (Matthews *et al.*, 1976). So it seems advisable to analyse the death rate *and* the functional outcome after 3 or 6 months and preferably 12 months.

Length of stay

The cost of staying in hospital is enormous and it has been proposed that this should be taken into account as a pragmatic criterion of the efficacy of treatment (Admani, 1978). Some criticism has been raised against this. Even in a one-centre trial there are many other factors beside the disability itself which can influence length of stay in hospital, notably family and social support, the availability of rehabilitation or chronic-care facilities, the interest of the physicians in the disease, etc. In multicentre trials these differences are magnified further.

Total cost

This is influenced by the non-specific factors just mentioned. In addition the calculation of the true savings that a treatment generates is difficult (Weinsten and Stason, 1977), and is not likely to be favourable here since stroke affects older, most often retired, people. Survival of severely disabled stroke patients will lead to continuing health expenses. On a personal basis, for patients working at the time of their stroke, 'loss of earnings' as a result of their illness represents another measure of outcome.

Neurological score

So far no acute stroke score has been generally accepted or formally validated. Of the various scores proposed in the literature (table A.6,

p. 316), only the one of Mathew *et al.* (1972) (table A.7, p. 317) has been used in several trials. The objective of a score is to summarise and sum up the neurological deficits in numbers which can be compared and analysed statistically. It is clear that to be simple and easy to use, a score cannot contain all the possible neurological abnormalities and a choice has to be made according to the design of the study.

We have designed a score summarising the deficits resulting from cerebral infarction in the middle cerebral artery territory which has been tested in terms of interobserver reliability (Orgogozo *et al.*, 1983). This score (table A.8, p. 318) gives more weight to the items representative of motor function. The other items are mainly prognostic predictors (Anderson *et al.*, 1975; Oxbury *et al.*, 1975; Miller and Miyamoto, 1979; Sheikh *et al.*, 1983). We have found that the interobserver agreement for each item is from 0.75 to 1, which is satisfactory, and from 0.93 to 0.99 for the total score. Its sensitivity and the predictive value of the initial score are the aim of an ongoing study.

A basic problem of the score approach is the large variance as the items are in fact not independent. The result is that a change in one affects some of the others, resulting in large changes in the total score. This intrinsic shortcoming decreases the power of the scale and its ability to detect small differences in outcome between groups. Conversely an analysis of the individual items results in an increase of the alpha risk. At the level of $p<0.05$ the risk of finding a significant difference by chance alone among 10 items is more than 45%. So an item-by-item analysis should be avoided, and a stroke trial should be large enough to compensate for the lack of power of the scoring system.

Activities of daily living (ADL)

The evaluation of independence is a more pragmatic measurement than a neurological score since it better reflects the *quality* of recovery in terms of return to the family, society, or even to work. It also gives an indication of the long-term cost of sequelae. Among the several disability scales which have been designed, some have been more widely used, and are listed in table A.9, p. 319. To be useful for a stroke trial a scale must be both objective and sensitive, must have a low interrater variability, and must correspond well to the question asked. As the items are added to give a global score, it is essential that some degree of weighting takes into account the relative importance of each item (for example walking is far more important for independence than 'brushing teesh' or 'combing hair'). Such a weighting is included in two widely used ADL scales: the Barthel Index (Mahoney and Barthel, 1965) and the Kenny scale (Schoening *et al.*, 1965).

The Barthel Index (Chapter 3; see also table A.10, p. 320) measures the actual abilities of the patient in 10 basic activities, chosen and weighted to reflect the amount of help needed. The maximum total score is 100, and the prognostic values of some thresholds (Granger *et al.*, 1977) have been established. A score of more than 20 at the onset, when the stroke is just completed, or of more than 40 at discharge to the rehabilitation centre, carries a good functional prognosis. Below that, the probability of deriving benefit from rehabilitation and the chances of returning home are low. A score of 60 or over means that the vast majority of these patients will have enough personal recovery to return home. Furthermore the same group has shown that the Barthel Index is a sensitive tool to follow progress during rehabilitation (Granger *et al.*, 1979). As a pilot study, J. F. Dartigues and J. M. Orgogozo (1982, unpublished observations) analysed the spontaneous (untreated) outcome of 68 patients with superficial MCA infarction, from days 15–30 to day 180 (6 months) with determination of the Barthel Index (BI) at and between these two target dates. The patients were selected according to an initial BI between 20 and 60. The mean difference between initial and final BI was:

$$\mathrm{BI}f - \mathrm{BI}i = 36.4 \ (\pm \ 18.7) \quad \text{Variance}: 349.8$$

With these figures the number of patients needed to detect a 25% mean improvement of the BI, with an alpha risk of 0.05 and a beta risk of 0.10, is 71 patients for each group (treated and control) which is reasonable. But with a more realistic improvement of 10% only, the number of patients required would be 428 in each group! In this same study the crossing of the threshold score of 60 has always been irreversible (except in the case of recurring stroke). This allows us to make an actuarial analysis of outcome using a score of 60 as the end-point. The log-rank method yields more statistical power than the classical comparison of mean differences, it gives credit for patients with temporary or partial follow-up, and is better suited to comparisons of temporal profiles of recovery (see chapter 3 by Maurer and Commenges). We also tested the interrater agreement for this scale (Orgogozo *et al.*, 1983). The concordance rate was 0.86 in Bordeaux in 20 patients, and 0.99 in London in 22 patients. In the first centre, the comparison was made between nurse and nurse-aid assessors, and in the second it was made between two ward nurses.

The Kenny Rehabilitation Institute Scale (Schoening *et al.*, 1965) includes 17 items belonging to six categories. This division is based upon the assumption that these categories are equivalent, each corresponding grossly to one hour of the patient's (and nursing staff's) time a day. This scale for self-care evaluation has a 5-point rating code which seems reasonably sensitive and accurate (Schoening and Iversen, 1968). However, it is likely that the 3- to 4-point code of the Barthel Index with its explicit definition yields a higher reproducibility.

A formal comparison of the sensitivity of the two above scales and of the Katz scale (Katz *et al.*, 1970) has been made by Donaldson *et al.* (1973), starting from a unified ADL form which can generate each of the three others. Their results show that the scales are equivalent for describing the evolution of the patients in 68% of the cases. The Katz scale, the least detailed of the three, is 19% less sensitive than the two others which reach an 89% agreement. Globally the Kenny scale is slightly more sensitive than the Barthel Index, but is also less easy to use.

Choice and use of judgement criteria for stroke outcome

This depends obviously on the object of the trial and on the expected effect of the treatment under trial. Apart from this, should the different methods of assessment be considered concurrent or complementary? Spence and Donner (1982) consider the use of the same scoring systems to measure severity at entry and to measure outcome as a weakness in design, and recommend the use of an initial severity neurological score to predict mortality, and of a separate outcome ADL score to reflect benefits of treatments. Even if this opinion is based on a correct (but only alluded to) criticism of the neurological score approach, we would argue the following two points.

(1) A complex set of criteria should be tested for its prognostic value before it can be claimed to be a better predictor than a single major factor, e.g. the level of consciousness or the severity of the motor deficit, and, if so, its predictive value is likely to apply only to the clinical model for which it was tested.
(2) Still more important is the question of pertinence. When the score used for the inclusion and stratification at the onset is also used for assessment of the outcome, one can be certain that the recorded improvement is an improvement in the symptoms and signs for which the patient was treated.

It is true that ADL scales better reflect the 'real life' benefits of a given treatment, so our recommendation is to use both a neurological and an ADL score for assessment. If a parallel trend towards improvement is shown, it will strongly suggest that the functional improvement is due to a better clearing of the neurological deficits and not to non-specific factors possibly unrelated to treatment. Comparing our neurological score and the Barthel Index we have shown that they are correlated up to a Barthel score of 60 (i.e. the threshold of independence): above that the BI may show improvements no longer detected by the neurological score (Orgogozo *et al.*, 1983). The opposite approach is to mix the same score neurologically and ADL items may be useful to show in a single (but complicated) form the status of a given patient, but certainly not to provide a valid quantitiative measure of outcome in a series of patients.

DURATION OF TREATMENT AND FOLLOW-UP

How long should treatment last?

Much of the damage occurs during the first minutes of brain ischaemia (Raichle, 1983). This includes loss of ion homeostasis, depletion in energy stores rapidly followed by an accumulation of lactic acid, and later on by uncoupling of cerebral blood flow and metabolism and breakdown of the blood/brain barrier. The battle is by no means lost after the first minutes or hours, since further events such as the accumulation of calcium, free radical release, inhibition of PGI 2 synthesis and accumulation of thromboxane A2 will contribute to a further deterioration in the situation, making brain infarction an evolving process over days and even weeks (Plum, 1983).

In humans CT- and PET-scanning studies have shown respectively that the breakdown of the blood/brain barrier and the uncoupling between blood flow and metabolism may last up to 1 month after the onset (Constant *et al.*, 1977; Tubman *et al.*, 1981; Baron *et al.*, 1981, 1983). The choice for the duration of treatment will depend upon the mechanism of its action, but in most cases it will be reasonable to treat for at least 3 or 4 weeks in order to cover the entire period of acute pathophysiological events.

Duration of follow-up

In almost all of the published acute stroke trials (see chapter 9), the duration of follow-up has been too short. There are three main reasons why the follow-up should be extended beyond the acute phase previously defined as up to 1 month:

(1) to make sure that preventing early deaths does not leave unacceptable long-term neurological and functional deficits;
(2) to increase the sensitivity and power of the analysis, as discussed by Spence and Donner (1982);
(3) to check whether using only differences in scores between assessments is a useful measure of efficacy in stroke.

Let us assume that a proportion of the patients under study recover completely in both treatment groups. This 'ceiling' effect will hide a possible benefit of treatment, and it may induce a bias since patients with more severe deficits at the onset will seem to have made more improvement than milder cases (they have more way to go to the ceiling), when in fact the *timing* of improvement is the important factor to look at (and also the *proportion* of patients with full recovery in this special case). The same is true for the more frequent case of partial recovery. Even if treatment does not make a difference to the final level of recovery, it may prove very useful if it significantly reduces the time at which this level is reached (which might mean earlier discharge from hospital).

For all these reasons, repeated assessments over a prolonged period of time are advisable. Our preliminary studies on the temporal course of MCA infarctions have led us to adopt the following schedule:

Neurological score + Barthel Index: Days 1 – 3 – 6 – 10 – 28 – 84 – 168

CONCLUSIONS

From what has been said, it is obvious that stroke trials are not easy. None of the difficulties that have been discussed is in itself unsolvable. Unfortunately their combination makes it particularly challenging to design a stroke trial 'beyond reproach'. It seems to us that a fair compromise can be reached, in particular between scientific credibility (which requires selection of highly specific cases), representativity (a drug good for all strokes would be a major help in daily practice), optimal power (1 − beta) and alpha risk values and feasibility of the trial. To demonstrate convincingly that a treatment has no effect in a well-defined category of stroke, good methodology involving a large number of patients is required. But such a negative result is worth while since it may lead to considerable savings and, for the more aggressive kinds of treatments, may prevent stroke victims being submitted to unnecessary risks and discomfort. Perhaps the major reproach that can be levelled at most of the published trials is that they have not attained this last objective. Future stroke trials should be designed in order to give at least this answer, and negative reports should be accepted more widely by medical journals. More optimistically we believe that the advances in both our understanding of the pathophysiology of stroke and the spread of methodological rigour among clinical investigators will result in positive answers, either with new drugs or with already known drugs in better selected patients.

ACKNOWLEDGEMENTS

We thank J. F. Dartigues for his helpful comments, M. Sugier for her contribution to the ADL scale discussion, and Sandoz Switzerland and its affiliates in France and the UK for supporting part of this work.

REFERENCES

Admani, A. K. (1978). New approach to treatment of recent stroke. *Brit. Med. J.,* **ii**, 1678–9.

Anderson, T. P., Bourestom, N., Greenberg, F. R. and Hildyard, V. G. (1975). Predictive factors in stroke rehabilitation. *Arch. Phys. Med. Rehabil.,* **56**, 545–53.

Astrup, J., Siesjo, B. K. and Symon, L. (1981). Thresholds in cerebral ischemia — The ischemic penumbra. *Stroke,* **12**, 723–5.

Baron, J. C., Bousser, M. G., Comar, D., Soussaline, E. and Castaigne, P. (1981). Non-invasive tomographic study of cerebral blood flow and oxygen metabolism *in vivo*: potentials, limitations and clinical applications. *Eur. Neurol.,* **20**, 273–84.

Baron, J. C., Delattre, J. Y., Bories, J., Bousser, M. G. and Castaigne, P. (1983). Comparison study of C.T. and positron emission tomographic data in recent cerebral infarction. *AJNR,* **4**, 536–40.

Christensen, M. S., Paulson, O. B., Olesen, J., Alexander, S. C., Skinhoj, E., Dam, W. H. and Lassen, N. A. (1973). Cerebral apoplexy (stroke) treated with or without prolonged artificial ventilation. Part I: Cerebral circulation, clinical course and causes of death. *Stroke,* **4**, 568–619.

Constant, P., Revou, A. M., Caillé, J. M., Vernhiet, J., Dop, A., *et al.* (1977). Aspects and evolution of cerebrovascular accidents. *J. Neuroradiol.,* **4**, 291–310.

Donaldson, W. S., Wagner, C. C. and Gresham, G. E. (1973). A unified ADL evaluation form. *Arch. Phys. Med. Rehabil.,* **54**, 175–85.

Granger, C. V., Dewis, L. S., Peters, N. C., Sherwood, C. C. and Barrett, J. E. (1979). Stroke rehabilitation: analysis of repeated Barthel Index measures. *Arch. Phys. Med. Rehabil.,* **60**, 14–17.

Granger, C. V., Sherwood, C. C. and Greer, D. S. (1977). Functional status measures in a comprehensive stroke care programme. *Arch. Phys. Med. Rehabil.,* **58**, 555–61.

Harrison, M. G. H., Pollock, S., Kendall, B. E. and Marshall, J. (1981). Effects of hematocrit on carotid stenosis and cerebral infarction. *Lancet,* **ii**, 114–15.

Joint Committee for Stroke Resources (1975). A classification and outline of cerebrovascular diseases II. *Stroke,* **6**, 564–626.

Katz, S., Downs, T. D., Cash, M. R. and Grotz, R. C. (1970). Progress in the development of the index of ADL. *Gerontologist,* **10**, 20–30.

Kurtzke, J. F. (1982). On the role of clinicians in the use of drug trial data. *Neuroepidemiol.,* **1**, 124–36.

Mahoney, F. I. and Barthel, D. W. (1965). Functional evaluation: Barthel Index. *Md. State Med. J.,* **14**, 61–5.

Mathew, N. T., Meyer, J. S., Rivera, V. M., Charney, J. Z. and Hartmann, A. (1972). Double blind evaluation of glycerol therapy in acute cerebral infarction. *Lancet,* **ii**, 1327–9. ·

Matthews, W. B., Oxbury, J. M., Grainger, K. M. R. and Greenhall, C. D. (1976). A blind controlled trial of Dextran 40 in the treatment of ischaemic stroke. *Brain,* **99**, 193–206.

Miller, A. S. and Miyamoto, A. T. (1979). Computed tomography: its potential as a predictor of functional recovery following stroke. *Arch. Phys. Med. Rehabil.,* **60**, 108–9.

Norris, J. (1976). Steroid therapy in acute cerebral infarction. *Arch. Neurol.,* **33**, 69–71.

Norris, J. and Hachinski,V. C. (1982). Comment on 'study design of stroke treatments'. *Stroke,* **13**, 527–8.

Olesen, J. and Paulson, O. B. (1971). The effect of intra-arterial Papaverine on the regional cerebral blood flow of patients with stroke or intracranial tumor. *Stroke*, **2**, 148–59.

Orgogozo, J. M., Capildeo, R., Anagnostou, C. N., Juge, O., Pere, J. J., Dartigues, J. F., Steiner, T. J., Yotis, A. and Clifford Rose, F. C. (1983). Mise au point d'un score neurologique pour l'évaluation clinique des infarctus sylviens. *Nouv. Presse. Med.*, **12**, 3039–44.

Oxbury, J. M., Greenhall, R. C. D. and Grainger, K. M. R. (1975). Predicting the outcome of stroke: acute stage after cerebral infarction. *Brit. Med. J.*, **iii**, 125–7.

Plum, F. (1983). What causes infarction in ischemic brain? The Robert Wartenberg Lecture (1983). *Neurol.*, **33**, 222–33.

Plum, F. and Posner, J. (1980). *Diagnosis of Stupor and Coma*. Davis, Philadelphia, 3rd edn.

Raichle, M. E. (1983). The pathophysiology of brain ischaemia. *Ann. Neurol.*, **13**, 2–10.

Schoening, M. A., Anderegg, L., Bergsltom, D., Fonda, M., Steinke, N. and Ulrich, P. (1965). Numerical scoring of self-care status of patients. *Arch. Phys. Med. Rehabil.*, **46**, 689–97.

Schoening, M. A. and Iversen, I. A. (1968). Numerical scoring of self-care status. A study of the Kenny self-care evaluation. *Arch. Phys. Med. Rehabil.*, **49**, 221–9.

Sheikh, K., Brennan, P. J., Meade, T. W. and Goldenberg, E. (1983). Predictors of mortality and disability in stroke. *J. Epidemiol. Commun. Health*, **37**, 70–74.

Sheikh, K., Smith, D. S., Meade, T. W., *et al.* (1979). Repeatability and validity of a modified activities of daily living (ADL) index in studies of chronic disabilities. *Int. Rehab. Med.*, **1**, 51–8.

Silver, F. L., Norris, J. W., Lewis, A. J. and Hachinski, V. C. (1984). Early mortality following stroke and prospective review. *Stroke*, **15**, 492–6.

Smith, A. L. (1977). Barbiturate protection in cerebral hypoxia. *Anesthesiol.*, **47**, 285–93.

Spence, J. D. and Donner, A. (1982). Problems in design of stroke treatment trials. *Stroke*, **13**, 94–9.

Tubman, D. E., Ethier, R., Melacin, D., Belanger, G. and Taylor, S. (1981). The computerized tomographic assessment of brain infarcts. *Can. J. Neurol. Sci.*, **8**, 121–6.

Von Arbin, M., Britton, M., De Faire, U., Helmers, C., Miah, K. and Murray, V. (1980). Validation of admission criteria to a stroke unit. *J. Chron. Dis.*, **33**, 215–20.

Weinsten, M. C. and Stason, W. B. (1977). Foundations of cost-effectiveness analysis for health and medical practices. *New Engl. J. Med.*, **293**, 716–21.

Yatsu, F. M. (1982). Acute medical therapy of stroke, *Stroke*, **13**, 524–6.

11
Methodology of clinical trials in Parkinson's disease. Part I: Analysis of previous clinical trials

X. LATASTE and L. J. FINDLEY

INTRODUCTION

In the last 15 years, the evolution of therapies proposed for the management of Parkinson's disease has represented a real challenge for clinicians to select the best methodology for their evaluation. Since the spectacular introduction of levodopa, accurate and reliable assessment techniques have been extensively developed for testing drug efficacy in parkinsonism. A large and growing body of literature on Parkinson's disease has been published since 1973, especially on the use of new drugs and their efficacy, with more agents than ever being evaluated in the last decade. However, less than 10% of the publications on the use of antiparkinsonian drugs in clinical trials included any form of control group (figure 11.1).

There still remains confusion and controversy about the management of parkinsonism. In spite of an extensive number of clinical studies, basic questions that are still unsolved include, for instance: When should levodopa be started? Should the maximum dosage be introduced from the onset? What are the role and place of dopamine-agonist drugs? Is there a place for monotherapy? In whom and when? Most neurologists would give a competent account on how they manage the disease themselves, but this may be quite different from that of other clinicians with similar experience (Fahn and Bressman, 1984; Grimes, 1984; Lieberman *et al.*, 1984; Muenter, 1984; Rascol *et al.*, 1984; Yahr, 1984). Should the treatment be continuous or intermittent? In view of the known long-term side-effects of levodopa, do 'avant-garde' modes of therapy such as sequential treatment, i.e. alternating levodopa and dopamine agonists, have a place in the management of patients with Parkinson's disease?

Number of publications

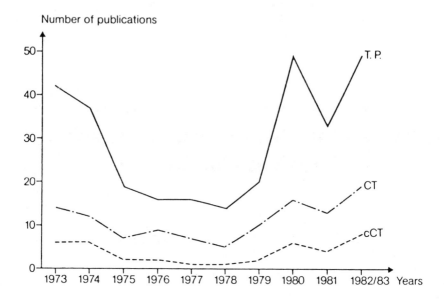

Figure 11.1 Parkinson's disease. Review of publications on antiparkinsonian drugs (source: *Index Medicus*) since 1973. TP, Therapeutic publications; CT, clinical trials; cCT, controlled clinical trials.

It was perhaps a disadvantage that levodopa was found to be so effective from the beginning, as this precluded early controlled studies (Cotzias *et al.*, 1967). In terms of evolutionary clinical pharmacology, perhaps it would have been preferable if several effective agents had been available together at the same time, an occurrence which would have forced a more critical evaluation of these drugs from the onset of their clinical use. The methodo- logical problems in the initial clinical trials of levodopa were emphasised with the introduction of newer and effective agents in the control of the disease. Instead of newer agents being evaluated to assess their efficacy as anti-parkinsonian drugs, they have been largely assessed as drugs which could cirvumvent the by then well-established long-term side-effects of chronic levodopa therapy, or as additional medication for patients already receiving levodopa (Fahn, 1982; Marsden *et al.*, 1982).

It is important to keep such historical facts in mind when reviewing the clinical trials in Parkinson's disease over the last two decades. For instance it is very obvious that successive trials have attempted to deal with the evolving long-term side-effects of levodopa by introducing measurements of dyskinesia, fluctuations in therapeutic response or dementia in the evalua- tion of newer 'add-on' antiparkinsonian drugs.

LITERATURE REVIEW: CRITICAL ANALYSIS

We have chosen 15 clinical trials taken from the period 1973 to 1983 which exemplify the typical approaches used to evaluate new treatments in Parkinson's disease. However, we decided to exclude some of the most widely quoted studies. These publications mainly report clinical experience with new drugs and should be considered as 'open clinical' studies rather than formal clinical trials (Calne *et al.*, 1974, 1979). Such open studies cannot be analysed as clinical trials because their objectives are not clearly specified. In these studies, the emphasis has largely been on drug activity, clinical response, and tolerance.

Studies have been conducted as investigational open trials in the early development of new therapy (i.e. Phase I trials). They generally provide the basis from which more sophisticated controlled trials can be carried out. With levodopa such an approach was never properly effected. Moreover all new antiparkinsonian drugs have usually been evaluated in an 'add-on' situation. Monotherapy studies, as they have been done, have usually been performed after 'add-on' therapeutical trials, and for logistic reasons such trials cannot be directly compared with levodopa as the standard medication. This situation has led to an increase in invalid retrospective comparative studies (Rinne, 1983).

We have selected 15 representative trials of different designs (e.g. open, single blind, double blind and/or cross-over) to include a large variety of assessment methodologies. This approach was performed to highlight the methodological problems attached to the evaluation of antiparkinsonian drugs. All the data of these trials have been collected in the format of a 'prospective' clinical trial. It should be emphasised that this means that the aims of the study have been carefully defined prior to data collection. The choice of these trials has not been entirely random: we have deliberately chosen accepted trials that have been the most widely quoted in the literature to underline the difficulty in the initial planning and subsequent reporting of the results of a new treatment for parkinsonism.

In each trial report, the criteria listed in table 11.1 have been reviewed, and specific comments will be presented according to these criteria. Concerning the conclusions of the study, our analysis was performed on the individual author(s)' conclusions relevant to each specific paper without any reference to other experiences. The overall summary of the clinical trials reviewed is presented in table 11.2. However, for the analysis of each individual study, the reader is referred to tables 11.3–17.

From table 11.2 the vast variations in the methodological logistics of the trials, which were all attempting to answer similar questions, can be appreciated.

Table 11.1 Criteria used for report analysis.

1. Author's aims

2. Criteria of selection
   (i) diagnosis of Parkinson's disease
   (ii) specific entry criteria

3. Number admitted to trial

4. Trial design
   (i) open
   (ii) single blind
   (iii) double blind
   (iv) double-blind cross-over with placebo and/or standard control
   (v) single centre (SC)
   (vi) multicentre

5. Patient group
   (i) age range
   (ii) duration of disease (years)
   (iii) *de novo*/prior therapy
   (iv) duration of previous levodopa (years)

6. Methods of assessment
   (i) subjective:
      clinical rating scale
      self-rating scale
      functional disability
   (ii) simple objective (e.g. drawing, peg-board, walking)

7. Duration of follow-up

8. Data analysis
   (i) patients included in analysis
   (ii) type of data:
      individual parameters
      global assessment
   (iii) type of analysis:
      descriptive
      inferential

9. Author's conclusions

Table 11.2 An overview of the general design characteristics of the 15 trials reviewed.

Number of publications	Number of patients	Number of test medications	Trial design*				Age	Disease duration	Previous treatment	Hoehn and Yahr	Groups
			Open	Single blind	DBPC	DBCO standard					
15	472 (6–119)	7	7	1	5	2 (40%)	9	9	7	5	1 (*de novo*) 7 (mixed) 7 (L-DOPA)

Methods of assessment			Duration of follow-up	Analysis	
Clinical	Functional	Objective		Data	Analysis
15	6	5	4 weeks to 1 year (mean = 3 months)	IND 10 Global 5	Descriptive 5 Inferential 10 (5)
Columbia 2/4 Webster 4 NYUPD 3 KCHPD 1 On-off 4	NWUDS 3 NYUPD 1 Webster 1 ADL 1				

Abbreviations: DBPC, double blind, placebo controlled; DBCO, double-blind cross-over with standard medication; IND represents separate symptoms global scoring. NYUPD, New York University Parkinson Disability Scale; KCHPD King's College Hospital Parkinson's Disease Scale; NWUDS North Western University Disability Scale; ADL activity of daily living.
†The number of trials with details of their entry criteria.

Table 11.3 Treatment of Parkinson's disease with levodopa combined with L-alpha methyldopa hydrazine, an inhibitor of extracerebral dopa-decarboxylase (Marsden *et al.*, 1973).

1. *Authors' aims*:	Comparison of levodopa with levodopa + PDI
2. Selection criteria	
(i) diagnosis	Not defined
(ii) specific criteria	None
3. Number admitted	30
4. Study design	Open (SC)
5. Patient group	
(i) age	49–74
(ii) duration of disease	Not given
(iii) *de novo*	12
(iv) previously treated	18 (levodopa)
(v) duration of previous levodopa	Not given
6. Methods of assessment	
(i) subjective:	
clinical rating scale (RS)	King's College Hospital RS
self-rating scale	None
functional disability	King's College Hospital RS
(ii) simple objective	None
7. Duration of follow-up	—
8. Data analysis	
(i) excluded data defined	Not given
(ii) type of data	Individual
(iii) type of analysis	Inferential (Student's test)
9. *Authors' conclusions*:	More rapid improvement, less side-effects

Comments. Often quoted. Diagnosis not defined. Population not defined. Open, retrospective comparison. Double-blind format more appropriate.

Table 11.4 Deprenyl in Parkinson's disease (Eisler *et al.*, 1981).

1. *Authors' aims*:	Double-blind cross-over: deprenyl vs. placebo
2. Selection criteria	
(i) diagnosis	None
(ii) specific criteria	None
3. Number admitted	11
4. Study design	Double-blind cross-over, placebo controlled (SC)
5. Patient group	
(i) age	31–78 (55.5)
(ii) duration of disease	Not given
(iii) *de novo*	2
(iv) previously treated	9
(v) duration of previous levodopa	1–6 years
6. Methods of assessment	
(i) subjective:	
clinical rating scale	Columbia (modified)
self-rating scale	None
functional disability	None
(ii) simple objective	None
7. Duration of follow-up	At least 4 weeks (?)
8. Data analysis	
(i) excluded data defined	2 (adverse drug reaction, ADR/ Deterioration)
(ii) type of data	Global (?)
(iii) type of analysis	Descriptive only
9. *Authors' conclusions*:	Limited advantages dominated by mood evaluation

Comments. No diagnosis. Heterogeneous groups. Duration not defined. Individual symptoms not analysed.

Table 11.4   Deprenyl in Parkinson's disease (Eisler *et al.*, 1981).

1. *Authors' aims*:	Double-blind cross-over: deprenyl vs. placebo
2. Selection criteria	
(i) diagnosis	None
(ii) specific criteria	None
3. Number admitted	11
4. Study design	Double-blind cross-over, placebo controlled (SC)
5. Patient group	
(i) age	31–78 (55.5)
(ii) duration of disease	Not given
(iii) *de novo*	2
(iv) previously treated	9
(v) duration of previous levodopa	1–6 years
6. Methods of assessment	
(i) subjective:	
clinical rating scale	Columbia (modified)
self-rating scale	None
functional disability	None
(ii) simple objective	None
7. Duration of follow-up	At least 4 weeks (?)
8. Data analysis	
(i) excluded data defined	2 (ADR/Deterioration)
(ii) type of data	Global (?)
(iii) type of analysis	Descriptive only
9. *Authors' conclusions*:	Limited advantages dominated by mood evaluation

Comments. No diagnosis. Heterogeneous groups. Duration not defined. Individual symptoms not analysed.

Table 11.5 Lisuride in Parkinsonism (Gopinathan *et al.*, 1981).

1. *Authors' aims*:	Comparison of lisuride vs. bromocriptine to evaluate serotonergic functions in basal ganglia
2. Selection criteria	
(i) diagnosis	Not defined (18 idiopathic post-encephalitic)
(ii) specific criteria	None
3. Number admitted	20
4. Study design	Double-blind cross-over placebo controlled (SC)
5. Patient group	
(i) age	19–73 (53)
(ii) duration of disease	Not given
(iii) *de novo*	2
(iv) previously treated	18
(v) duration of previous levodopa	Not given
6. Methods of assessment	
(i) subjective:	
clinical rating scale	Columbia (modified)
self-rating scale	None
functional disability	None
(ii) simple objective	Reaction time/motor test
7. Duration of follow-up	40 days
8. Data analysis	
(i) excluded data defined	2 (ADR)
(ii) type of data	Individual
(iii) type of analysis	Descriptive and inferential (no statistical reference)
9. *Authors' conclusions*:	Lisuride effective treatment similar to bromocriptine

Comments. Nothing related to serotonin in basal ganglia. Diagnosis not defined. Probably heterogeneous group, short treatment. Small population. No evidence of randomised placebo. Not strictly double blind. At end comparison low vs. high dose in non-comparable experimental conditions.

Table 11.6 'Sustained bromocriptine therapy in previously untreated patients with Parkinson's disease' (Lees and Stern, 1981).

1. *Authors' aims*:	Long-term efficacy of bromocriptine in *de novo* retrospective comparison with levodopa
2. Selection criteria	
(i) diagnosis	Not given
(ii) specific criteria	Not given
3. Number admitted	50
4. Study design	Open
5. Patient group	
(i) age	Not given
(ii) duration of disease	2 (mean) years
(iii) *de novo*	50
(iv) previously treated	None
(v) duration of previous levodopa	Not given
6. Methods of assessment	
(i) subjective:	
clinical rating scale	Webster scale
self-rating scale	None
functional disability	NWU rating scale
(ii) simple objective	None
7. Duration of follow-up	$\geq$ 1 year and up to 5 years
8. Data analysis	
(i) excluded data defined	Not given
(ii) type of data	Global
(iii) type of analysis	Descriptive
9. *Authors' conclusions*:	Bromocriptine produces sustained improvement; tendency for deterioration after two years comparable to levodopa

Comments. Diagnosis not mentioned. Groups not clearly defined (no age ranges). Analysis used global score and was descriptive. Retrospective comparison is questionable.

Table 11.7 'Lisuride versus bromocriptine treatment in Parkinson's disease: a double-blind study' (Le Witt *et al.*, 1982).

1. *Authors' aims*:	Comparison of clinical efficacy of toxicity pergolide vs. bromocriptine
2. Selection criteria	
(i) diagnosis	Not given
(ii) specific criteria	Some (e.g. cerebrovascular disease)
3. Number admitted	27
4. Study design	Double-blind cross-over controlled-randomised vs. standard (SC)
5. Patient group	
(i) age	45–72 (59)
(ii) duration of disease	1–29 (11) years
(iii) *de novo*	2
(iv) previously treated	25 (levodopa)
(v) duration of previous levodopa	Not given
6. Methods of assessment	
(i) subjective:	
clinical rating scale	Columbia (modified)
self-rating scale	ADR only
functional disability	None
(ii) simple objective	RT/MT gait
7. Duration of follow-up	Unclear (7- to 10-week period)
8. Data analysis	
(i) excluded data defined	3 (2 ADR + 1 CD)
(ii) type of data	Individual + global
(iii) type of analysis	Descriptive + inferential
9. *Authors' conclusions*:	No difference in efficacy, tolerance in favour of pergolide

Comments. No diagnostic criteria. Heterogeneous group with mixed levodopa problems. Retrospective comparison of lisuride vs. pergolide not justified.

Table 11.8 'Bromocriptine: low dose therapy in Parkinson's disease' (Teychenne *et al.*, 1982).

1. *Authors' aims*:	Evaluation of low-dose therapeutic effects of bromocriptine
2. Selection criteria	
(i) diagnosis	Not defined
(ii) specific criteria	None
3. Number admitted	29
4. Study design	Double-blind placebo-controlled cross-over (SC)
5. Patient group	
(i) age	47–85
(ii) duration of disease	5.3 (*de novo*)/8.5 (levodopa) years
(iii) *de novo*	11
(iv) previously treated	14
(v) duration of previous levodopa	Not defined
6. Methods of assessment	
(i) subjective:	
clinical rating scale	Columbia
self-rating scale	
functional disability	
(ii) simple objective	Gait/finger movements
7. Duration of follow-up	Mean 10 months
8. Data analysis	
(i) excluded data defined	4 (3 ADR/1 Inefficacy)
(ii) type of data	Individual
(iii) type of analysis	Inferential (sign test)
9. *Authors' conclusions*:	Low-dose bromocriptine is as effective as high-dose

Comments. Diagnosis not defined. Heterogeneous groups with mixed previously treated and untreated. Conclusion stated depends on retrospective analysis. They are not comparable studies and therefore statement is partially invalid. The conclusion should be 'low-dose of bromocriptine can produce a significant improvement'.

Table 11.9 'Pergolide mesylate and idiopathic Parkinson's disease' (Tanner *et al.*, 1982).

1. *Authors' aims*:	Evaluation of safety and efficacy of pergolide
2. Selection criteria	
(i) diagnosis	Not defined
(ii) specific criteria	Loss efficacy to levodopa or dose-limiting side-effects
3. Number admitted	23
4. Study design	Open (SC)
5. Patient group	
(i) age	Not mentioned
(ii) duration of disease	5–23 (13) years
(iii) *de novo*	—
(iv) previously treated	23
(v) duration of previous levodopa	3–12 (8.8) years
6. Methods of assessment	
(i) subjective:	
clinical rating scale	NYUPDS
self-rating scale	'On–off'
functional disability	NWUDS
(ii) simple objective	None
7. Duration of follow-up	6 months
8. Data analysis	
(i) excluded data defined	2 (unrelated to drug)
(ii) type of data	Individual
(iii) type of analysis	Inferential (Student's test)
9. *Authors' conclusions*:	Effective therapeutic benefit to patients with idiopathic Parkinson's disease and exhibiting problems in response to chronic levodopa therapy

Comments. No diagnosis. Wide duration of disease and previous treatment. Only valid conclusion on 'on–off'. Retrospective comparisons with bromocriptine and lergotrile. Is this study an extension of another trial (see Lees and Stern, 1981)? To prevent confusion the authors should have indicated this.

Table 11.10 'Further studies with pergolide in Parkinson's disease' (Lieberman *et al.*, 1982)

1. *Authors' aims*:	Pergolide response in diurnal oscillations in performance
2. Selection criteria	
(i) diagnosis	Not defined (are they parkinsonians?)
(ii) specific criteria	None
3. Number admitted	56
4. Study design	Single blind (SC)
5. Patient group	
(i) age	35–84 (63.3)
(ii) duration of disease	1–31 years
(iii) *de novo*	1
(iv) previously treated	55
(v) duration of previous levodopa	1 month to 13 years (8.9 years)
6. Methods of assessment	
(i) subjective:	
clinical rating scale	NYUDS
self-rating scale	—
functional disability	—
(ii) simple objective	None
7. Duration of follow-up	1 day to 34 months
8. Data analysis	
(i) excluded data defined	13 (ADR)
(ii) type of data	Individual
(iii) type of analysis	Descriptive
9. *Authors' conclusions*:	Pergolide is a useful treatment; maximum improvement in 2 months; severity and duration of 'on–off' reduced

Comments. Diagnosis not defined (or mentioned). Undoubtedly heterogeneous groups (e.g. pergolide given alone or in association). In spite of in-depth symptom scoring, the only comment is on 'on–off' effect; tolerance of drug not discussed.

Table 11.11 'Treatment of Parkinson's disease with 8-alpha-amino-ergoline, CU 32-085' (Schneider *et al.*, 1983).

1. *Authors' aims*:	Not clearly stated
2. Selection criteria	
(i) diagnosis	Not given
(ii) specific criteria	None
3. Number admitted	24
4. Study design	Open (SC)
5. Patient group	
(i) age	42–81
(ii) duration of disease	1–27 years
(iii) *de novo*	5
(iv) previously treated	19
(v) duration of previous levodopa	Not given
6. Methods of assessment	
(i) subjective:	
clinical rating scale	Webster
self-rating scale	None
functional disability	(Weighed Webster)
(ii) simple objective	Pegboard gait
7. Duration of follow-up	3 months
8. Data analysis	
(i) excluded data defined	5 (3 ADR/2 CD)
(ii) type of data	Individual + global
(iii) type of analysis	Inferential + descriptive (Student's test)
9. *Authors' conclusions*:	Beneficial effect; retrospective comparison with bromocriptine: few side-effects

Comments. Diagnosis and groups poorly defined. Mixed population. Open study. Few comments on efficacy on individual symptoms. Relatively short duration. The treatment of Webster scores by factor loading with small numbers in individual patient groups results in 'artefactual' statistics.

Table 11.12 'Controlled trial of pergolide mesylate in Parkinson's disease and progressive supranuclear palsy'(Jankovic, 1983).

1. *Author's aims*:	Evaluation in PD and supranuclear palsy
2. Selection criteria	
(i) diagnosis	Not defined for PD
(ii) specific criteria	None
3. Number admitted	22
4. Study design	Open (initially)/double-blind placebo-controlled cross-over (SC)
5. Patient group	
(i) age	37–77 (62.9)
(ii) duration of disease	2–18 (9.2) years
(iii) *de novo*	—
(iv) previously treated	22
(v) duration of previous levodopa	0.25–10.5 years
6. Methods of assessment	
(i) subjective:	
clinical rating scale	Hoehn and Yahr
self-rating scale	'On–off' (own scale)
functional disability	None
(ii) simple objective	None
7. Duration of follow-up	Not defined (> 12 weeks): mean 43 weeks (?)
8. Data analysis	
(i) excluded data defined	4 (2 ADRs/2 compliance)
(ii) type of data	Individual
(iii) type of analysis	Inferential (Wilcoxon)
9. *Author's conclusions*:	Pergolide useful in treatment of levodopa-induced fluctuation; 8 patients had total withdrawal of levodopa

Comments. No definition of disease. Heterogeneous group for treatment and duration. Complex trial design; own scale not comparable with other standard scales.

Table 11.13 'On–off effects in Parkinson's disease: a controlled investigation of ascorbic acid therapy' (Reilly *et al.*, 1983).

1. *Authors' aims*:	Effects of ascorbic acid on levodopa-induced dyskinesia and 'on–off' phenomenon
2. Selection criteria	
(i) diagnosis	Not defined
(ii) specific criteria	Dyskinesia + 'On–off'
3. Number admitted	6
4. Study design	Double-blind placebo-controlled cross-over (SC)
5. Patient group	
(i) age	47–78 (67)
(ii) duration of disease	4–26 (11) years
(iii) *de novo*	—
(iv) previously treated	6
(v) duration of previous levodopa	3–9 (6) years
6. Methods of assessment	
(i) subjective:	
clinical rating scale	Webster (3 items)
self-rating scale	Dyskinesia + functional performance (own scale)
functional disability	None
(ii) simple objective	None
7. Duration of follow-up	1 month (stable therapy)
8. Data analysis	
(i) excluded data defined	None
(ii) type of data	Global only
(iii) type of analysis	Descriptive
9. *Authors' conclusions*:	No effect

Comments. Diagnosis not defined. Probable heterogeneous group. Inappropriate number, too short duration. Scaling and individual symptoms not analysed. Invalid conclusion.

Table 11.14 'A 6-month trial of pergolide mesylate in the treatment of idiopathic Parkinson's disease' (Klawans *et al.*, 1983).

1. *Authors' aims*:	Evaluation of safety and efficacy of pergolide over 6 months' treatment
2. Selection criteria	
(i) diagnosis	Not defined
(ii) specific criteria	Only exclusion criteria (given)
3. Number admitted	16 (2 additional excluded?)
4. Study design	Open
5. Patient group	
(i) age	Not given
(ii) duration of disease	5–22 (12.6) years
(iii) *de novo*	—
(iv) previously treated	16
(v) duration of previous levodopa	3–11 (8) years
6. Methods of assessment	
(i) subjective:	
clinical rating scale	NYUPDS
self-rating scale	—
functional disability	NWUDS (gait only)
(ii) simple objective	None
7. Duration of follow-up	6 months
8. Data analysis	
(i) excluded data defined	None
(ii) type of data	Individual + global
(iii) type of analysis	Inferential (Student's and sign tests)
9. *Authors' conclusions*:	Sustained beneficial effect on symptoms and 'on–off' phenomena

Comments. No diagnosis defined. Wide range of duration of disease and previous treatment. Trial only valid for 'on–off'. Retrospective comparison with bromocriptine and lergotrile. Any conclusion on efficacy and tolerance invalid.

Table 11.15 'Pergolide treatment in Parkinsonism' (Ilson *et al.*, 1983).

1. *Authors' aims*:	To report on initial experiences with pergolide
2. Selection criteria	
(i) diagnosis	Not given ('Parkinsonism')
(ii) specific criteria	No longer responding to levodopa
3. Number admitted	11
4. Study design	Open (5 patients) double-blind placebo-controlled cross-over (6 patients)
5. Patient group	
(i) age	27–73 (55)
(ii) duration of disease	5.5–34.5 years
(iii) *de novo*	—
(iv) previously treated	11
(v) duration of previous levodopa	4–11.5 (8) years
6. Methods of assessment	
(i) subjective	
clinical rating scale	Columbia
self-rating scale	'On–off'
functional disability	ADL (Schwab)
(ii) simple objective	None
7. Duration of follow-up	Incomplete (6 weeks?)
8. Data analysis	
(i) excluded data defined	4 (ADR)
(ii) type of data	Global assessment
(iii) type of analysis	Descriptive (%) inferential (Student's test) for 'on–off'
9. *Authors' conclusions*:	Pergolide is a valuable adjuvant to levodopa

Comments. Diagnostic group not defined. Confused trial design with small population. Little data on placebo period. Not clear if it is a double-blind format. Conclusions only valid to assess drug effects upon 'fluctuating' patients. Extension of this trial to 19 patients did not further clarify the situation and can be criticised as above.

Table 11.16 'Lisuride treatment in Parkinson's disease: clinical and pharmacokinetic studies' Le Witt *et al.*, 1983).

1. *Authors' aims*:	Comparison of lisuride vs. bromocriptine
2. Selection criteria	
(i) diagnosis	Not given
(ii) specific criteria	None
3. Number admitted	28
4. Study design	Double-blind cross-over 'add-on' therapy (SC)
5. Patient group	
(i) age	Not given
(ii) duration of disease	2–18 years
(iii) *de novo*	—
(iv) previously treated	28
(v) duration of previous levodopa	Not given
6. Methods of assessment	
(i) subjective:	
clinical rating scale	Columbia (modified)
self-rating scale	None
functional disability	None
(ii) simple objective	Gait + RT
7. Duration of follow-up	2 months (each period)
8. Data analysis	
(i) excluded data defined	2 (Inefficacy)
(ii) type of data	Individual
(iii) type of analysis	Inferential (?)
9. *Authors' conclusions*:	Both drugs equally effective

Comments. No definition of diagnosis, disease stage; problems related to current therapy not defined, as well as effect of test medications. Short duration of treatment. Limited drug doses but large individual dose requirements: statement not clearly defined. No reference to method of assessment. No correlation between objective and clinical data. No statistical methodology stated. Conclusions of authors invalid.

Table 11.17 'Experiences with lisuride in the treatment of Parkinson's disease' (Ulm, 1983).

1. *Author's aims*:	Open study experienced with lisuride
2. Selection criteria	
(i) diagnosis	Not defined
(ii) specific criteria	None
3. Number admitted	119
4. Study design	Open (SC)
5. Patient group	
(i) age	42–84 (61.8)
(ii) duration of disease	9 years
(iii) *de novo*	Not mentioned (?)
(iv) previously treated	Not mentioned (?)
(v) duration of previous levodopa	Not defined
6. Methods of assessment	
(i) subjective:	
clinical rating scale	Webster + 'on–off' scale
self-rating scale	None
functional disability	None
(ii) simple objective	None
7. Duration of follow-up	Not defined
8. Data analysis	
(i) excluded data defined	35 (No clear statement)
(ii) type of data	Mainly global
(iii) type of analysis	Descriptive
9. *Author's conclusions*:	Useful treatment (70% with convincing results)

Comments. We are not convinced that this study is entirely prospective: no diagnosis. Heterogeneous group. No end-point. No definition of global assessment and dyskinesia. 35 patients excluded: why? Exclusion data unclear. Author states in introduction: 'Following observations are based on open studies, and without double-blind comparison, it is not possible to draw valid conclusions.' Why carry out such a trial?

In the 15 trials considered, the patient population varies from 6 to 119. If one considers in terms of clinical trials that the double-blind format is the 'gold standard', then, although these trials were carefully selected, only 40% would be acceptable on this criterion. More florid anomalies in trial design are apparent in the review of table 11.2 especially in the groups of patients selected. In seven trials, the groups of patients were mixed: some were previously untreated and others were already on levodopa. In only one study was the new therapy applied as monotherapy in *de novo* parkinsonian patients. From the 14 studies in which patients were receiving levodopa, no mention has been made of the duration of treatment with levodopa.

It is clear in these trials that the possible effect of chronic exposure to levodopa on the responsiveness to other antiparkinsonian drugs or the exhibition of long-term side-effects of levodopa has not been adequately considered. This may indeed invalidate some of the conclusions reached by the clinicians.

Considering the methods of assessment in the selected trials (clinical, functional or/and objective), the large variety in the rating scales used reflects the lack of a well-accepted and reliable methodology in assessing signs and symptoms of parkinsonism. None of these scales, either clinical or functional, has been objectively validated, and no comparability study has so far been carried out. The deficiencies in the methods of assessment make it impossible for any kind of comparison between trials of the effectiveness of the different tested medications to be made, and call into question the accepted qualitative assessments of Parkinson's disease.

As a final comment on our analysis, in only one-third of the trials described were statistical methods used to evaluate the results obtained.

CONCLUSIONS

Our critical evaluation on trials performed in Parkinson's disease was easy to do and could be done in any other disease group. It does not represent a criticism of the authors and workers involved, and in no way denigrates the amount of effort used to collect the results. Rather, its aim is to highlight the difficulties and deficiencies of such trials so that the next generation of antiparkinsonian drugs can receive a reliable evaluation from the onset. It is clear that we need a more standardised approach to improve trial methodology. We are sure that anyone who is engaged in clinical trials would agree that the more 'perfect' trial may not be the one that is the most practical for the clinical situation. However, we feel strongly that a more standardised approach would produce more valuable information in terms of helping us to manage the individual patient with Parkinson's disease.

REFERENCES

Calne, D. B., Leigh, P. N., Bamji, A. N., Teychenne, P. F. and Greenacre, J. K. (1974). Treatment of Parkinson on bromocriptine. *Lancet,* **2**, 1355–6.

Calne, D. B., Stern, G. M. and Laurence, D. R. (1979). L-Dopa in post-encephalitic parkinsonism. *Lancet,* **1**, 744–6.

Cotzias, G. C., Van Woert, M. H. and Schiffer, L. M. (1967). Aromatic amino acids and modification of parkinsonism. *New Engl. J. Med.,* **276**, 374–9.

Eisler, T., Teravainen, H., Nelson, R., Krebs, H., Weis, V., Lake, C. R., Ebert, M. H., Whetzel, N., Murphy, D. L., Kopin, I. J. and Calne, D. B. (1981). Deprenyl in Parkinson's disease. *Neurology,* **31**, 19–23.

Fahn, S. (1982). Fluctuations of disability in Parkinson's disease: pathological aspects. In Marsden, C. D. and Fahn, S. (eds), *Movement Disorders.* Butterworth Scientific, London, pp. 96–122.

Fahn, S. and Bressman, S. B. (1984). Should levodopa therapy for parkinsonism be started early or late? Evidence against early treatment. *Can. J. Neurol. Sci.,* **11** (1), 200–5.

Gopinathan, G., Teravainen, H., Dambrosia, J. M., Ward, C. D., Sanes, J. N., Stuart, W. K., Evarts, E. V. and Calne, D. B. (1981). Lisuride in parkinsonism. *Neurology,* **31**, 371–6.

Grimes, J. D. (1984). Bromocriptine in Parkinson's disease: results obtained with high and low dose therapy. *Can. J. Neurol. Sci.,* **11** (1), 225–8.

Ilson, J., Fahn, S., Mayeux, R., Cote, L. J. and Snider, S. R. (1983). Pergolide treatment in parkinsonism. In Fahn, S., Calne, D. B. and Shoulson, I. (eds), *Advances in Neurology, vol. 37: Experimental Therapeutics of Movement Disorders.* Raven Press, New York, pp. 85–94.

Jankovic, J. (1983). Controlled trial of pergolide mesylate in Parkinson's disease and progressive supranuclear palsy. *Neurology,* **33**, 505–7.

Klawans, H. L., Tanner, C. M., Glatt, S. and Goetz, C. G. (1983). A 6-month trial period of pergolide mesylate in the treatment of idiopathic Parkinson's disease. In Fahn, S., Calne, D. B. and Shoulson, I. (eds), *Advances in Neurology, vol. 37: Experimental Therapeutics of Movement Disorders.* Raven Press, New York, pp. 75–83.

Lees, A. J. and Stern, G. M. (1981). Sustained bromocriptine therapy in previously untreated patients with Parkinson's disease. *Res. Clin. Forums,* **3** (2) 29–35.

Le Witt, P. A., Gopinathan, G., Ward, C. D., Sanes, J. N., Dambriosia, J. M., Durso, R. and Calne, D. B. (1982). Lisuride versus bromocriptine treatment in Parkinson's disease: a double-blind study. *Neurology,* **32**, 69–72.

Le Witt, P. A., Burns, R. S. and Calne, D. B. (1983). Lisuride treatment in Parkinson's disease: clinical and pharmacokinetic studies. In Fahn, S., Calne, D. B. and Shoulson, I. (eds), *Advances in Neurology, vol. 37: Experimental Therapeutics of Movement Disorders.* Raven Press, New York, pp. 131–40.

Lieberman, A. N., Goldstein, M., Gopinathan, G., Leibowitz, M., Neophytides, A., Walker, R., Heisser, E. and Nelson, J. (1982). Further studies with pergolide in Parkinson's disease. *Neurology,* **32**, 1181–4.

Lieberman, A., Gopinathan, G., Hassouri, H., Neophytides, A. and Goldstein, M. (1984). Should dopamine agonists be given early or late? A review of nine years' experience with bromocriptine. *Can. J. Neurol. Sci.,* **11**, 233–7.

Marsden, C. D., Barry, P. E., Parkes, J. D. and Zilkha, K. J. (1973). Treatment of Parkinson's disease with levodopa combined with L-alpha-methyldopahydrazine, an inhibitor of extracerebral dopa-decarboxylase. *J. Neurol. Neurosurg. Psychiatr.,* **36**, 10–14.

Marsden, C. D., Parkes, J. D. and Quinn, N. (1982). Fluctuations in disability in Parkinson's disease — clinical aspects. In Marsden, C. D. and Fahn, S. (eds), *Movement Disorders*. Butterworth Scientific, London, pp. 96–122.

Muenter, M. D. (1984). Should levodopa therapy be started early or late? *Can. J. Neurol. Sci.,* **11** (1), 195–9.

Rascol, A., Montastruc, J. L. and Rascol, O. (1984). Should dopamine agonists be given early or late in the treatment of Parkinson's disease? *Can. J. Neurol. Sci.,* **11** (1), 229–32.

Reilly, D. K., Hershey, L., Rivera-Calimlin, L. and Shoulson, I. (1983). On–off effects in Parkinson's disease. A controlled investigation of ascorbic acid therapy. In Fahn, S., Calne, D. B. and Shoulson, I. (eds), *Advances in Neurology, vol. 37: Experimental Therapeutics of Movement Disorders*. Raven Press, New York, pp. 51–9.

Rinne, U. K. (1983) Dopamine agonists in the treatment of Parkinson's disease. In Fahn, S., Calne, D. B. and Shoulson, I. (eds), *Advances in Neurology, Vol. 37: Experimental Therapeutics of Movement Disorders*. Raven Press, New York, pp. 141–50.

Schneider, E., Hubener, K. and Fischer, P. A. (1983). Treatment of Parkinson's disease with 8-alpha-amino-ergoline, Cu 32-085. *Neurology, 33*, 468–72.

Tanner, C. M., Goetz, C. G., Glantz, R. H., Glatt, S. L. and Klawans, H. L. (1982). Pergolide mesylate and idiopathic Parkinson's disease. *Neurology, 32*, 1181–4.

Teychenne, P. F., Berstrud, D., Racy,A., Elton, R. L. and Vern, B. (1982). Bromocriptine: low-dose therapy in Parkinson's disease. *Neurology, 32*, 577–83.

Ulm, G. (1983). Experiences with lisuride in the treatment of Parkinson's disease. In Calne, D. B., Horowski,R., McDonald, R. J. and Wuhke, W. (eds), *Lisuride and Other Dopamine Agonists*. Raven Press, New York, pp. 463–72.

Yahr, M. B., (1984). Limitations of long-term use of anti-parkinson drugs. *Can. J. Neurol. Sci.,* **11** (1), 191–4.

12

Methodology of clinical trials in Parkinson's disease.
Part II: Future trials—Recommendations

L. J. FINDLEY and X. LATASTE

As long as one uses only symptoms for the basis of a classification, it will vary like our spirits, each person will construct a framework according to the way in which he sees these same symptoms.

Bichat, 1802

INTRODUCTION

From the previous chapter, it will be appreciated that a large number of fundamental questions remain unanswered in spite of the various clinical trials published on the therapeutic management of Parkinson's disease. Some of the deficiencies in trial methodology have already been highlighted. The purpose of this chapter is to put forward the elements of an ideal trial format including a consideration of the more obvious aspects of the disorders which have often been neglected in trial design. The proposals should be considered as a framework on which future trials should be based rather than as a dogmatic statement on precisely how an individual trial can be carried out. In addition, we would expect to be provocative in order to stimulate debate so that a consensus might be called on what is the best format for clinical trials in Parkinson's disease.

DIAGNOSIS AND PATIENT SELECTION

In none of the clinical trials we have considered in our analysis was the disease group prospectively defined. It is clear that idiopathic Parkinson's disease is not a homogeneous entity even though as yet it is impossible to separate different patient groups in terms of basic pathology (Marshall, 1984). However, clinically we recognise distinct groups: for instance the young hemi-tremulous patient with relatively non-progressive disease is clinically different from the akinetic rigid, rapidly dementing, elderly patient. The recognition of such clinical types is important in terms of therapeutic response. It is well established that tremor is less responsive to levodopa than bradykinesia (Boshes, 1976). It thus seems logical to assume that, within these patient groups, differences in response to new or existing drugs are to be expected. Any future clinical trial must define prospectively and precisely the patients intended for the study.

At the present time, it is difficult to know the best way of defining such patient groups. Unfortunately the International Classification of Disease (ICD, 1977) is not helpful in the diagnosis of Parkinson's disease (Barbeau *et al.*, 1981) in terms of trial methodology (table 12.1). Most of the comprehensive classifications used are based on the pathophysiological findings which would clearly not be available in a prospective trial situation (table 12.2; Duvoisin, 1984).

In consideration of the above comments, we are forced to accept a classification of patients based on symptoms and clinical signs to define the patients prospectively in the form of a cumulative numbering system (Capildeo *et al.*, 1981). This system would include, for example: clinical features (major/minor); type of parkinsonism, e.g. idiopathic, postencephalitic, etc; effects of previous drug therapy; disability status; and current therapy.

From such systems of cumulative numbering, patient groups can be more precisely and clearly defined. A simple example is given in table 12.3. It will be appreciated that the total cumulative score clearly defines a single clinical type without overlap into other groups.

Table 12.1 International classification of disease, 9th revision (WHO, 1977).

332   Parkinson's disease

332.0 Paralysis agitans (parkinsonism or Parkinson's disease):
       NOS
       idiopathic
       primary

332.1 Secondary parkinsonism:
       due to drugs
       syphilitic (094.8)

Notes: NOS = 'not otherwise specified'; 094.8 = alternative code for syphilis.

The use of this system has other advantages. It can be directly computerised for selection and/or stratification of patients at entry. It is important that the individual patient's point of entry into the trial (the point of assessment when the cumulative numbering is applied) should be carefully defined. If, for instance, the trial has to be a monotherapy study, it should be performed after a wash-out period. In a trial in which the test medication is added on, an initial controlled phase must be planned to ensure that the previous treatment is optimum so that as far as possible problems of pre-existing overdosage or underdosage, fluctuations in response or apparent dyskinesia do not contaminate the evaluation of the new treatment.

Table 12.2   A classification of parkinsonism (adapted from Duvoisin, 1984).

1. Parkinson's disease
   (a) Classic Lewy body disease
   (b) With alzheimerisation
   (c) Juvenile onset

2. Post-encephalitic
   (a) Encephalitis lethargica
   (b) Other encephalitides
   (c) Luetic mesencephalitis

3. Iatrogenic

4. Symptomatic
   (a) Structural lesions — congenital, acquired, neoplastic
   (b) Post-traumatic
   (c) Toxic — metabolic

5. Multiple system degeneration:
   strionigral degeneration
   the olivopontocerebellar atrophies
   progressive supranuclear palsy
   the Shy–Drager syndrome
   Wilson's disease
   Hallervorden–Spatz disease
   Creutzfeld–Jakob disease
   phenotypic variants of various genetic disorders
   Parkinson dementia complex
   pallidonigral degeneration

6. Pseudoparkinsonism:
   multiple cerebral infarctions
   normal pressure hydrocephalus
   acquired hepatocerebral degeneration

Table 12.3 Example of a cumulative index in Parkinson's disease (adapted from R. Capildeo, 1981). A clinical evaluation of drug *x* should be performed in patients with hemi-Parkinson's disease, with dominant rigidity and tremor, who are receiving chronic levodopa and exhibiting 'on–off' phenomena. Such a patient population should be defined with the cumulative index shown here.

Clinical feature		1 + 2 tremor rigidity	= 3
Clinical feature (minor)		8 + 16 facies posture	= 24
Type of parkinsonism		1 idiopathic	= 1
Effect of drug therapy		Levodopa/'on–off'	32
Disability	*a* right	1 + 2 tremor rigidity	= *a*3
Current therapy		Dopaminergic agonists	4

[*Editor's note*: Each item in a series of short tables is identified by a number according to the decimal system, e.g. 1, 2, 4, 10, etc. The addition of these numbers gives a total which can easily be broken down into the salient numbers and hence the individual items. For example, the total score indicates severity by the number of items affected and higher numbers indicate a greater degree of severity than lower numbers.]

Additional criteria for selection can and will be added to the basic cumulative numbering index. Two obvious criteria will be the age at onset of parkinsonian symptoms and the duration and/or the cumulative amount of previous therapy (table 12.4).

TRIAL DESIGN

The type of trial design is closely dependent upon the basic question being asked and the development stage of the new drug. The early evaluation of a therapy should be carried out in patients in the form of a short-term evaluation of efficacy and tolerance (Phase I trials). This approach must conform with the accepted format for clinical trials and therefore should be double blind and placebo controlled, either in previously untreated patients or in an add-on situation. For ethical reasons, the patients should benefit from the tested active treatment from the start of the study. A 'randomised placebo substitute' phase can be planned after the active phase of treatment while maintaining the double-blind conditions.

Table 12.4   Criteria for defining a patient group.

- Cumulative index
- Age of onset
- Duration of previous treatment
- Cumulative amount of previous therapy

When two active treatments have to be compared either in *de novo* or in 'add-on' therapy, we would propose a randomised, double-blind, parallel-group design. A cross-over design for this type of trial would at first sight appear to be more appropriate. However, certain problems would arise. First, the wash-out period in between the two cross-over periods should be long enough so that there is no overlapping in the evaluation of therapeutic response. No 'within-patients' comparison is possible, as the clinical status of the patients at cross-over has been altered from entry, not only by the progression of the disease, but also by the effects of previous trial treatment. Trials in Parkinson's disease with a cross-over format can only be used if the different phases of treatment can be analysed separately as two parallel-group studies (table 12.5).

Experience with levodopa over the last 15 years has shown that the long-term side-effects have become an increasing problem with chronic use of the drug. In addition, as patients are living longer, it is difficult to differentiate between the effect of long-term treatment and the natural course of the disease process (e.g. dementia). There is no information as yet on whether new antiparkinsonian agents such as bromocriptine will have long-term side-effects. It is apparent that any prospective study in the treatment of Parkinson's disease must include long-term evaluation in clearly defined patient populations, using a randomised blind allocation with careful pretreatment stratification, blind observer assessment and regular follow-up.

From the rigidity of definition and selection we are advocating, it is evident that it would not be possible for one centre, however large, to select enough patients to undertake a realistic clinical trial. Therefore we are forced to admit that all future trials in Parkinson's disease attempting to answer fundamental questions will have to be multicooperative with possible central computerised control. This would require the setting up of national or international groups of clinical researchers with the appropriate degree of experience to coordinate such, of necessity, large and complicated trials. In order to increase the validity of such studies and to maintain the interest of all participants, a steering committee would be required, ideally allowing all participant groups a share in the executive function on a rotational basis.

Table 12.5 Cross-over trial design in Parkinson's disease. (Comparative evaluation of two active treatments, either *de novo* or add-on. Randomised double-blind cross-over study (with appropriate stratification according to indices).)

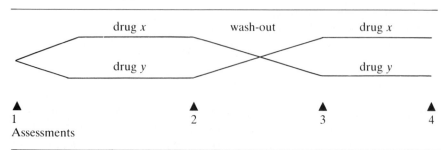

METHODS OF ASSESSMENT

Parkinson's disease is a disease complex in which a large number of theoretical and practical considerations on how best to assess the clinical deficit have been published (Marsden and Schachter, 1981; Larsen *et al.*, 1983; Ward *et al.*, 1983). Since the introduction of levodopa, a wide number of subjective clinical rating systems have been developed and are continuing to be developed, suggesting that no single system is completely satisfactory. These scales attempt to measure symptoms, signs and/or functional disability. The most common ones are listed in table 12.6. (See also Annex 1–XV.)

The complications observed in parkinsonian patients under chronic levodopa therapy have necessitated the development of additional rating scales evaluating dyskinesias, fluctuating responses and 'on–off' phenomena, especially for add-on studies (table 12.7) (AIMS, 1976; Kartzinel and Calne, 1976; Marsden and Parkes, 1976; Lees *et al.* 1977; Lieberman *et al.* 1980; Schachter *et al.*, 1980). Detailed perusal of the large number of systems of evaluation will convince the reader that there is no common agreement on what is the best or most suitable mode of assessment. Indeed it is now becoming apparent that cross-comparison cannot be made from trials using one system of assessment of disability to trials using different systems. However, this is frequently done in the literature.

In the paper by Diamond and Markham (1983), the most interesting study, four commonly used rating scales have been demonstrated to measure quite different aspects of parkinsonian disability. From this it can be concluded that results from different studies may only be valid for comparative analysis if the scales used in the trials are identical.

Table 12.6   Clinical rating scale in Parkinson's disease.

	Symptoms and signs	Functional disability	Reference
Karnofsky *et al.*		●	Karnofsky *et al.*, 1951
Massachusetts General Hospital Rating Scale		●	England and Schwab 1956
Northwestern University Disability Scale		●	Canter *et al.*, 1961
Hoehn and Yahr Staging Scale		●	Hoehn and Yahr, 1967
Webster Rating Scale	●		Webster, 1968
New York University Rating Scale	●	●	Alba *et al.*, 1968
Klawans and Garvin	●		Klawans and Garvin, 1969
Columbia University Rating Scale	●		Duvoisin, 1970
King's College Hospital Rating Scale	●	●	Parkes *et al.*, 1970
Parkinson's Disease Information Center	●		Cotzias *et al.*, 1970
Rinne *et al.*	●		Rinne *et al.*, 1970
Cornell weighed scale	●	●	McDowell *et al.*, 1970
Anden *et al.*	●	●	Anden *et al.*, 1970
Parkinson weighed scale	●	●	Treciokas *et al.*, 1971
Birkmayer and Neumayer	●		Birkmayer and Neumayer, 1972
Potvin and Tourtelotte (unspecific)	●		Potvin and Tourtelotte, 1975

continued overleaf

	Symptoms and signs	Functional disability	Reference
Lhermitte *et al.*	●	●	Lhermitte *et al.*, 1978
UCLA disability scale	●	●	Diamond *et al.*, 1978
New York University Parkinson's disease scale	●	●	Lieberman *et al.*, 1980
Modified Hoehn and Yahr's scale		●	Larsen *et al.*, 1983

In addition to rating scales, simple objective assessments (e.g. the pegboard test, walking time, writing time) may give useful clinical information. Complex objective measurements however (e.g. on-line computer analysis of movements, telemetry, spectral analysis of tremor) are available. These experimental complex measurements will have a place in routine clinical trials. However, they do have a place in laboratory-based investigations looking for the precise and specific action of drugs in small numbers of well-defined patients.

In all trials we foresee that there must be a method of assessing the stage of the disease, a rating scale of symptoms and signs which can be quickly and conveniently applied giving reliable results, and also some measurements of the patient's functional disability in his normal environment. In addition in specific trials, assessment of fluctuations of symptoms and dyskinesia and mood changes will have to be made. We would propose the methods of assessment listed in table 12.8 as suitable for trials in Parkinson's disease.

DURATION OF FOLLOW-UP

In short-term trials, a minimum of two months on optimum dosage will be required.

DATA ANALYSIS

As emphasised in the review of published trials (chapter 11), the statistical methods used to analyse the results are rarely defined in the methods of the report. We firmly advocate that *all* prospective studies should state the

Table 12.7 Rating scale developed for adverse drug effects of chronic levodopa.

	Dyskinesia	*'On–off'*	*Reference*
King's College Hospital	●	●	Marsden *et al.*, 1976
Kartzinel and Calne	●	Mean daily	Kartzinel and Calne, 1976
AIMS scale	●		AIMS, 1976
Lees *et al.*		Mean hourly	Lees *et al.*, 1977
Lieberman	●	Total off	Lieberman *et al.*, 1980
Schachter		Total off	Schachter *et al.*, 1980
Sandoz Parkinson's scale	●	Total off	Unpublished

Table 12.8 Proposal for a standardised method of assessment for a trial in Parkinson's disease.

- ● Modified Hoehn and Yahr staging scale (Larsen *et al.*, 1983)
- ● Webster rating scale (symptoms/signs) (Webster, 1968)
- ● Patient's self-assessment of functional disability (VAS)*
- ● Dyskinesia, 'on–off' rating scale (Canter *et al.* 1961)
- ● Beck or Zung index for depressive symptoms

*VAS, Visual analogue scale.

number of assessments planned over the study period and mention all exclusions of data. Inferential analysis (i.e. statistical methods) should be carefully chosen and well defined in the planning phase of the trial. Statistical advice must be taken in advance to ensure that a sufficient number of well-defined patients have entered the study to answer the questions being asked (Hills and Armitage 1979; Vere, 1979). We emphasise the importance of multicooperative studies with properly defined population sizes to increase the power of the final conclusions.

CONCLUSIONS

The methodological approaches in clinical trials in Parkinson's disease suggested in this chapter will improve our ability to evaluate existing and newer antiparkinsonian drugs and lead ultimately to better therapeutic management of the individual patient. We hope that our proposals will encourage more discussions on specific aspects of the methodology, to generate a more general consensus for future trials and solve the outstanding clinical problems facing us. Recently, at a meeting of North American and European neurologists, an attempt was made to formulate a unified rating scale for Parkinson's disease that will be universally acceptable. This scale is currently being evaluated and offers the possibility of greater uniformity in the approach to the assessment of disability in patients with Parkinson's disease.

ANNEX I TO XI   COMMONLY USED CLINICAL RATING SCALES IN PARKINSON'S DISEASE

I	Hoehn and Yahr, clinical stage (1967) and Modified Hoehn and Yahr clinical stage rating (1983)
II	Webster rating scale (1968)
III	Columbia University rating scale (1970)
IV	Modified Columbia University rating scale (1981)
V	Modified Columbia University rating scale — version 5 (1983)
VI	King's College Hospital rating scale (1970)
VII	New York University rating scale (1980)
VIII	Northwestern University Disability Scale (1961)
IX	ADL (Activities of Daily Living) (1980)
X	Modified Schwab and England ADL scale (1983)
XI	Rinne *et al.* rating scale (1983)
XII	ADR to levodopa (1983)
XIII	Dyskinesia rating scale on–off (Sandoz, 1984)
XIV	AIMS (1982)
XV	AIMS (1983) Yahr

REFERENCES

AIMS (1976). In Guy, W. (ed.), *ECDEU Assessment Manual for Psychopharmacology,* Department of Health, Education and Welfare, Rockville, Maryland, pp. 534–7.

Alba, A., Trainor, F. S., Ritter, W. and Dacso, M. M. (1968). A clinical disability rating for parkinsonian patients. *J. Chron. Dis.*, **21**, 507–22.

Anden, N. E., Carlsson, A., Kerstell, J., Magnusson, T., Olsson, R., Roose, B. E., Steen, B., Steg, G., Svangorg, A., Thieme, G. and Werdinius, B. (1970). Oral L-dopa treatment of parkinsonism. *Acta Med. Scand.*, **187**, 247–55.

Barbeau, A., Duvoisin, R. C., Gerstenbrand, F., Lakke, J. P. W. F., Marsden, C. D. and Stern, C. (1981). Classification of extrapyramidal disorders. *J. Neurol. Sci.*, **51**, 311–27.

Birkmayer, W. and Neumayer, E. (1972). Die moderne medikamentose Behandlung des Parkinsonismus. *Z Neurol.*, **202**, 257–64.

Boshes, B. (1976). In Birkmayer, W. and Hornykiewicz, O. (eds) *Advances in Parkinson's Disease*. Roche, Basle, p. 303.

Canter, C. J., De La Torre, R. and Mier, M. (1961). A method of evaluating disability in patients with Parkinson's disease. *J. Nerv. Mental Dis.*, **133**, 143–7.

Capildeo, R., Haberman, S. and Rose, F. C. (1981). The classification of parkinsonism. In Rose, F. C. and Capildeo, R. (eds), *Research Progress in Parkinson's Disease*. Pitman Medical, London, pp. 17–24.

Cotzias, G. C., Papavasiliou, P. S., Fehling, C., Kaufman, B. and Mena, I. (1970). Similarities between neurologic effects of L-dopa and apomorphine. *New Engl. J. Med.*, **282**, 31–3.

Diamond, S. G. and Markham, C. H. (1983). Evaluating the evaluation: or how to weigh the scales of parkinsonian disability. *Neurology*, **33**, 1098–9.

Diamond, D. G., Markham, C. H. and Treciokas, L. J. (1978). A double-blind comparison of Levodopa, Madopar and Sinemet in Parkinson's disease. *Ann. Neurol.*, **3**, 267–72.

Duvoisin, R. C. (1970). The evaluation of extrapyramidal disease. In De Ajuriagerra, J. (ed.), *Monoamines, Noyaux Gris Centraux et Syndrome de Parkinson*, Masson, Paris, pp. 313–25.

Duvoisin, R. C. (1984). Parkinson's disease: acquired or inherited? *Can. J. Neurol. Sci.*, **11** (1), 151–5.

England, A. C. and Schwab, R. S. (1956). Postoperative evaluation of 26 selected patients with Parkinson's disease. *J. Am. Geriat. Soc.*, **4**, 1219–32.

Hills, M. and Armitage, P. (1979). The two-period cross-over clinical trial. *Brit. J. Clin. Pharmacol.*, **8**, 7–20.

Hoehn, N. M. and Yahr, M. D. (1967). Parkinsonism: onset, progression and mortality. *Neurology*, **17**, 427–42.

Karnofsky, D. A., Burchenal, J. H., Armistead, G. C., Southam, C. M., Bernstein, J. L., Craver, L. F. and Rhoads, C. P. (1951). Triethylene nealamine in the treatment of neoplastic disease. *Arch. Int. Med.*, **87**, 477–516.

Kartzinel, R. and Calne, D. B. (1976). Studies with bromocriptine. Part I. On–off phenomena. *Neurology*, **26**, 508–10.

Klawans, H. L. and Garvin, J. S. (1969). Treatment of parkinsonism with levodopa. *Dis. Nerv. Syst.*, **30**, 737–46.

Larsen, A. T., Le Witt, P. A. and Calne, D. B. (1983). Theoretical and practical issues in assessment of deficits and therapy in parkinsonism. In Calne, D. B., (eds), *Lisuride and Other Dopamine Agonists*. Raven Press, New York, pp. 363–73.

Lees, A. J., Shaw, K. M., Kohout, L. J., Stern, G. M., Elsworth, J. D., Sandler, M. and Youdim, M. B. H. (1977). Deprenyl in Parkinson's disease. *Lancet*, **2**, 791–5.

Lhermitte, F., Agid, Y. and Signoret, J. L. (1978). Onset and end-of-dose levodopa-induced dyskinesia. Possible treatment by increasing the daily dose of levodopa. *Arch. Neurol.*, **35**, 261–3.

Lieberman, A., Dziatolowski, M., Gopinathan, G., Kopersmith, M., Neophytides, A. and Korein, J. (1980). Evaluation of Parkinson's disease. In Goldstein, M. (ed.), *Ergot Compounds and Brain Function: Neuro-endocrine and Neuropsychiatric Aspects.* Raven Press, New York, pp. 277–86.

McDowall, F., Lee, J. E., Swift, T., Sweet, R. D., Ogsbury, J. S. and Tesslet, J. T. (1970). Treatment of Parkinson's syndrome with dihydroxyphenyl alanine (L-dopa), *Ann. Int. Med.*, **72**, 29–35.

Marsden, C. D. and Parkes, J. D. (1976). On–off effects in patients with Parkinson's disease on chronic levodopa therapy. *Lancet*, **1**, 292–6.

Marsden, C. D. and Schachter, M. (1981). Assessment of extrapyramidal disorders. *Brit. J. Clin. Pharmacol.*, **11**, 129–51.

Marshall, A. (1984). Pathology of tremor. In Findley, L. J. and Capildeo, R. (eds), *Movement Disorders: Tremor*, Macmillan, London, pp. 95–123.

Parkes, J. D., Zilkha, K. J., Calver, D. M. and Knill Jones, R. P. (1970). Controlled trial of amantadine hydrochloride in Parkinson's disease. *Lancet*, **1**, 259–62.

Potvin, A. R. and Tourtelotte, W. W. (1975). The neurological examination: advancement in its quantification. *Arch. Phys. Med. Rehab.*, **56**, 425–37.

Rinne, U. K., Sonninen, V. and Siirtola, J. (1970). L-dopa treatment in Parkinson's disease. *Eur. Neurol.*, **4**, 348–69.

Schachter, M., Marsden, C. D., Parkes, J. D., Jenner, P. and Testa, B. (1980). Deprenyl in the management of response fluction in patients with Parkinson's disease on levodopa. *J. Neurol. Neurosurg. Psychiatr.*, **43**, 1016–21.

Treciokas, L. J., Ansel, R. D. and Markham, C. H. (1971). One to two years' treatment of Parkinson's disease with levodopa. *Calif. Med.*, **114**, 7–16.

Vere, D. W. (1979). Validity of cross-over trials. *Brit. J. Clin. Pharmacol.*, **8**, 5–6.

Ward, C. D., Sanes, J. N., Dambriosia, J. M. and Calne, D. B. (1983). Methods for evaluating treatment in Parkinson's disease. In Fahn, S., Calne, D. B. and Shoulson, I. (eds), *Advances in Neurology, vol. 37: Experimental Therapeutics of Movement Disorders.* Raven Press, New York, pp. 1–7.

Webster, D. D. (1968). Clinical analysis of the disability in Parkinson's disease. *Mod. Treat.*, **5**, 257–82.

WHO (1977). *Manual of the International Statistical Classification of Diseases, Injuries and Causes of Death*, 9th Revision, World Health Organization, Geneva.

13
Vascular disease and dementia: an introduction

M. J. G. HARRISON

INTRODUCTION

In trials of therapy for dementia the problem is again the heterogeneity of the clinical material and the lack of certainty of diagnosis without patholological confirmation. An important subgroup among the demented population is that made up of individuals whose deterioration is due to cerebrovascular disease.

In the past, dementia was often uncritically attributed to 'arteriosclerosis' if the patient was of the age group where vascular disease is common. It is clearly important in the interpretation of trials involving dementia that patients with vascular disease as the underlying cause are clearly identified. It is also important that treatment aimed at this group is not confused by the inclusion of patients with Alzheimer's disease. In this introduction a few comments about the differential diagnosis are pertinent.

Trials of vasodilators or other drugs affecting vascular changes in cases of vascular dementia also need to be founded on a clear understanding of the pathogenesis of dementia in vascular disease, and this too will be considered.

It is believed that Alzheimer's disease represents a quantitative departure from normal. There appears to be a threshold effect. Thus the presence (or absence) of 12 or more plaques per microscopic field correctly classifies 85% of senile dementia patients and 90–100% of individuals with no evidence of deterioration (Roth, 1980). Tomlinson et al. (1968, 1970) demonstrated a similar threshold for vascular damage as a cause of mental deterioration. In nine patients thought to have dementia related to vascular disease they found 60–412 ml of infarction in their post-mortem brains. Only one non-demented control had more than 60 ml of brain softening, and none more than 100 ml. Patients with Alzheimer's disease defined by the presence

259

of many plaques, neurofibrillary tangles, etc. had only minute softening if any, except for two individuals with 40–50 ml infarction. They decided that 50 ml might represent the threshold, generalised mental deterioration being likely in patients with more extensive ischaemic softening. A more rigorous cut-off point might have been 100 ml (Brust, 1983).

Unfortunately, pathological series cannot give a reliable indication of the prevalence of infarction as a cause of dementia since these series are of selected cases. It is of interest that in the series of Tomlinson *et al.* (1968, 1970) 50% had Alzheimer's disease, 17% vascular damage and 18% a mixed picture.

CLINICAL EVIDENCE

Based on the clinical features of the patients described by Roth and his group (1980), Hachinski *et al.* (1974) devised a clinical 'ischaemic score' based on weighted features obtained from the history or examination. A score below 4 was thought to be indicative of Alzheimer's or other degenerative disease, and a score of 7 or more implied a vascular cause for dementia. Rosen *et al.* (1980) in a recent prospective clinicopathological study have verified the score (table 13.1).

Table 13.1 Pathological verification of the 'ischaemic score' diagnosis of cause of dementia (from Rosen *et al.*, 1980).

	Alzheimer's (5)	*Multi-infarct* (4)	*Mixed* (5)
Ischaemic score	2–5	7–13	8–14

Using clinical features from the ischaemic score such as an abrupt onset, stepwise deterioration, a history of stroke and focal signs (which occurred in none of the Alzheimer's cases in Rosen's, albeit small, study), Marsden and Harrison (1972) estimated that about 10% of demented patients were suffering from the effects of multiple cerebral infarcts.

PATHOPHYSIOLOGY

Cerebral blood flow declines with age (Thomas *et al.*, 1979), a finding that at first sight appears to confirm the widely held belief that normal age changes and dementia in ageing subjects are due to an insufficient blood supply to the brain. There is, however, a parallel reduction in cerebral metabolic rate for oxygen and glucose so the inference must be that flow declines secondary to a reduced metabolic demand (there being a tight couple between metabolism and flow). Measures of oxygen extraction using PET scanning with $O_2{}^{15}$ and $CO_2{}^{15}$ reveal that evidence of high oxygen extraction implying a blood flow too low for the prevailing regional metabolic need is extremely rare in demented subjects (Frackowiak *et al.*, 1981). This suggests that their reduced cerebral metabolism is rarely if ever due to critical underperfusion (and incidentally that vasodilators will only cause ineffectual luxury perfusion). Further support for this contention comes from the finding that aged and demented subjects still show an increase in CBF in response to an increase in inspired $pACO_2$. Increases also occur with arousal and during the carrying out of specific mental tasks (Lassen and Ingvar, 1980), making it unlikely that the low blood flow at rest is limiting function.

Patients with dementia due to multiple cerebral infarcts show proportionately greater degrees of cerebral blood flow impairment (Harrison *et al.*, 1979). Kuhl (1983) has confirmed that regional glucose metabolism is also reduced in demented patients. Those with multi-infarct dementia showed patchy regional glucose metabolism compatible with multifocal rather than diffuse metabolic disturbances.

The evidence from physiological studies is thus that chronic ischaemia does not cause dementia. When dementia occurs in association with cerebrovascular disease, it is due to the occurrence of multiple infarcts whose presence can often be detected by CT scanning, EEG or angiography.

CT SCANNING

A recent comparison by Loeb (1980) has shown that patients identified clinically as having multi-infarct dementia frequently have low-density areas compatible with areas of infarction, whereas patients with Alzheimer's disease more usually show simple atrophy. Some patients with multi-infarct dementia as defined clinically had simple atrophy, presumably due to the small size of their infarcts, a contention supported by PET-scan evidence of patchy metabolic derangement in such cases (Kuhl, 1983). It is anticipated that NMR scanning may prove an even more sensitive way of detecting multiple small infarcts.

ELECTROENCEPHALOGRAPHY

Harrison *et al.* (1979) showed that patients with multi-infarct dementia more often showed focal or lateralising EEG abnormalities than did patients with clinical evidence of a primary degenerative Alzheimer type of dementia.

ANGIOGRAPHY

The same study (Harrison *et al.*, 1979) examined the angiographic features of patients with multi-infarct dementia and Alzheimer's disease. The former group showed areas of delayed filling or hyperacmia indicative of infarction, and there was evidence of more extensive atheromatous disease of small vessels in such cases. The cause of this particular distribution of atheroma could not be determined since there was no simple association with hypertension.

CONCLUSION

Thus though cerebral blood flow declines with age and in dementia, there is no evidence that it causes critical ischaemia of the brain. When dementia is due to vascular disease, there is evidence pathologically, clinically, angiographically and on electroencephalography and CT scanning of the presence of multiple areas of infarction. Clinical surveys suggest that vascular disease is only responsible for some 10–15% of cases of dementia. The ischaemic score method of diagnosing cases of multi-infarct dementia is at present the best method of defining patient groups for inclusion in trials, and CT scans and EEGs are useful confirmatory tests. NMR scans may prove helpful too, but are unlikely to be available for such trials for some time.

The evidence from PET scans is that true chronic ischaemia is not found in demented patients so the logic of trials of vasodilators is suspect. Measures aimed at metabolic function or at the prevention of further infarcts would appear more fruitful avenues to follow.

REFERENCES

Brust, J. C. M. (1983). Vascular dementia — still overdiagnosed. *Stroke,* **14**, 298–300.

Frackowiak, R. S. J., Pozzilli, C., Legg, N. J., Du Boulay, G. H., Marshall, J., Lenzi, C. L. and Jones, T. (1981). Regional cerebral oxygen supply and investigation in dementia. *Brain,* **104**, 753–78.

Hachinski, V. C., Lassen, N. A. and Marshall, J. (1974). Multi-infarct dementia. A cause of mental deterioration in the elderly. *Lancet,* **2**, 207–10.

Harrison, M. J. G., Thomas, D. J., Du Boulay, G. H. and Marshall, J. (1979). Multi infarct dementia. *J. Neurol. Sci.,* **40**, 97–103.

Kuhl, D. E. (1983). The effects of ageing and stroke on patterns of local cerebral glucose utilization. In Reivich, M. (ed.), *Cerebrovascular Diseases, Thirteenth Princeton Conference.* Raven Press, New York.

Lassen, N. A. and Ingvar, D. H. (1980). Blood flow studies in the ageing normal brain and in senile dementia. In Amaducci, L. *et al.* (eds), *Aging,* vol. 13. Raven Press, New York, pp. 91–8.

Loeb, C. (1980). Clinical diagnosis of multi infarct dementia. In Amaducci, L. *et al.* (eds), *Aging,* vol. 13. Raven Press, New York, pp. 251–60.

Marsden, C. D. and Harrison, M. J. G. (1972). Outcome on investigation of patients with presenile dementia. *Brit. Med. J.*, **2**, 249–52.

Rosen, W. G., Terry, R. D., Fuld, P. A., Katzman, R. and Peck, A. (1980). Pathologic verification of ischaemic score in differentiation of dementias. *Ann. Neurol.*, **7**, 486–8.

Roth, M. (1980). Aging of the brain and dementia: an overview. In Amaducci, L. *et al.* (eds), *Aging,* vol. 13. Raven Press, New York, pp. 1–21.

Thomas, D. J., Zilkha, E., Redmond, S., Du Boulay, G., Marshall, J., Ross Russell, R. W. and Symon, L. (1979). An intravenous 133xenon clearance technique for measuring cerebral blood flow. *J. Neurol. Sci.*, **40**, 53–63.

Tomlinson, B. E., Blessed, G. and Roth, M. (1968). Observations on the brains of non-demented old people. *J. Neurol. Sci.*, **7**, 331–56.

Tomlinson, B. E., Blessed, G. and Roth, M. (1970). Observations on the brains of demented old people. *J. Neurol. Sci.*, **11**, 205–42.

14
Methodology of clinical trials in dementia. Part I: Analysis of previous trials

J. M. S. PEARCE, M. G. WALLACE and R. CAPILDEO

INTRODUCTION

With increasing life expectancy, dementia is rapidly becoming one of the greatest problems facing modern society: catastrophic for the patient, and a severe burden for the family, community and state. In a recent report from the UK, a College Committee on Geriatrics of the Royal College of Physicians has calculated that between 1976 and 1988 the over-65 population is projected to increase by 7% nationally. This conceals, however, a real increase of 25% in the over-75s who will then form 6.4% of the total population. Thus, in the UK, a health district of 250 000 people will have to provide services for 3000 elderly people suffering from dementia.

The most frequent cause of dementia is Alzheimer's disease, accounting for more than 50% of cases. The disabilities associated with this type of dementia (memory loss, confusion, disorientation, lack of self-care) are frequently accepted by relatives and the community as being part of and seen as an inevitable consequence of growing old. It is generally believed that there is little that can be done to treat such cases who are tolerated by the family until they exceed reasonable limits, so that it is more often a social crisis rather than a medical one which brings dementia to the notice of the general practitioner.

Definition of dementia

The Royal College of Physicians (1981) has defined dementia as follows:

The global impairment of higher cortical function including memory, the capacity to solve the problems of day-to-day living, the performance of

265

learned perceptuomotor skills, the correct use of social skills and control of emotional reactions, in the absence of gross clouding of consciousness. The condition is often irreversible and progressive.

Acute confusional states

It is important to distinguish an acute confusional state from dementia. The former occurs in old people as a result of physical illness, metabolic disturbance, or drug intoxication. These are usually short-term disorders, accompanied by clouding of consciousness and a fluctuating level of awareness, and will respond to sedation and treatment of the underlying cause.

Primary and secondary dementia

Dementia is either 'primary', due to intrinsic brain degeneration, or 'secondary', caused by an underlying physical disease. Presenile dementia (age of onset before 65 years of age) was first described by Alzheimer in 1907.

Senile dementia of the Alzheimer type (SDAT) and multi-infarct dementia

It is now accepted that the pathological processes of presenile and senile dementia are identical, which explains the use of the term 'senile dementia of the Alzheimer type (SDAT)'. It is characterised by brain atrophy, and the presence of neurofibrillary tangles and senile plaques. Multi-infarct dementia is less common, and the brain at post-mortem will contain many small areas of infarction, unevenly distributed, hence the term. The old concept of progressive diffuse cerebral arteriosclerosis as a cause for this condition is no longer tenable.

Secondary dementia

Secondary dementia, as already stated, can be caused by an underlying physical disease. It is important that all cases of dementia be investigated as thoroughly as possible, for perhaps 20% of all dementias have a treatable cause (Katzman, 1981). The most common causes of secondary dementia are listed in table 14.1.

Pseudodementia and depression

Pseudodementia is the name given to those patients who present with a clinical picture indistinguishable from dementia, but on investigation are found to have no organic brain impairment.

Table 14.1 Some causes of secondary dementia

Trauma	*Intoxications*
Acute and delayed effects of head injury	Barbiturates, bromides
Punch-drunk syndrome	Alcoholism
Subdural haematoma	Amphetamines and hallucinogens
	Organic poisons, solvents (glue sniffing)
Anoxia	
Hypoperfusion states	*Metabolic*
	Hypothyroidism
Infections	Hypopituitarism
Brain abscess	Hypercalcaemia
Sequelae of meningitis/encephalitis	Cushing's disease
Fungal meningitis (e.g. torulosis)	Renal failure and dialysis dementia
Subacute sclerosing panencephalitis	Hepatic encephalopathy
Neurosyphilis	
Creutzfeldt-Jakob disease	*Dynamic*
	Communicating ('normotensive') or
Deficiency states	obstructive hydrocephalus
Vitamin B_{12}, folic acid	
Pellagra	
Wernicke-Korsakoff's syndrome	*Vascular*
(thiamine)	Multi-infarcts — embolic, thrombotic,
	lacunar
Neoplasms	Arteritides
Primary or metastatic carcinoma or	Angioma
lymphoma	Binswanger's encephalopathy
Carcinomatous meningitis	

The incidence of depression in the elderly is high, and its wide-ranging effects, including pseudodementia, are potentially reversible. It is therefore clearly important to differentiate between these two conditions (see table 14.2).

Investigation of dementia

It would be impossible to investigate thoroughly all those patients who show signs of early mental and cognitive impairment. The investigation of dementia is regarded as being typical of that carried out in most modern neurological departments (see table 14.3).

DRUG TRIALS IN DEMENTIA

Of the many different groups of drugs which have been employed over several decades to attempt to relieve the symptoms of dementia or to correct the primary causal disease, none has proved convincingly successful. There

Table 14.2 Differentiating depression from dementia (adapted from Katzman 1981).

	Depression	*Dementia*
Onset	Usually rapid	Insidious
Mood	Stable, but depressed and apathetic	Labile: apathetic then normal
Mental impairment	Pseudodementia, or no cognitive deficits	Cognitive deficits
History	May be previous or family history	No previous or family history necessary
Duration	Generally self-limited	Chronic and progressive

are, however, many papers which claim to show benefits in mental function and in behaviour in certain selected areas. Most of these trials can be criticised on methodological grounds, and careful scrutiny of the trials shows defects which to some extent are inherent in the population studied. The varied nature of the underlying pathological process or processes, the common occurrence of mixed vascular and Alzheimer changes and the common unknown factors of premorbid intelligence, of personality and resilience are usually unknown. Each of these factors may well determine the apparent response to drug treatment. In most patients included in trials, precise information of this sort is lacking.

Yesavage *et al.* (1979) published a review of 102 clinical trials in dementia which they analysed according to the following criteria:

(1) Was the sample size adequate?
(2) Were the patients demented or 'simply depressed'?
(3) Was the study double blind?
(4) Were the groups well matched?
(5) Were objective methods of outcome used?
(6) Was the duration of the trial adequate?
(7) Was the dosage of medication adequate?

Using these criteria, 53 out of the 102 clinical trials reviewed were considered as 'well-designed' controlled trials. Of these 53 trials, 48 showed a positive result (90.5%), i.e. showing a significant improvement of the patients under active treatment, and five were negative (9.5%), i.e. no statistical significance between treatment and placebo groups.

Table 14.3 Investigation of dementia

Investigation	Possible results
Blood count and film	Anaemia and macrocytosis of vitamin B_{12} or folate deficiency
ESR	Connective tissue disorders
Chest radiography	Bronchial neoplasm, cardiac lesions
Plasma urea	Uraemia
Liver function tests	Hepatocellular failure
VDRL, TPI, TPHA	Neurosyphilis
Serum B_{12} and Schilling test	Vitamin B_{12} deficiency
Red blood cell folate	Folate deficiency
Serum T3, T4, TSH	Hypothyroidism
Skull radiography	Pineal shift, calcified mass, erosion of posterior clinoids or bone in space-occupying lesion
CSF	Chronic meningitides or neurosyphilis
EEG	Slowing in primary cerebral atrophies and metabolic encephalopathies; focal change in space-occupying lesion
ECG	Arrhythmias, rheumatic and ischaemic heart disease, other sources of embolism
Angiography	Carotid and cerebral vascular stenoses, occlusions, subdural haematoma, tumours
CT scanning or NMR in selected cases	Central and cortical atrophy, other focal lesions, infarcts, tumours, haematomas

We have taken 16 out of these 53 trials which we consider to be 'the best' of these and analysed each according to preset criteria. Comments concerning the relevance of analysis of the results were subsequently excluded on a variety of grounds, chiefly because of the lack of definition of the patient group, the criteria of selection, method of assessment, numbers entered into the trial, etc. The individual analysis of each of these trials is given in tables 14.4–19.

Table 14.4 'An ergot alkaloid preparation (Hydergine) versus placebo for treatment of symptoms of cerebrovascular insufficiency: double-blind study' (Jennings, 1972).

1. Type of study	Double blind, Hydergine versus placebo
2. Patient group	'Cerebrovascular insufficiency'
3. Criteria of selection	Moderate degree 'confusion, impairment recent memory, mental alertness or deviation from normal mood'
4. Number of patients assessed	Not specified
5. Number admitted to trial	50
6. Treatment groups	26 placebo/24 Hydergine (3.0 mg daily)
7. Judgement criteria	Clinical status checklist (17 symptoms)
8. Duration of treatment	12 weeks
9. Duration of follow-up	Not specified
10. Complications	None reported

11. *Author's conclusions*: 'Hydergine group improved significantly in respect to "confusion, depression, uncooperativeness, fatigue, anorexia, dizziness".'

Comments. This trial can be criticised on the following four points: (2) Patient group is not adequately defined. (3) Patients with depression probably included. (4) Number of patients assessed is not specified. (9) Duration of follow-up is not specified.

Table 14.5'A double-blind investigation of Hydergine in the treatment of cerebro-vascular insufficiency in the elderly' (Rao and Norris, 1972).

1. Type of study	Double blind, Hydergine versus placebo
2. Patient group	Mild to moderate 'cerebrovascular insufficiency'
3. Criteria of selection	19-symptom checklist/overall clinical impression
4. Number of patients assessed	Not specified
5. Number admitted to trial	60 (57 completed trial)
6. Treatment groups	28 placebo/29 Hydergine (3.0 mg/day)
7. Judgement criteria	19-symptom checklist/overall clinical impression
8. Duration of treatment	12 weeks
9. Duration of follow-up	Not specified
10. Complications	None reported

11. *Authors' conclusions*: 'Hydergine provided significant relief of symptoms related to patient's physical, social and psychological functioning.' 12 symptoms out of 19 improved.

Comments. This trial can be criticised on the following three points: (2) Patient group is not adequately defined. (4) Number of patients assessed is not specified. (9) Duration of follow-up is not specified.

Table 14.6 'A clinical trial comparing "Hydergine" with placebo in the treatment of cerebrovascular insufficiency in elderly patients' (McConnachie, 1973).

1. Type of study	Double blind, Hydergine versus placebo
2. Patient group	Mild to moderate 'cerebrovascular insufficiency due to arteriosclerosis'
3. Criteria of selection	Crichton Royal Behavioural Rating Scale
4. Number of patients assessed	Not specified
5. Number admitted to trial	58 (52 completed trial)
6. Treatment groups	26 placebo/26 Hydergine (1.5 mg t.d.s.)
7. Judgement criteria	Crichton Royal Behavioural Rating Scale
8. Duration of treatment	12 weeks
9. Duration of follow-up	Not specified
10. Complications	4 Hydergine group: 2 broncho-pneumonia, 1 fractured femur, 1 refusal to comply; 2 placebo group, 2 deaths, 1 cerebral haemorrhage and 1 myocardial infarction

11. *Author's conclusions*: 'Significant statistical difference in favour of Hydergine was achieved in 3 or 4 symptom complexes.'

Comments. This trial can be criticised on the following three points: (2) Patient group is not adequately defined. (4) Number of patients assessed is not specified. (9) Duration of follow-up is not specified.

Table 14.7 'Two trials comparing "Hydergine" with placebo in the treatment of patients suffering from cerebrovascular insufficiency' (Rehman, 1973).

1. Type of study	Double blind, Hydergine versus placebo
2. Patient group	Cerebral arteriosclerosis/senile dementia
3. Criteria of selection	Crichton Royal Behavioural Rating Scale. Rating of 2 or 3 in 7 out of 10 factors.
4. Number of patients assessed	Not specified
5. Number admitted to trial	43 (30 completed trial)
6. Treatment groups	15 placebo/15 Hydergine (1.5 mg t.d.s.)
7. Judgement criteria	Crichton Royal Behavioural Rating Scale
8. Duration of treatment	12 weeks
9. Duration of follow-up	Not specified
10. Complications	None reported (6 patients died during course of study, concurrent illnesses, 3 in each group)

11. *Author's conclusions*: 'Hydergine group showed greater improvement over placebo, significant at $p = 0.01$ (over 10 symptoms).'

Comments: Cross-over study showed equivocal results because of inadequate 'wash-out' period and has therefore not been analysed. This trial can be criticised on the following 5 points: (2) Patient group is not adequately defined. (4) Number of patients assessed is not specified. (5) 13 (of 43) withdrawn as a result. (6) Patient groups are too small. (9) Duration of follow-up is not specified.

Table 14.8   'A double blind evaluation of "Hydergine" and placebo in the treatment of patients with organic brain syndrome and cerebral arteriosclerosis in a nursing home' (Thibault, 1974).

1. Type of study	Double blind, Hydergine versus placebo
2. Patient group	'Cerebral arteriosclerosis/chronic brain syndrome'
3. Criteria of selection	18-symptom scale
4. Number of patients assessed	Not specified
5. Number admitted to trial	49 (48 completed trial)
6. Treatment groups	26 placebo/22 Hydergine (6 mg daily 1 month, 3 mg daily 2 months)
7. Judgement criteria	18-symptom scale
8. Duration of treatment	12 weeks
9. Duration of follow-up	Not specified
10. Complications	None reported

11. *Author's conclusions*: 'Areas of significant improvement with Hydergine were "restlessness, appearance, initiative, fatiguability, sleep difficulties, dizziness, appetite, mobility, irritability, mood, memory, interest in activities and degree of nursing time".'

Comments. An initial higher dosage was used (viz. 6 mg as opposed to 3 mg). This trial can be criticised on the following three points: (2) Patient group is not adequately defined. (4) Number of patients assessed is not specified. (9) Duration of follow-up is not specified.

Table 14.9 'Mental decline in the elderly: pharmacotherapy (ergot alkaloids versus papaverine)' (Rosen, 1975).

1. Type of study	Double-blind, Hydergine versus papaverine
2. Patient group	'Mental ageing'
3. Criteria of selection	Moderate degree impairment 6 or more out of 15 symptoms on rating scale
4. Number of patients assessed	60
5. Number admitted to trial	60 (53 completed trial)
6. Treatment groups	27 papaverine (300 mg daily)/26 Hydergine (3 mg daily)
7. Judgement criteria	Overall clinical impression/global change rating/assessment of clinical status/mental status checklist
8. Duration of treatment	12 weeks
9. Duration of follow-up	Not specified
10. Complications	No side-effects

11. *Author's conclusions*: 'Hydergine group improved twice as much as those given papaverine, "confusion, dizziness, unsociability, depressive mood, mental status".'

Comments. This trial can be criticised on the following three points: (2) Patient group is not adequately defined. (4) Number of patients assessed is not specified. (9) Duration of follow-up is not specified.

Table 14.10   'Relieving select symptoms of the elderly' (Nelson, 1975).

1. Type of study	Double-blind, Hydergine versus papaverine
2. Patient group	'Select symptoms of the elderly'
3. Criteria of selection	Moderate degree impairment, 6 or more of 15 symptoms on rating scale
4. Number of patients assessed	Not specified
5. Number admitted to trial	68 (45 completed trial)
6. Treatment groups	20 papaverine (300 mg daily)/Hydergine (3 mg daily)
7. Judgement criteria	Mental status checklist
8. Duration of treatment	12 weeks
9. Duration of follow-up	Not specified
10. Complications	4 patients: 3 papaverine group; 1 Hydergine group. (Non-specific, e.g. headache (1), nausea (1).)

11. *Author's conclusions*: 'Hydergine group significantly improved compared with papaverine in 6 symptoms: recent memory, orientation, self-care, depression, confusion and emotional lability.'

Comments. This trial can be criticised on the following five points: (2) Patient group is not adequately defined. (4) Number of patients assessed is not specified. (5) 23 (of 68) withdrawn from analysis because of 'protocol violations', 9 Hydergine/14 papaverine. (6) As result of 'drop-outs', patient groups are too small. (9) Duration of follow-up is not specified.

Table 14.11 'A double-blind clinical trial of naftidrofuryl in cerebrovascular disorders' (Robinson, 1972).

1. Type of study	Double blind, naftidrofuryl versus placebo
2. Patient group	'Cerebrovascular disorders'
3. Criteria of selection	Proforma: intellectual and emotional functioning, speech and memory
4. Number of patients assessed	80
5. Number admitted to trial	57 patients evaluated (6 excluded, 17 'normal')
6. Treatment groups	29 placebo/28 naftidrofuryl (50 mg t.d.s.)
7. Judgement criteria	According to proforma (see 3)
8. Duration of treatment	2 months
9. Duration of follow-up	Not specified
10. Complications	None reported

11. *Author's conclusions*: 'Naftidrofuryl was significantly superior to placebo at $p = 0.05$. Quite evidently a considerable placebo effect was present in this trial.'

Comments. This trial can be criticised on the following five points: (2) Patient group is not adequately defined. (3) Criteria of selection and (8) judgement criteria are not specified. (9) Duration of follow-up is not specified. (11) On the published data, author's conclusion is not tenable.

Table 14.12   'Naftidrofuryl — a double-blind cross-over study in the elderly' (Judge and Urquhart, 1972).

1. Type of study	Double blind, cross-over, naftidrofuryl versus placebo
2. Patient group	'Elderly subjects with severe intellectual impairment'
3. Criteria of selection	Proforma derived from Longmore disability score, modified Robinson intelligence test.
4. Number of patients assessed	Not specified
5. Number admitted to trial	24
6. Treatment groups	24 placebo/24 naftidrofuryl (300 mg/day)
7. Judgement criteria	According to proforma
8. Duration of treatment	8 weeks on each
9. Duration of follow-up	16 weeks
10. Complications	Placebo group: 1 severe headache, 2 died bronchopneumonia. Active group: 1 cerebral infarction

11. *Authors' conclusions*: 'Significant improvement in intellectual function occurred with the drug and this effect was prolonged (at least 12 weeks).'

Comments. This trial can be criticised on the following two points: (2) The patient group is not adequately defined. They were, according to authors, 'severely affected intellectually'. (4) Number of patients assessed is not specified.

Table 14.13 'Double blind trial of naftidrofuryl in the treatment of cerebral arteriosclerosis' (Gerin, 1974).

1. Type of study	Double blind, naftidrofuryl versus placebo
2. Patient group	'Cerebral arteriosclerosis'
3. Criteria of selection	Proforma: orientation, memory, general behaviour, social contacts
4. Number of patients assessed	Not specified
5. Number admitted to trial	20 (18 completed)
6. Treatment groups	10 placebo/10 naftidrofuryl (300 mg day)
7. Judgement criteria	According to proforma (see 3)
8. Duration of treatment	2 months
9. Duration of follow-up	Not specified
10. Complications	'Few, relatively mild'

11. *Author's conclusions*: 'Social behaviour and recent memory improved significantly with the active drug but not with placebo.'

Comments. This trial can be criticised on the following seven points: (2) The patient group is not adequately defined. (4) Number of patients assessed is not specified. (5) Number of patients admitted to the trial is too few. (6) The treatment groups are too small. (9) Duration of follow-up is not specified. (10) Complications are not specified. (11) Author's conclusions are untenable.

Table 14.14   'Double blind evaluation of naftidrofuryl in treating elderly confused hospitalised patients' (Cox, 1975).

1. Type of study	Double blind, naftidrofuryl versus placebo
2. Patient group	'Elderly, confused, hospitalised patients' (confusional states with impairment in orientation, social adjustment, mental and physical status)
3. Criteria of selection	Clinical assessment, occupational and nursing assessments
4. Number of patients assessed	Not specified
5. Number admitted to trial	Not specified. 32 completed trial. 3 excluded due to aphasia
6. Treatment groups	Not specified (16 in each group?)
7. Judgement criteria	(See 3)
8. Duration of treatment	2 months
9. Duration of follow-up	Not specified
10. Complications	No side-effects reported

11. *Author's conclusions*: 'Naftidrofuryl patients significantly improved on all three assessments. No improvement was found for the placebo treated patients.'

Comments. Author comments 'there was considerable variation between assessors', interpreted as 'measuring different aspects of the patient's condition'. There are too many unspecified points to make constructive comment.

Table 14.15 'Vertebrobasilar arterial insufficiency with dementia. Controlled trial of treatment with betahistine' (Rivera *et al.*, 1974).

1. Type of study	Double blind cross-over betahistine versus placebo
2. Patient group	'Vertebrobasilar insufficiency associated with dementia'
3. Criteria of selection	History/neurological examination/neuropsychological tests
4. Number of patients assessed	85
5. Number admitted to trial	50
6. Treatment groups	21 placebo/29 betahistine (32 mg daily)
7. Judgement criteria	Neurological rating scale
8. Duration of treatment	12 weeks
9. Duration of follow-up	Not specified
10. Complications	None reported

11. *Authors' conclusions*: 'Significant improvement with betahistine therapy . . . verbal and non-verbal cognition, memory, language use, spatial construction, perception.'

Comments. This trial can be criticised on the following two points: (2) From the data presented it would be difficult to know whether the patients are a homogeneous group. (9) Duration of follow-up is not specified.

Table 14.16 'Bencyclan — a new vasodilator drug — in the treatment of patients with ischaemic cerebral infarction' (Fogelholm *et al.*, 1974).

1. Type of study	Double blind, bencyclan versus placebo
2. Patient group	'Ischaemic cerebrovascular disease'
3. Criteria of selection	Ischaemic hemispherical infarction, 4 months before beginning of trial. Confirmed by CSF, EEG, angiography, brain scan
4. Number of patients assessed	Not specified
5. Number admitted to trial	60 (58 completed trial)
6. Treatment groups	29 placebo/29 bencyclan (300 mg daily)
7. Judgement criteria	Neurological examination, psychological tests
8. Duration of treatment	6 weeks
9. Duration of follow-up	Not specified
10. Complications	3 placebo: 2 dizziness, 1 diarrhoea; 3 active: 1 dyspepsia, 1 syncopal, 1 sleeping problems

11. *Authors' conclusions*: 'Little proof that bencyclan, at least in doses used, differs from placebo in its effects on symptoms, signs of ischaemic cerebrovascular disease.'

Comments. The authors made every attempt to define their patient group. The trial can be criticised on the following two points: (2) Number of patients assessed is not specified. (9) Duration of follow-up is not specified.

Table 14.17 'Treatment of the cerebral manifestations of arteriosclerosis with cyclandelate' (Young *et al.*, 1974).

1. Type of study	Double blind cross-over, cyclandelate versus placebo
2. Patient group	'Cerebral arteriosclerosis'
3. Criteria of selection	8 clinical criteria, including hypertension, focal neurological signs, recent stroke, epilepsy or drop attacks, retinal arteriosclerosis, confusion at night, etc.
4. Number of patients assessed	Not specified
5. Number admitted to trial	24 (21 completed trial)
6. Treatment groups	21 placebo/21 cyclandelate (400 mg q.d.s. daily)
7. Judgement criteria	'Simple behavioural scales' (ADL) Modified Weschler IQ scale
8. Duration of treatment	12 months
9. Duration of follow-up	12 months
10. Complications	No serious side-effects

11. *Authors' conclusions*: 'Patients deteriorated to a statistically significant extent on placebo. This decline was absent on cyclandelate.' (IQ performance, comprehension and vocabulary tests)

Comments. This trial was of interest because of the way in which the patient group was defined (based on previous studies where diagnosis was confirmed in 90% at post-mortem) and for the duration of follow-up. The authors state that deterioration was most marked when placebo was given in the second 6 months, 'suggesting that cyclandelate may have a prophylactic function in arresting decline in mental performance'.

Table 14.18 'Vasopressin studies in Alzheimer's disease' (Tamminga *et al.*, 1982).

1. Type of study	Double blind, vasopressin versus placebo
2. Patient group	'Mild to moderate symptoms of Alzheimer's disease'
3. Criteria of selection	Wechsler Adult Intelligence Scale and Wechsler Memory Scale
4. Number of patients assessed	Not specified
5. Number admitted to trial	14
6. Treatment groups	7 placebo/7 vasopressin (16 units intranasally/day)
7. Judgement criteria	Weschler Adult Intelligence Scale and Weschler Memory Scale
8. Duration of treatment	10 days
9. Duration of follow-up	17 days
10. Complications	None

11. *Authors' conclusions*: vasopressin failed to enhance memory or learning in human subjects with Alzheimer's disease but reaction time was improved

Comments. Placebo group was given placebo intranasal spray. This trial can be criticised on the following points: (4) Number of patients assessed is not specified. (5) Number of patients admitted to trial is too small. (6) Patient groups are too small. (9) Duration of follow-up is probably too short.

Table 14.19 'No effect from double-blind trial of physostigmine and lecithin in Alzheimer's disease' (Wettstein, 1983).

1. Type of study	Double blind cross-over, physostigmine and lecithin
2. Patient group	Mild to severe Alzheimer's disease
3. Criteria of selection	After Eisdorfer and Cohen
4. Number of patients assessed	Not specified
5. Number admitted to trial	8
6. Treatment groups	8 placebo/8 physostigmine (3–10 mg orally) and lecithin (18 g daily)
7. Judgement criteria	Psychological test battery
8. Duration of treatment	12 weeks
9. Duration of follow-up	Not specified
10. Complications	2 patients (treated group) with severe nausea and 1 with diarrhoea

11. *Author's conclusions*: 'No improvement in behaviour, recent memory or other neuropsychological functions occurred.'

Comments. This trial can be criticised on the following 5 points: (4) Number of patients assessed is not specified. (5) Number admitted to trial is too small. (7) Psychological test battery changed according to patient's abilities. (9) Duration of follow-up not specified. (11) Author's conclusions are not tenable.

Of the 16 trials analysed

● all were double-blind
● 14 were against placebo, and two were drug comparisons (Hydergine versus papavcrine, physostigmine versus lecithin)
● patient group ranged from: cerebrovascular insufficiency, 'mild to moderate', cerebral arteriosclerosis, chronic brain syndrome, 'mental ageing', 'select symptoms of the elderly', 'cerebrovascular disorders', 'elderly subjects with severe intellectual impairment', vertebrobasilar insufficiency with dementia to 'mild to moderate Alzheimer's disease' (two)
● the number of patients assessed prior to inclusion in the study is not generally given
● the numbers are small: 8, 14, 21, 29, up to 60
● judgement criteria varied enormously
● duration of treatment and duration of follow-up were usually the same. Average follow-up was 8–12 weeks with only one study following-up for 12 months.
● complications and drop-outs appear to be remarkably few.

There are clearly major methodological problems with each of these studies.

Only two large multicentre studies have been reported. Wallace *et al.* (1983) carried out a multicentre general practitioner study to see whether a simple questionnaire, the Abbreviated Mental Test (Qureschi and Hodkinson, 1974) (see table A.11, p. 321) could be used by a nurse to detect early signs of mental impairment. If the subject scored 7 out of 10 or less, the result was checked by the family doctor. If the result was the same, then the subject was assessed on a 6-symptom rating scale adapted from the Crichton Geriatric Behavioural Rating Scale (see table A.12, p. 322). Patients with dementia were then entered into a pilot study to test the efficacy of a new formulation of Hydergine, a 4.5 mg tablet given once daily.

There were 118 patients who failed to complete the 12-week treatment period. Of the 266 patients who completed the study, a significant improvement occurred in all the symptom areas. The aims of this study were specific, and since it was an uncontrolled study the therapeutic efficacy of the new treatment is viewed with the usual caution. That such a study could be carried out in general practice has been shown and opens the door for new trials to be done from a general-practice base. A detailed analysis of this study is to be found in Wallace *et al.* (1983).

In a large multicentre trial from Italy, more than 500 patients were randomised in a double-blind, placebo-controlled study using Hydergine 4.5 mg daily. At the end of 1 year, 204 patients were still being treated, 111 on Hydergine and 93 on placebo. The initial results show that at the beginning of the study the effects of Hydergine and placebo were similar, but as time went on the placebo effect clearly began to decrease, whereas the effect of Hydergine became more obvious especially after 3 months, and improvement was maintained for up to 1 year. As well as clinical assessments, a battery of psychometric tests was also used. Improvement was recorded in several parameters: improved sociability and initiative, less emotional lability, improved long- and short-term memory, space–time orientation, attention and mental alertness.

The overall clinical assessment showed that the relatives were more aware of improvement than the investigators, provoking the conclusion that patients became more acceptable to the relatives by fitting more easily into their social environment (see table A.13, p. 323). An interim report on this study has been published by Lazari *et al.* (1983).

Based on these studies, certain constructive criticisms can be made.

Selection of patients

Many studies from geriatric centres have been dominated by very old patients with advanced dementia and almost total social dependency. Ideally, trials should include patients with a definite cognitive impairment, but at a relatively early stage so that any improvement attributable to the drug may be seen.

An attempt should be made to separate the cases with different pathological processes, and this necessitates strict selection criteria which, in turn, means stringent diagnostic investigation. Attempts should be made to differentiate between those patients with multi-infarct dementia and those with Alzheimer dementia (see chapter 13 by Harrison). Mixed cases ought to be excluded as well.

Trial design

A major problem has been the lack of control subjects. This has occurred in up to 50% of trials of vasodilators, for instance (Yesavage *et al.*, 1979). It is desirable that placebo be given to control subjects matched carefully for the disease process, its radiological correlates, sex and age.

Elderly patients improve when more attention is paid to them under the conditions imposed by clinical trials, and this itself produces an appreciable placebo effect.

Double-blind controlled studies are ideal, but problems of ethical acceptability are raised, and it is necessary to have informed consent from close relatives and friends. Cross-over studies have rarely been used despite the fact that they increase the statistical power of a comparison between treatments of a completely randomised design with an equal number of subjects. However, cross-over studies require longer periods of treatment, and this may increase the number of drop-outs and also may necessitate wash-out periods to prevent carry-over effects. There is probably also a place for open pilot studies with carefully selected criteria of progress for new drugs. If any dramatic benefit is shown, then it is necessary to proceed to a lengthy double-blind controlled trial using carefully matched subjects. Smaller groups of patients included in pilot trials allow a better and more careful selection, which will produce a more homogeneous population. There is also an important role for pharmacological investigations of selected functions, as has been shown in the use of Physostigmine in memory tests.

Measurement of benefit

Another difficulty is the lack of accepted measurements of improvement. Many rating scales have been used. The shorter ones or mini-mental function tests are limited by the very small area of mental function which they cover, most being devoted to orientation, current general knowledge and tests of short-term memory. The vitally important cognitive functions and assessment of abstraction and reasoning are often omitted. Behavioural scales too are of limited value, indicating in general the overall result of social functioning rather than any possible benefit to selected areas of impaired mental function. None the less, behavioural scales do give a measure of social acceptability, and gross changes in performance are certainly of clinical significance. The more commonly used scales are listed in table 14.20. (For review see Lezak, 1985.)

Analysing the different clinical trials, one finds that nearly 90% concern new scales for assessment of dementia. The use of different scales makes comparison between different studies difficult and often impossible. There

Table 14.20   Tests used in dementia.

Psychological tests
Weschler Adult Intelligence Scale
Raven's Progressive Matrices
Bender: Gestalt Test
Babcock Sentence Completion
Critical Flicker Fusion

Behavioural scales
Crichton Royal Behaviour Rating Scale
Mental Status Checklist
Sandoz Clinical Assessment — Geriatric
Brief Psychiatric Rating Scale
Nurses'
Relatives'   Observation Scale (inpatients)

---

are marked differences in sensitivity between the different rating schemes, and it is desirable that uniform criteria be agreed to enable suitable comparisons to be made between different investigators. Pooling of data from different centres poses problems of its own, largely due to variability in criteria and the skill and methods of eliciting observations.

The major problem is to formulate agreed tests covering both psychological and behavioural criteria as well as agreed clinical and radiological observations.

CEREBRAL VASODILATORS

Of the many drugs used, this group of substances has been most frequently employed (see table 14.21). The original rationale was that dementia might result from impaired cerebral blood flow caused by narrowing of arteries. Drugs which could dilate these vessels were expected to improve blood flow and consequently produce a mental improvement. This thesis is based on a

Table 14.21 Drugs used in treatment of dementia.

Primary vasodilators
Cyclandelate (Cyclospasmol)
Papaverine (Pavabid)
Isoxsuprine (Vasodilan, Duvadilan, Defencin)
Cinnarizine (Stugeron)

Drugs with mixed action
Dihydroergotoxin, co-dergocrine mesylate (Hydergine)
Nafronyl, naftidrofuryl oxalate (Praxilene)
Pyritinol plus Pyridylcarbinol (Decaden)
Pentifylline (Cosaldon, Trental)

---

fallacy. In Alzheimer's disease of both presenile and senile types, the impaired cerebral blood flow is now thought to be the consequence rather than the cause of the disease. If blood flow could be increased, it would be unlikely to improve the primary degeneration of neurones. In multi-infarct dementia, vasodilators could not be expected to reverse atherosclerotic changes nor to improve perfusion through occluded vessels or through infarcted tissue. Vasodilators could theoretically act on anastomotic communications around the periphery of areas of infarction, but there is a real risk of a 'steal' effect which could hinder rather than help the clinical features.

Cerebral vasodilators have not achieved any measure of clinical success in practice. These drugs fall into two classes:

(1) those with vasodilator action alone;
(2) those with mixcd vasodilator and metabolic actions.

Yesavage and colleagues have reviewed these drugs (Yesavage *et al.*, 1979).

Cyclandelate (Cyclospasmol)

Only seven of 18 studies reviewed showed satisfactory clinical methods. Six showed some positive results but only three reported practical benefit. A review of four of the double-blind cross-over studies concluded that cyclandelate was no more effective than placebo, and claims that the drug produced a slowing of cognitive decline as compared with placebo are unconvincing. The drug remains controversial but there is little evidence of its general efficacy.

Papaverine (Pavabid)

Of 13 studies nine were rated satisfactory in their methods. Six showed some effect but only one claimed practical benefit. Trials comparing papaverine with dihydroergotoxin found the latter drug to be superior.

Isoxuprine (Vasodilan, Duvadilan, Defencin)

Only three of the five trials of this drug were rated satisfactory and two claimed some improvement in cognitive function. No satisfactory study reported any practical benefit on clinical grounds.

Cinnarizine (Stugeron)

Three of eight studies of this drug were rated satisfactory in terms of methodology and two of these claim significant practical benefits. Unfortunately the clinical conditions treated were very varied and did not have any direct relevance to patients with dementia.

DRUGS WITH MIXED VASODILATOR AND METABOLIC ACTIONS

Dihydroergotoxin, co-dergocrine mesylate (Hydergine)

Of 33 studies 21 were rated satisfactory and all of these trials claimed significant improvement in behavioural or psychological measurements. In 18 improvement was considered to be of practical importance. Dosage may be important, and better results have been obtained with 4.5 mg per day than for lower dose regimes. In their review Yesavage and colleagues claimed that overall this drug has the best confirmed efficacy.

Nafronyl, naftidrofuryl oxalate (Praxilene)

All eight clinical trials used test scales which showed improvement, and seven trials claimed practical benefits. The degree of improvement, however, suggests the need for much more detailed and larger studies before any general claim for clinical use can be supported.

Pyritinol plus Pyridylcarbinol (Decaden)

This pyridoxine derivative is claimed to improve cerebral metabolism, glucose uptake and blood flow. Only one trial produced positive evidence of benefit.

Pentifylline (Cosaldon, Trental)

This caffeine-like drug is a stimulant and is said to relax smooth muscle and may also increase cerebral glucose uptake. It is combined with niacin. Only one satisfactory study was reported and this claimed practical benefit, but obviously the drug needs more extensive trials.

The very varied pharmacology of these drugs claiming metabolic effects on the brain may be questioned. Sometimes referred to as 'cerebral activators', it is thought that by improving the utilisation of oxygen and glucose by the brain they will be of practical benefit.

Dihydroergotoxin is an alpha-blocker, but has complex actions on dopamine, noradrenalin and serotonin. Naftidrofuryl (Praxilene) is claimed to increase the brain concentration of ATP and to reduce lactic acid. Oxpentifylline (Trental) is conjugated with a nicotinic acid derivative and may increase cerebral glucose uptake. Cyclandelate (Cyclospasmol) has a direct action on smooth muscle, but its value in vascular dementia has not been convincingly shown and its side-effects of flushing, rashes and nausea can be objectionable. It does not reduce cerebral perfusion, which suggests that if it has a cerebral action it may be more than that attributable to vasodilatation.

The Swiss Federal Insurance Office is currently considering a report from the Federal Medicines Commission (the CFM) on 'cerebrally active' products. The CFM, as a result of its evaluation, classified the substances as follows with respect to their cerebral activity

Category A: demonstrated clinical activity — co-dergocrine
Category B: probable clinical activity — naftidrofuryl
Category C: marginal or uncertain clinical activity — cyclandelate, pentifyl-line, piracetam, pyritinol, vincamine
Category D: no clinical activity yet demonstrated — bencyclan, cinnarizine, *Ginkgo biloba* extract, ginseng, etc., flunarizine, hexobendine + oxyethyl theophylline + etamivan, isoxuprine, meclofenamate, nicergoline, buphemine, papaverine, cerebral phospholipids, pirisudanol, pyrindol, car-bamate, raubasin, suloctidil, viquidil, vitamins, etc. (*Scrip*, 1985).

CONCLUSIONS

In a disease that is insidious in onset, that pursues a progressively degenerat-ing course, and for which no cure is yet known, doctors and the lay public may be excused a feeling of pessimism. Hollister (1983) puts the matter into perspective by commenting:

> the question finally comes down to whether or not one should take a totally pessimistic view of drug treatment of senile dementia or whether one should be more optimistic. A pessimist would either not use any psychotherapeutic drugs at all, or would use only those directed at providing symptomatic treatment.
>
> An optimist would use symptomatic treatment to the fullest possible extent and then would try to go a bit further by trying an adequate course of drug aimed at altering the progression of the illness. His optimism would not lead him to expect that a shambling, perplexed oldster would suddenly be transformed into a spry and alert person: rather he would settle for much less. He would use such drugs as he would any others, increasing the dose to one that produces either unpleasant side effects or the desired beneficial effects. He would not be discouraged too early in treatment, probably settling for no less than three months of treatment and possibly treating for as long as six months before deciding on its value.
>
> Physicians are not expected to cure every patient. They are expected to provide as much as they can for the relief of suffering and disability. Rather than risk doing less than the utmost for the patient with senile dementia I would choose to be an optimist. I would not deceive myself or the patient about what to expect, nor would I pursue an obviously futile course indefinitely. Meanwhile, I should be most humble about what we know of senile dementia, the final affliction of life for many patients.

REFERENCES

Cox, J. R. (1975). Double-blind evaluation of naftidrofuryl in treating elderly confused hospitalised patients. *Gerontol. Clin.*, **17**, 160–67.

Fogelholm, R., Waltimo, O., Putkonin, A. R. and Lansonen, R. (1974). Bencyclan — a new vasodilator drug — in the treatment of patients with ischaemic cerebral infarction. *Ann. Clin. Res.*, **6**, 93–6.

Gerin, J. (1974). Double-blind trial of naftidrofuryl in the treatment of cerebral arteriosclerosis. *Brit. J. Clin. Pract.*, **28**, 177–8.

Hollister, L. (1983). Clinical trials of co-dergocrine in senile dementia. *Brit. J. Clin. Prac.*, Suppl. **30**, 41–5.

Jennings, W. G. (1972). An ergot alkaloid preparation (Hydergine) versus placebo for treatment of symptoms of cerebrovascular insufficiency: double-blind study. *J. Am. Geriatr. Soc.*, **20**, 407–12.

Judge, T. G. and Urquhart, A. (1972). Naftidrofuryl — a double-blind cross-over study in the elderly. *Current Med. Res. Opinion*, **1**, 166–72.

Katzman, R. (1981). Early detection of senile dementia. *Hosp. Prac.*, **16**, No. 15, 61.

Lazzari, R., Franzese, A., Cheirichetti, S. M., Vibelli, C., Rudelli, G., Passeri, M. and Cucinotta, D. (1983). Multicentre double-blind placebo-controlled long-term clinical trial of Hydergine in chronic senile cerebral insufficiency: an interim report. In Agnoli, A., Crepaldi, G., Spano, P. E. and Trabucci, M. (eds), *Aging Brain and Ergot Alkaloids*, Raven Press, New York, 347–71.

Lezak, M. D. (1985). Neuropsychological assessment. In Vinken, P. J., Bruyn, G. W. and Klawans, H. L. (eds), *Handbook of Clinical Neurology*, Volume 1 No. 45, Elsevier, Amsterdam and New York, 515–30.

McConnachie, R. (1973). A clinical trial comparing 'Hydergine' with placebo in the treatment of cerebrovascular insufficiency in elderly patients. *Current Med. Res. Opinion*, **1**, 463–8.

Nelson, J. J. (1975). Relieving select symptoms of the elderly. *Geriatrics*, **30**, 133–42.

Qureschi, K. N. and Hodkinson, H. M. (1974). Evaluation of a ten-question mental test in the institutionalised elderly. *Age Aging*, **3**, 152–6.

Rao, D. B. and Norris, J. R. (1972). A double-blind investigation of Hydergine in the treatment of cerebrovascular insufficiency in the elderly. *Johns Hopkins Med. J.*, **130**, 317–24.

Rehman, S. A. (1973). Two trials comparing 'Hydergine' with placebo in the treatment of patients suffering from cerebrovascular insufficiency. *Current Med. Res. Opinion*, **1**, 456–62.

Rivera, V. M., Meyer, J. S., Baer, P. E., Faibish, G. M., Mathew, N. T. and Hartmann, A. (1974). Vertebrobasilar arterial insufficiency with dementia. Controlled trial of treatment with betahistine. *J. Amer. Geriatr. Soc.*, **22**, 397–406.

Robinson, K. (1972). A double-blind clinical trial of naftidrofuryl in cerebrovascular disorders. *Med. Dig.* Dec., 50–55.

Rosen, H. J. (1975). Mental decline in the elderly: pharmacotherapy (ergot alkaloids verus papaverine). *J. Amer. Geriatr. Soc.*, **23**, 169–74.

Scrip (Leading Article) (1985). 1037,8.

Tamminga, C. A., Durso, R., Fedro, P. and Chase, T. N. (1982). Vasopressin studies in Alzheimer's disease. *Psycho. Pharmacol. Bull.*, **18**, 48–9.

Thibault, A. (1974). A double-blind evaluation of 'Hydergine' and placebo in the treatment of patients with organic brain syndrome and cerebral arteriosclerosis in a nursing home. *Current Med. Res. Opinion*, **2**, 482–7.

Wallace, M. G., Capildeo, R. and Rose, F. C. (1983). Multicentre general practitioner trial of Hydergine in dementia using a screening programme. In Agnoli, A., Crepaldi, G., Spano, P. E. and Trabucci, M. (eds), *Aging Brain and Ergot Alkaloids,* Raven Press, New York, 339–46.

Wettstein, A. (1983). No effect from double-blind trial of physostigmine and lecithin in Alzheimer's disease. *Ann. Neurol.,* **12**, 210–12.

Yesavage, J. A., Tinklenburg, J. R., Hollister, L. E. and Berger, P. A. (1979). Vasodilators in senile dementias — a review of the literature. *Arch. Gen. Psychiatr.,* **36**, 220–23.

Young, J., Hall, P. and Blakemore, L. (1974). Treatment of the cerebral manifestations of arteriosclerosis with cyclandelate. *Brit. J. Psychiat.,* **124**, 177–80.

15
Methodology of clinical trials in dementia. Part II: Future trials— Recommendations

J. F. DARTIGUES

INTRODUCTION

In a large review of the 102 clinical trials in dementia (Yesavage *et al.*, 1979) 53 of the clinical trials were considered to be 'well-designed' studies (see chapter 14). Of these 53 trials, 48 were positive. It is therefore surprising that, despite these apparently satisfactory figures, the number of controlled trials in dementia has considerably decreased since 1975. Furthermore the medical community at large has not accepted the above-mentioned results as real proof of advancement in the treatment of dementia. The reasons for this have been summarised by Hughes *et al.* (1976):

Because of the small magnitude of the improvement to be expected and the absence of indications of long-term benefits, it would seem that at present vasodilators are of minor clinical value in the treatment of dementia. Further studies with better methodologies and longer follow-up periods . . . may lead to more favourable conclusions.

In fact there remain a lot of drawbacks in the 53 'well-designed' trials analysed by Yesavage *et al.*, and the first one is: what is the aim of the study? Is it to demonstrate the action of one drug during 12 weeks on five or six mental functions in demented patients? Or is it to demonstrate that one drug can change the malignant course of dementia? We can accept the first aim as a first step, but the second aim should be the true objective and it seems that it has never been achieved so far.

295

METHODOLOGY

When considering the second aim for further studies, we must analyse two important aspects of the methodology: inclusion and assessment criteria.

Inclusion criteria

The principal problem for the inclusion of patients in a study is what is meant by dementia. The patients described as 'not normal' or 'not simply depressed' must not be included, and it is necessary to eliminate from the trial the so-called treatable causes of dementia, especially communicating hydrocephalus and endocrine or metabolic disorders (National Institute on Aging Task Force, 1980; Small and Jarvik, 1983). The difficulty is that these conditions are often not easy to recognise and their explicit diagnosis requires either costly ancillary procedures, or much time, or both.

The use of the stringent criteria proposed by the dementia study group of the World Federation of Neurology in 1982 could be an answer to that problem, but a long-standing mental deterioration is probably less likely to be improved by a treatment than one that is just beginning, due to the larger extent of the lesions and to the occurrence of complications with time.

Assessment criteria

For the assessment of the outcome of patients with dementia it may appear that the survival rate is one of the best criteria of long-term practical benefit for the following reasons.

● The criterion is objective, has good reliability and is practicable for multicentre trials.
● If one analyses the death rate reported in a few publications (Roth, 1955; Shah *et al.*, 1969; Hare, 1978; Blessed and Wilson, 1982; Naguib and Levy; 1982) at six months after admission in a psychiatric or geriatric ward, and then two years after this admission (table 15.1), it is clear that it is high enough to be a sensitive criterion.
● The death rate can be analysed with longitudinal models using the *Life Table Method* (Kaplan and Meyer, 1958). This type of analysis (Elandt-Johnson and Johnson, 1979) has been applied to the problem of dementia using data published by Todorov *et al.* (1975). With the sample studied, the death rate at two years after the 'age of diagnosis' was 32%, at four years it was 60%, at six years 75%, at eight years 80%, and at ten years 90%. However, this sample comprised only autopsied cases. Figures 15.1 and 15.2 represent the same kind of analysis made by the author from data reported by Shah *et al.* (1969). Comparison between two or more curves (Peto and Peto, 1972), and adjustment and use of multivariate

Table 15.1   Death rates (%) at 6 months and at 2 years after admission in demented patients in chronic care institutions.

	Type of dementia	*6 months*	*2 years*
Roth (1955)	Senile	60	80
Roth (1955)	Multi-infarct	30	75
Shah *et al.* (1969)	All	35	65
Hare (1978)	All	16	
Blessed and Wilson (1982)	Senile	30	70
Blessed and Wilson (1982)	Multi-infarct	35	60
Naguib and Levy (1982)	All	25	70

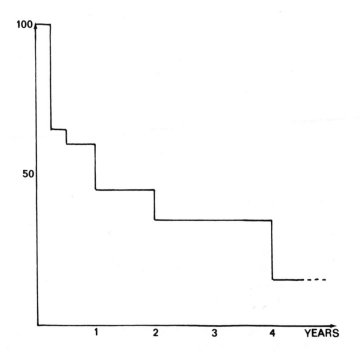

Figure 15.1   Actuarial rate of survival (%) in dementia (calculated by the author from Shah *et al.*, 1969).

models (Cox, 1972) are possible, and the greater sensitivity of the survival curves method allows significant differences to be shown even with small samples.

● Death rate is the only criterion which has been well studied when considering the prognosis of dementia. This has an important advantage for stratification, adjustment matching or multivariate analysis since the

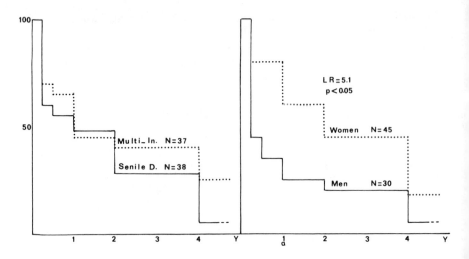

Figure 15.2   Actuarial rates of survival in dementia derived from the data of Shah *et al.* (1969) according to different types of dementia and sex.

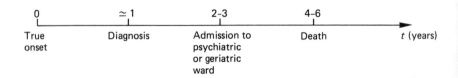

Figure 15.3   Natural history of dementia — average course.

main prognostic factors are known: age at onset (Heston *et al.* 1981), type of dementia (Go *et al.*, 1978), mental dysfunction (Naguib and Levy, 1982), parieto-temporal dysfunction (Naguib and Levy, 1982), and early course of mental dysfunction (Hare, 1978).

   The use of this parameter raises two important questions, one concerning validity, and the other the time of entry in the trial.

Validity

The use of death rates appears to be valid according to the results of Kay (1962) on the causes of death in demented patients in Newcastle upon Tyne. The death rate per year per 1000 demented patients is ten times greater than in the general population adjusted for age. Even if the death is not due to the cerebral lesion itself, it is directly related to the severity of the handicap of the patients, e.g. bronchopneumonia in the bedridden patients.

Time of entry into the trial

The problem of the time of entry into the trial and the duration of the follow-up is more difficult to answer. If we represent the natural history of dementia (figure 15.3) according to the data from Go *et al.* (1978) and Heston *et al.* (1981), it seems quite clear that if a trial is started when the diagnosis of dementia is made by a neurologist or the general practitioner, then the duration of follow-up must be at least 5 years. If the trial begins on admission to a psychiatric hospital or a geriatric ward, a follow-up period of two years will be sufficient.

However, if the death rate appears to be the easiest criterion of assessment to be used, the quality of life is probably more important from a human and economic point of view. For its evaluation, Yesavage *et al.* (1979) and more recently Cook and James (1981) have recommended the use of the Crichton Behavioural Rating Scale (1961) and of the Sandoz Clinical Assessment Geriatric Scale (1978) which is discussed in this book by Maurer and Commenges (see chapter 3). More recently, the Mini Mental Status (1978) has been proposed, a clinical score method which seems to be very simple to use and to have a high inter-rater reliability.

CONCLUSIONS

For the future, improvements in the medical treatment of dementia may become possible if the following conditions are fulfilled:

● Dementia should be considered as a major public health problem, because of its high prevalence, more than 5% after 60 years (Mortimer and Schuman, 1981), and because of its great human, social and financial cost. Better funding is by no means synonymous with better research, but it may contribute a lot. The problem is that in the countries that could afford it the national health agencies may not be very enthusiastic about supporting research that can lead to prolonged survival of substantially disabled patients in a non-productive age group.
● A better knowledge of the descriptive epidemiology of dementia and of its aetiological and prognosis factors is necessary. To achieve this, collaboration between neurologists, psychiatrists, gerontologists and epidemiologists would be the best way, leading hopefully to some effective preventive actions.
● Research into methodological aspects specific to this problem should aim at finding the appropriate statistical models for analysing the dynamic nature of the disease process causing dementia.
● Results in basic research could help define new types of drug treatment

able to stabilise or even reverse the pathological process of dementia. Perhaps a combination of treatments acting at different neurochemical levels could do better than only one, and this hypothesis should be tested with satisfactory study designs.

● The last, more challenging, condition which I wish to suggest would be to move away from the largely irrelevant scoring and scaling systems which have been used so far, and to replace — or at least supplement — them by more pragmatic and sensitive ways of detecting long-term benefits in dementia patients, i.e. quality of life, autonomy and death rate. The pragmatic aim then will be to avoid or delay as much as possible referral to chronic care institutions or facilities, which represent the ultimate catastrophe in terms of loss of human dignity for the patients and in terms of costs for the community.

REFERENCES

Blessed, G. and Wilson, D. (1982). The contemporary natural history of mental disorder in old age. *Brit. J. Psychiatr.,* **141**, 59–67.

Cook, P. and James, I. (1981). Cerebral vasodilators. (Two parts): *New Engl. J. Med.,* **305**, 1508–13; **305**, 1560–4.

Cox, D. R. (1972). Regression model and life-tables. *J. Roy. Stat. Soc.* (B), **134**, 187–220.

Elandt-Johnson, R. C. and Johnson, N. L. (1979). Survival models and data analysis. In Bradley, R. A., Hunter, J. S., Kendall, D. G. and Watson, G. S. (eds), *Wiley Series in Probability and Mathematical Statistics*, Wiley Interscience, New York.

Go, R. C. P., Todorov, A. B., Elston, R. C. and Constantinidis, J. (1978). The malignancy of dementia. *Ann. Neurol.,* **3**, 559–61.

Hare, M. (1978). Clinical check list for diagnosis of dementia. *Brit. Med. J.,* **2**, 266–7.

Heston, L. L., Maestri, A. R., Anderson, E. and White, J. (1981). Dementia of the Alzheimer type. *Arch. Gen. Psychiatr.,* **38**, 1085–90.

Hughes, J. R., Williams, J. G. and Currier, R. D. (1976). An ergot alkaloid preparation (hydergine) in the treatment of dementia. Review of the clinical literature. *Am. Geriat. Soc.,* **24**, 490–7.

Kaplan, E. L. and Meyer, P. (1958). Non parametric estimations from incomplete observations. *J. Am. Stat. Assoc.,* **53**, 457–81.

Kay, D. W. K. (1962). Outcome and cause of death in mental disorders of old age: a long-term follow-up of functional and organic psychosis. *Acta. Psychiatr. Scand.,* **38**, 249–76.

Mortimer, J. A. and Schuman, L. M. (1981). *Epidemiology of Dementia,* Oxford University Press, Oxford.

Naguib, M. and Levy, R. (1980). CT scan in senile dementia. *Brit. J. Psychiatr.,* **141**, 618–20.

Naguib, M. and Levy, R. (1982). Prediction of outcome in senile dementia. A computed tomography study. *Brit. J. Psychiatr., 140*, 263–7.

National Institute on Aging Task Force (1980). Senility reconsidered. *J. Am. Med. Assoc., 244*, 259–63.

Peto, R. and Peto, J. (1972). Asymptotically efficient rank invariant test procedures. *J. Roy. Stat. Soc. (A), 135*, 185–206.

Roth, M. (1955). The natural history of mental disorder in old age. *J. Ment. Sci., 102*, 281–301.

Shah, K. V., Banks, G. D. and Merskey, M. (1969). Survival in atherosclerotic and senile dementia. *Brit. J. Psychiatr., 115*, 1283–6.

Small, G. W. and Jarvik, L. F. (1983). The dementia syndrome. *Lancet, 2*, 1443–5.

Todorov, A. B., Go, R. C. P., Constantinidis, J. and Elston, R. C. (1975). Specificity of the clinical diagnosis of dementia. *J. Neurol. Sci., 26*, 81–98.

Yesavage, J. A., Tinklenberg, J. R., Hollister, L. E. and Berger, P. A. (1979). Vasodilators in senile dementia. *Arch. Gen. Psychiatr., 36*, 220–3.

APPENDIX

Table A.1 Headache diary as used in proplylactic migraine drug trials (see p. 107)

Weekday and date	Monday /	Tuesday /	Wednesday /	Thursday /	Friday /	Saturday /	Sunday /
NAME:	REMEMBER TO ANSWER ALL QUESTIONS WITH HEADACHE						
Severity of headache 1 = bothering 2 = cannot work 3 = must go to bed	1 2 3	1 2 3	1 2 3	1 2 3	1 2 3	1 2 3	1 2 3
Was the headache half-sided?	+ –	+ –	+ –	+ –	+ –	+ –	+ –
Was the pain pulsating?	+ –	+ –	+ –	+ –	+ –	+ –	+ –
Was the attack associated with:							
Nausea?	+ –	+ –	+ –	+ –	+ –	+ –	+ –
Vomiting?	+ –	+ –	+ –	+ –	+ –	+ –	+ –
Hypersensitivity to light or sound?	+ –	+ –	+ –	+ –	+ –	+ –	+ –
Other visual disturbances?	+ –	+ –	+ –	+ –	+ –	+ –	+ –
How many hours did the attack last?							
Did you have your period?	+ –	+ –	+ –	+ –	+ –	+ –	+ –
Name and amount of tablets, suppositories or injections taken for headache							
Medicine taken for other reasons							
Did you feel that it was a migraine attack?	+ –	+ –	+ –	+ –	+ –	+ –	+ –
Other information, possible side effects of drugs							

Table A.2 Patient's diary card from a trial of Migravess (see p. 107)

Date of migraine attack: Day _____ Month _____ Year _____

Time of onset of attack: Hour _____ Minute _____

Time of taking medication: Hour _____ Minute _____

Symptoms at time of taking medication (place a × in the appropriate box)

Headache	Mild	☐	Moderate	☐	Severe	☐
Nausea	None	☐	Mild	☐	Moderate	☐	Severe ☐
Diarrhoea		Yes	☐	No	☐
Photopsia		Yes	☐	No	☐
Phonophobia		Yes	☐	No	☐
Photophobia		Yes	☐	No	☐

Did you vomit?   Yes ☐   No ☐

If yes, at what time? Hour _____ Minute _____

Did the tablets make the

1. Headache Worse ☐ Unchanged ☐ Better ☐ Disappear ☐
2. Nausea   Worse ☐ Unchanged ☐ Better ☐ Disappear ☐

Did you go to sleep?   Yes ☐   No ☐

Did you notice any unexpected symptoms after taking the tablets?

Yes ☐   No ☐

If yes, please describe the symptoms:

_____

_____

_____

At what time did the

1. Headache disappear: Hour _____ Minute _____ or when alseep? ☐
2. Nausea disappear: Hour _____ Minute _____ or when asleep? ☐

Did you need to take any other medication to cure the attack?

Yes ☐   No ☐

If yes, what drug did you take?

At what time did you take the further medication?

Hour _____ Minute _____ am/pm

Did you notice any unexpected symptoms after this further medication?

Yes ☐   No ☐

If yes, please describe the symptoms:

When you have completed this diary card please post as soon as possible in the stamped, addressed envelope provided.

Table A.3 Registration card for patients in a trial of nimodipine for classical migraine attacks (see p. 107)

1. Date of attack: Day _____ Month _____ Year _____

2. Start of the prodromes: Hour _____ Minute _____

3. Time of intake of the capsules: Hour _____ Minute _____

4. Describe the prodromes that were present when you took the capsules

	Right side		Left side	
	YES	NO	YES	NO
Zig-zag lines	☐	☐	☐	☐
Spots of light	☐	☐	☐	☐
Part of the visual area fails	☐	☐	☐	☐
Other visual disturbances	☐	☐	☐	☐

5. When did the prodromes disappear? Hour _____ Minute _____

6. Did a headache develop?   NO ☐   YES ☐   Right side ☐
   Left side ☐
   Both sides ☐

7. If yes, what time was it? Hour _____ Minute _____

8. Did you have to stop work?   Yes ☐   or
   No ☐

9. Did you have to go to bed?   Yes ☐
   No ☐

10. Did you take other drugs to stop the attack?

    Yes ☐   No ☐

    If yes, which drug?_____

11. What time was it when you took the other drug? Hour _____ Minute _____

12. What time was it when the headache disappeared? Hour _____ Minute _____

13. Did the headache stop when you went to sleep?

    No ☐   Yes ☐   Hour _____ Minute _____

14. Did you notice unexpected symptoms after intake of the capsules?

Yes ☐   No ☐

If yes, please describe these symptoms:

_____

_____

_____

_____

Table A.4 UK Carotid Surgery Trial: notification form (see p. 169)

Complete after telephone randomisation (0865–40972, 0830–1630) and send the top copy as soon as possible (without stamp) to the Clinical Trial Service Unit, FREEPOST, Oxford OX2 6BR. Also inform the GP of the patient's entry into the trial.

PATIENT: Full name (not just initials) _____ Sex _____

Date of birth: Day _____ Month _____ Year _____

HISTORY (at day of randomisation)

(i) Cerebrovascular:

Fill in ALL boxes in the relevant column(s)

	TIA <24 hours	Amaurosis fugax <24 hours	Minor stroke <one week	Non-disabling major stroke	Retinal artery occlusion
Date of first episode					
Date of most recent episode (not >3/12 ago)					
Duration of longest episode					
Duration of shortest episode					
No. episodes in last 3/12					
Carotid (C), hemiphenomena (H) or vertebrobasilar (VB)		C			C
Which side of brain/eye (L, R, or both)					

Are there any residual neurological signs? (tick one)   Yes ☐   No ☐

Date(s) of any *disabling* major stroke in the past _____

(ii) Date(s) of any myocardial infarct in the past _____

(iii) Dates and details of any arterial surgery _____

(iv) What drugs are being taken regularly and why? _____

(v) Current situation (tick box if applicable)

Daily smoking in past year ☐   Angina ☐

Enlarged heart (X-ray) ☐   Treated hypertension ☐

Cardiac failure ☐   Treated hyperlipidaemia ☐

Treated diabetes ☐

Peripheral vascular disease ☐

Retinal emboli (ever) ☐

(vi) Describe any other relevant conditions (e.g. cardiac valvular disease, etc.) _____

Height _____ Weight _____ BP ____/____ (Phase IV)

BLOOD TESTS: Urea (specify units) _____

HB _____ GLUCOSE _____ (circle: fasting or random)

PCV _____ CHOLESTEROL _____ (circle: fasting or random)

Legible name of neurologist _____ Date of randomisation _____

(1) Enclose original ECG or photocopy (any original will be returned)

(2) *CT-scan*: Please reproduce report below:

Date of scan _____

(3) *Angiography* (if possible biplanar views of both carotid arteries) Please reproduce radiologist's report in full noting the *side* and extent of angiogrpahy.

Date of angiogram _____

	R-ICA	L-ICA
Origin of ICA		
ulceration? yes		
or no		
% diameter stenosis		

Send at least two views of carotid artery in the neck (for each side) plus any film showing significant intracranial or arch/great vessel disease.

(4) *SURGERY*

	Right carotid endarterectomy	Left carotid endarterectomy
Exact date		
Duration of surgery (minutes)		
Local or general anaesthesia?		
Stump pressure if measured		
Occlusion time (minutes)		
Thrombus present (yes, or no)		
Ulceration present (yes, or no)		
Degree of stenosis (mild, moderate, or severe)		
Anticoagulation during surgery? (yes, or no)		
EEG monitoring? (yes, or no)		
Operation was easy? average? or difficult?		
Post-operative hypertension (yes, or no)		
Post-operative hypotension (yes, or no)		

Was there any complication during or after (within hospital) surgery? If so please specify _____

Legible name of surgeon _____

Table A.5   UK–TIA Study: Follow-up and/or death (see p. 169)

To be completed as soon as informed of death, or as near to the scheduled follow-up as possible, and the top copy then sent immediately (without stamp) to Clinical Trial Service Unit, FREEPOST, Oxford OX2 6BR, along with a one-week packet of tablets from this patient's previous batch, if in aspirin trial.

PATIENT: Full   name _____   Randomisation code _____ (aspirin trial)

1. *If dead*, date Day _____ Month _____ Year _____ and underlying cause of death (brief details)

   _____

   EVEN IF PATIENT HAS DIED, PLEASE ATTEMPT TO COMPLETE THE FOLLOWING (except BP)

2. Date of previous report Day _____ Month _____ Year _____

3. Strokes (>24 hours): Describe all previously unresolved strokes (i.e. with persistent symptoms at the previous report) and all *new* strokes (i.e. with onset since the last report)

Date of onset Day Month Year	Uncertain (U) or definite (D) stroke	Haemorrhage (H), infarct (I) or NK	Exact duration of symptoms (or enter 'still persisting', or 'until death')

4. Myocardial infarcts: Give dates and details of any possible MIs since previous report_____

   _____

   If there were any possible strokes or MIs, to whom do we write for clinical details?_____

   _____

5. Other diseases noted since previous report (✓if definite, ? if diagnosis uncertain)

   ☐ Angina   ☐ TIA (24 hour)   ☐ Retinal artery occlusion

   ☐ Peripheral vascular disease   ☐ Amaurosis fugax   ☐ Gastric intestinal bleeding

   Describe any other noteworthy illnesses and operations (particularly carotid surgery)_____

   _____

6. BP _____ / _____ (phase IV)

7. Current drugs with indications_____

_____

_____

8. Have anticoagulants been used since last report? Yes ☐ No ☐

9. Has venesection been used since last report? Yes ☐ No ☐

10. Is the patient smoking regularly? Yes ☐ No ☐

11. Has patient described any *side effects* from the trial tablets and if so what? (aspirin trial)_____

_____

12. Compliance (aspirin trial)

Since last report has the patient been taking the trial tablets

Fairly regularly ☐   Irregularly ☐   Stopped ☐   tick one box

4   2   4   1
regular regular enteric enteric none

Trial tablets taken yesterday ☐ ☐ ☐ ☐ ☐   tick one box

Trial tablets now prescribed ☐ ☐ ☐ ☐ ☐   tick one box

Reasons for stopping, or changing the regime since last follow-up_____

_____

Urine sent to biochemist? ☐ Yes ☐ No

If not, why not?_____

Legible name of investigator _____ Date of follow-up _____

Table A.6 Neurological scores used for stroke trials (see p.214)

Items	Mathew et al. (1972)	Bauer and Tellez (1973)	Gilsanz et al.(1975)	Kaste et al. (1976)	Larsson et al. (1976)	Matthews et al. (1976)	Admani (1978)	Woollard et al. (1978)	Dartigues (1980)	Norris and Hachinski (1982)
Consciousness	0–8 (:2)	0–7	0–9 (:3)	0–3 (×20)	0–6 (:2) ⎱	5–0	—	0–50 (:10)	0–9 (:3)	0–4 (×25)
Mental status including confusion	0–6 (:2)	0–38	0–9 (:3)	0–3 (×10)	0–6 (:2) ⎰		0–28	—	0–6 (:3)	0–57
Language	0–23	0–4	0–9 (:3)	0–3 (×7)	0–6 (:2)	?	0–12	—	0–9 (:3)	0–4 (×10)
Visual fields	0–3	—	0–6 (:3)	—	0–3	±	—	—	—	0–2 (×3)
Deviation of gaze	0–3	—	0–6 (:3)	—	0–3	3–0	—	0–20 (:10)	—	0–2 (×2)
Face paresis	0–3	—	0–6 (:3)	—	0–6 (:2)		—	—	—	0–3
Arm paresis	0–5	{0–11	0–6 (:2)	0–3 (×10)	0–4	4–0	0–4	0–15 (:3) }	0–9 (:3)	0–4 (×3.5)
Leg paresis	0–5	}	0–6 (:2)	0–3 (×10)	0–4	4–0	0–4	0–15 (:3)	—	0–4 (×2.5)
Sensory loss	0–3	0–3	0–9 (:3)	0–3	—	—	0–20	—	0–6 (:3)	0–24
Reflexes	0–3	0–3	0–6 (:3)	—	0–8 (:2)	—	—	—	—	—
Tonus	—	—	—	—	—	—	—	—	0–9 (:3)	—
Gait	—	—	—	0–6 (×20)	—	3–0 ⎱	0–24	—	0–6 (:3)	—
Incontinence	—	—	—	—	—	± ⎰	0–8	—	—	—
Autonomy	0–28 (:7)	0–5	0–9 (:3)	—	—	3–0	0–28	—	0–9 (:3)	—
Cranial nerves	—	—	—	0–3 (×3)	—	±	—	—	—	—
Incoordination	—	—	—	—	—	—	0–12	—	—	0–3 (×3)
Dysarthria	—	—	—	—	—	—	—	—	—	0–3 (×2)
Dysphagia	—	—	—	—	—	—	—	—	—	0–3 (×4)
Intracranial pressure	—	—	—	—	—	—	—	—	0–9 (:3)	—
TOTAL	100	68	75	273	54	Counts	114	100	72	285

(:n). Intervals between consecutive notes; (×n). weighting factors for the total score.

References

Admani (1978) *Brit. Med. J.*, **2**, 1678–9; Bauer and Tellez (1973) *Stroke*, **4**, 547–55; Dartigues (1980) quoted in Bidabe et al. (1982) *Agressologie*, **23**, 35–41; Gilsanz et al. (1975) *Lancet*, **1**, 1049–51; Kaste et al. (1976) *Brit. Med. J.*, **2**, 1409–10; Larsson et al. (1976) *Lancet*, **1**, 832–4; Mathew et al. (1972) *Lancet*, **2**, 1327–9; Matthews et al. (1976) *Brian*, **99**, 196–206; Norris and Hachinski (1982) *Stroke*, **13**, 527–8; Woollard et al. (1978) *Stroke*, **9**, 218–22.

Table A.7 Neurological evaluation for double-blind glycerol therapy in patients with acute stroke[a] (see p. 214)

Factor	Score
Mentation	
Level of consciousness:	
Fully conscious	8
Lethargic but mentally intact	6
Obtunded	4
Stuporous	2
Comatose	0
Orientation:	
Oriented × 3	6
Oriented × 2	4
Oriented × 1	2
Disoriented	0
Speech	
Reitan test	0–23
Cranial nerves	
Homonymous hemianopsia	
Intact	3
Mild	2
Moderate	1
Severe	0
Conjugate deviation of eyes	
Intact	3
Mild	2
Moderate	1
Severe	0
Facial weakness	
Intact	3
Mild	2
Moderate	1
Severe	0
Motor power (each limb separately)	
Normal strength	5
Contracts against resistance	4
Elevates against gravity	3
Gravity eliminated	2
Flicker	0
No movements	0
Performance or disability status scale	
Normal	28
Mild impairment	21
Moderate impairment	14
Severe impairment	7
Death	0

Reflexes

Normal	3
Asymmetrical or pathological reflexes	2
Clonus	1
No reflexes elicited	0

Sensation

Normal	3
Mild sensory abnormality	2
Severe sensory abnormality	1
No response to pain	0

[a]From Mathew *et al*. (1972) *Lancet*, **2**, 1327–9.

Table A.8   Acute Stroke Trial : Neurological Assessment (see p. 215)

Consciousness	0: normal; 1: drowsy; 2: stupor; 3: coma
Confusion	0: none; 1: mild; 2: severe
Communication	0: normal; 1: difficult; 2: impossible
Visual fields	0: normal; 1: inattention; 2: homonymous hemianopia
Gaze deviation	0: normal; 1: failure of gaze; 2: forced deviation
Facial paresis	0: normal; 1: mild; 2: severe
Arm function	0: MRC5; 1: MRC4; 2: MRC3 or less
Hand function	0: normal; 1: skilful; 2: useful; 3: useless
Arm tone	0: normal; 1: spastic; 2: flaccid
Leg function	0: MRC5; 1: MRC4; 2: MRC3; 3: MRC2 or less
Leg tone	0: normal; 1: spastic; 2: flaccid
Sensory disturbance	0: normal; 1: inattention or mild disturbance; 2: severe disturbance
Urinary incontinence	0: never; 1: occasional; 2: always/catheterised

Table A.9 Autonomy scales in neurology (see p. 215)

Items	Carroll (1962)	Towsend (1963)	Mahoney and Barthel (1965)	Dinnerstein et al. (1965)	Gordon and Kohn (1966)	Linn (1967)	New et al. (1968)	Schoening and Iversen (1968)	Katz et al. (1970)	Sheikh et al. (1979)
Dressing	+	+	+	+	+	+	+	+	+	+
Bathing	+	+	+	+	+	+	+	+	+	+
Personal grooming	+		+	+	+	+		+	+	+
Feeding	+	+	+	+	+	+	+	+	+	+
Toilet	+		+	+	+		+	+	+	+
Bed				+	+			+		
Transfers	+	+	+	+			+			
Wheelchair	+					+				
Ambulation	+	+	+	+		+		+	+	+
Stairs climbing	+	+	+					+		+
Sphincter control	+	+	+					+		+
Communication				+		+	+			
Writing				+		+	+			
Telephone						+	+			
Varia		+		+			+			

References

Carroll (1962) *J. Chron. Dis.*, **15**, 179–88; Dinnerstein *et al.* (1965) *Arch. Phys. Med. Rehabil.*, **46**, 579–84; Gordon and Kohn (1966) *J. Chron. Dis.*, **19**, 3–16; Katz *et al.* (1970) *Gerontologist*, **10**, 20–30; Linn (1967) *J. Amer. Geriat. Soc.*, **15**, 211–214; Mahoney and Barthel (1965) *Md. State Med. J.*, **14**, 61–5; New *et al.* (1968) *Soc. Sci. Med.*, **2**, 185–200; Schoening and Iversen (1968) *Arch. Phys. Med. Rehabil.*, **49**, 221–9; Sheikh *et al.* (1969) *Int. Rehabil. Med.*, **1**, 51–8; Towsend (1963) in Williams *et al.* (Eds) *Process in Aging*, New York, Atherton Press.

Table A.10 Barthel Index (see p. 215)

Tick the appropriate answer (one answer only for each item). If the performance of the patient is inferior to that described below, don't fill in the box.

Feeding	10	☐	Independent. Able to apply any necessary device. Feeds in reasonable time
	5	☐	Needs help, i.e. for cutting
Bathing	5	☐	Performs without assistance
Personal toilet (grooming)	5	☐	Washes face, combs hair, brushes teeth, shaves (manages plug if electric razor)
Dressing	10	☐	Independent. Ties shoes, fastens fasteners, applies braces
	5	☐	Needs help but does at leat half of task within reasonable time
Bowel control	10	☐	No accidents. Able to use enema or suppository, if needed
	5	☐	Occasional accidents or needs help with enema or suppository
Bladder control	10	☐	No accidents. Able to care for collecting device if used
	5	☐	Occasional accidents or needs help with device
Toilet transfers	10	☐	Independent with toilet or bedpan. Handles clothes, wipes, flushes or cleans pan
	5	☐	Needs help for balance, handling clothes or toilet paper
Chair/bed transfers	15	☐	Independent, including locks of wheelchair and lifting footrests
	10	☐	Minimum assistance or supervision
	5	☐	Able to sit but needs maximum assistance to transfer
Ambulation	15	☐	Independent for 50 yards. May use assistive devices, except for rolling walker
	10	☐	With help for 50 yards
	5	☐	Independent with wheelchair for 50 yards, only if unable to walk

Stair climbing   10 ☐   Independent. May use assistive devices

                  5 ☐   Needs help or supervision

TOTAL SCORE: ☐

Table A.11   Abbreviated mental test questionnaire (see p. 286)[a]

Age	☐	Score 1 for a correct answer. 0 if incorrect. If the patient scores 8 or less, refer them to the General Practitioner who will repeat the test.
Time (to nearest hour)	☐	
Address for recall at end of test — this should be repeated by the patient to ensure it has been heard correctly, e.g.: 42 West Street	☐	
Year	☐	
Where do you live (name of town or road)?	☐	
Recognition of two persons	☐	
Date of birth (day and month sufficient)	☐	
Year of First World War	☐	
Name of present monarch	☐	
Count backwards 20–1	☐	
Total	☐	

[a]After Qureshi and Hodkinson (1974) *Age & Aging*, **3**, 152–6.

Table A.12 Six-symptom rating scale (see p. 287)[a]

How to use this rating scale: Six symptoms commonly presenting in early senile dementia are listed down the left-hand side of the chart. The rating scale is from 0 (normal) to 4 (extremely severe impairment). Place the score for each symptom in the space provided, and add up the scores for the total score box.

Memory for recent events ☐

Confusion ☐

Self-care ☐

Sociability ☐

Mood—depression ☐

Dizziness ☐

Total ☐

[a]After Robinson (1961) *Geront. Clin.*, **3**, 247.

Table A.13 Relatives' assessment form (see p. 287)

Please fill in the boxes with a × or a ✓

Have you noticed any changes in your relative's memory?

Does he/she become forgetful?	No ☐	Often ☐	Occasionally ☐
Does he/she become confused?	No ☐	Often ☐	Occasionally ☐

Can he/she wash and dress properly	Yes ☐	No ☐
with a little help?	Yes ☐	No ☐
Can he/she do their own housework?	Yes ☐	No ☐
Can he/she prepare a cooked meal?	Yes ☐	No ☐
Can he/she use a telephone?	Yes ☐	No ☐
Can he/she do their own shopping?	Yes ☐	No ☐
Can he/she handle their own finances?	Yes ☐	No ☐
Can he/she use public or private transport?	Yes ☐	No ☐
Can he/she organise and take own medicine?	Yes ☐	No ☐

Has he/she any friends nearby?	Yes ☐	No ☐
Does he/she talk with them?	Yes ☐	No ☐
Can he/she get out to visit friends?	Yes ☐	No ☐

Does he/she seem sad? ☐ or depressed? ☐

Or is he/she usually bright and cheerful?	Yes ☐	No ☐
Does he/she eat well?	Yes ☐	No ☐
Does he/she have dizzy spells?	Yes ☐	No ☐
Can he/she use the toilet properly?	Yes ☐	No ☐
Are there occasions when the bed or clothing is wet?	Yes ☐	No ☐
Does he/she sleep well at night?, or	Yes ☐	No ☐
Does he/she wander about the house at night?	Yes ☐	No ☐

Index

325

DATE DUE